Advances in the Diagnosis and Treatment of Pediatric Infectious Diseases

Editor

CHANDY C. JOHN

PEDIATRIC CLINICS OF NORTH AMERICA

www.pediatric.theclinics.com

April 2013 • Volume 60 • Number 2

ELSEVIER

1600 John F. Kennedy Boulevard • Suite 1800 • Philadelphia, Pennsylvania, 19103-2899

http://www.theclinics.com

THE PEDIATRIC CLINICS OF NORTH AMERICA Volume 60, Number 2
April 2013 ISSN 0031-3955, ISBN-13: 978-1-4557-7134-9

Editor: Kerry Holland
Developmental Editor: Donald Mumford

The Pediatric Clinics of North America (ISSN 0031-3955) is published bimonthly by Elsevier Inc., 360 Park Avenue South, New York, NY 10010-1710. Months of issue are February, April, June, August, October, and December. Periodicals postage paid at New York, NY and additional mailing offices. Subscription prices are $191.00 per year (US individuals), $462.00 per year (US institutions), $259.00 per year (Canadian individuals), $614.00 per year (Canadian institutions), $308.00 per year (international individuals), $614.00 per year (international institutions), $93.00 per year (US students and residents), and $159.00 per year (international and Canadian residents and students). To receive students/resident rare, orders must be accompanied by name of affiliated institution, date of term, and the signature of program/residency coordinator on institution letterhead. Orders will be billed at individual rate until proof of status is received. Foreign air speed delivery is included in all *Clinics* subscription prices. All prices are subject to change without notice. **POSTMASTER:** Send address changes to *The Pediatric Clinics of North America*, Elsevier Health Sciences Division, Subscription Customer Service, 3251 Riverport Lane, Maryland Heights, MO 63043. **Customer Service: 1-800-654-2452 (US and Canada). From outside of the US and Canada: 1-314-447-8871. Fax: 1-314-447-8029. For print support, E-mail: JournalsCustomerService-usa@elsevier.com. For online support, E-mail: JournalsOnlineSupport-usa@elsevier.com.**

Reprints. For copies of 100 or more, of articles in this publication, please contact the Commercial Reprints Department, Elsevier Inc., 360 Park Avenue South, New York, NY 10010-1710. Tel.: 212-633-3812; Fax: 212-462-1935; E-mail: reprints@elsevier.com.

The Pediatric Clinics of North America is also published in Spanish by McGraw-Hill Inter-americana Editores S.A., Mexico City, Mexico; in Portuguese by Riechmann and Affonso Editores, Rua Comandante Coelho 1085, CEP 21250, Rio de Janeiro, Brazil; and in Greek by Althayia SA, Athens, Greece.

The Pediatric Clinics of North America is covered in *MEDLINE/PubMed (Index Medicus), Excerpta Medica, Current Contents, Current Contents/Clinical Medicine, Science Citation Index, ASCA, ISI/BIOMED*, and *BIOSIS*.

Printed and bound by CPI Group (UK) Ltd, Croydon, CR0 4YY
Transferred to Digital Printing, 2013

PROGRAM OBJECTIVE

The goal of the *Pediatric Clinics of North America* is to keep practicing physicians and residents up to date with current clinical practice in pediatrics by providing timely articles reviewing the state-of-the-art in patient care.

TARGET AUDIENCE

All practicing pediatricians, physicians and healthcare professionals who provide patient care to pediatric patients.

LEARNING OBJECTIVES

Upon completion of this activity, participants will be able to:

1. Recall the advances in the diagnosis and treatment of pediatric infectious diseases such as Rocky Mountain Spotted Fever, Acute Sinusitis, Neonatal Infectious Diseases, Otitis Media and Congenital Cytomegalovirus Infection.
2. Review travel-related infections in children.
3. Describe infections in internationally adopted children and childhood parasitic infections endemic to the United States.

ACCREDITATION

The Elsevier Office of Continuing Medical Education (EOCME) is accredited by the Accreditation Council for Continuing Medical Education (ACCME) to provide continuing medical education for physicians.

The EOCME designates this journal-based CME activity for a maximum of 11 *AMA PRA Category 1 Credit(s)*™. Physicians should claim only the credit commensurate with the extent of their participation in the activity.

All other health care professionals completing continuing education credit for this activity will be issued a certificate of participation.

DISCLOSURE OF CONFLICTS OF INTEREST

The EOCME assesses conflict of interest with its instructors, faculty, planners, and other individuals who are in a position to control the content of CME activities. All relevant conflicts of interest that are identified are thoroughly vetted by EOCME for fair balance, scientific objectivity, and patient care recommendations. EOCME is committed to providing its learners with CME activities that promote improvements or quality in healthcare and not a specific proprietary business or a commercial interest.

The planning committee, staff, authors and editors listed below have identified no financial relationships or relationships to products or devices they or their spouse/life partner have with commercial interest related to the content of this CME activity:

Meagan A. Barry; Itzhak Brook, MD, MSc; Andres Camacho-Gonzalez, MD; John Christenson, MD; Nicole Congleton; Judith Eckerle, MD; Thomas Fox, MD; Kerry Holland; Cynthia Howard, MD, MPHTM; Chandy John, MD, MS; Indu Kumari; Sandy Lavery; John Manaloor, MD; Jill McNair; Markus Paakkonen, MD; Heikki Peltola, MD, PhD; Michael Pichichero, MD; Swetha Pinninti, MD; Mark Schleiss, MD; Paul Spearman, MD; Barbara Stoll, MD; Elizabeth Swanson, DO; Pui-Ying Iroh Tam, MD; Jill Weatherhead, MD; and Laila Woc-Colburn, MD.

The planning committee, staff, authors and editors listed below have identified financial relationships or relationships to products or devices they or their spouse/life partner have with commercial interest related to the content of this CME activity:

Peter Hotez, MD has an employment affiliation with the National School of Tropical Medicine at Baylor College of Medicine.
David Kimberlin, MD has received research grants from GSK and Cellex.
Charles Woods, MD has industry funded research from Pfizer and sits on a data safety monitoring board for Cerexa.

UNAPPROVED/OFF-LABEL USE DISCLOSURE

The EOCME requires CME faculty to disclose to the participants:

1. When products or procedures being discussed are off-label, unlabelled, experimental, and/or investigational (not US Food and Drug Administration (FDA) approved); and
2. Any limitations on the information presented, such as data that are preliminary or that represent ongoing research, interim analyses, and/or unsupported opinions. Faculty may discuss information about pharmaceutical agents that is outside of FDA-approved labelling. This information is intended solely for CME and is not intended to promote off-label use of these medications. If you have any questions, contact the medical affairs department of the manufacturer for the most recent prescribing information.

TO ENROLL

To enroll in the *Pediatric Clinics of North America* Continuing Medical Education program, call customer service at 1-800-654-2452 or sign up online at http://www.theclinics.com/home/cme. The CME program is available to subscribers for an additional annual fee of USD 261.

METHOD OF PARTICIPATION

In order to claim credit, participants must complete the following:

1. Complete enrolment as indicated above.
2. Read the activity.
3. Complete the CME Test and Evaluation. Participants must achieve a score of 70% on the test. All CME Tests and Evaluations must be completed online.

CME INQUIRIES/SPECIAL NEEDS

For all CME inquiries or special needs, please contact elsevierCME@elsevier.com.

Contributors

EDITOR

CHANDY C. JOHN, MD, MS
Professor of Pediatrics and Medicine; Director, Divisions of Global Pediatrics and Pediatric Infectious Diseases, Department of Pediatrics, University of Minnesota Medical School, Minneapolis, Minnesota

AUTHORS

MEAGAN A. BARRY
Interdepartmental Program in Translational Biology and Molecular Medicine; BCM Medical Scientist Training Program, National School of Tropical Medicine, Baylor College of Medicine, Houston, Texas

ITZHAK BROOK, MD, MSc
Departments of Pediatrics and Medicine, Georgetown University School of Medicine, Washington, DC

ANDRES CAMACHO-GONZALEZ, MD, MSc
Assistant Professor of Pediatrics, Division of Pediatric Infectious Diseases, Emory Department of Pediatrics, Children's Healthcare of Atlanta, Emory University, Atlanta, Georgia

JOHN C. CHRISTENSON, MD
Professor of Clinical Pediatrics, Ryan White Center for Pediatric Infectious Disease, Riley Hospital for Children, Indiana University School of Medicine, Indianapolis, Indiana

JUDITH K. ECKERLE, MD
Assistant Professor, Division of Global Pediatrics, Department of Pediatrics, University of Minnesota Medical School, Minneapolis, Minnesota

THOMAS G. FOX, MD
Assistant Professor of Clinical Pediatrics, Ryan White Center for Pediatric Infectious Disease, Riley Hospital for Children, Indiana University School of Medicine, Indianapolis, Indiana

PETER J. HOTEZ, MD, PhD
Interdepartmental Program in Translational Biology and Molecular Medicine; Departments of Pediatrics, Molecular Virology and Microbiology, National School of Tropical Medicine, Baylor College of Medicine, Houston, Texas

CYNTHIA R. HOWARD, MD, MPHTM
Associate Professor, Division of Global Pediatrics, Department of Pediatrics, University of Minnesota Medical School, Minneapolis, Minnesota

PUI-YING IROH TAM, MD
Division of Pediatric Infectious Diseases, Department of Pediatrics, University of Minnesota, Minneapolis, Minnesota

CHANDY C. JOHN, MD, MS
Professor of Pediatrics and Medicine; Director, Divisions of Global Pediatrics and Pediatric Infectious Diseases, Department of Pediatrics, University of Minnesota Medical School, Minneapolis, Minnesota

DAVID W. KIMBERLIN, MD
Professor of Pediatrics, Division of Pediatric Infectious Diseases, The University of Alabama at Birmingham, Birmingham, Alabama

JOHN J. MANALOOR, MD
Assistant Professor of Clinical Pediatrics, Ryan White Center for Pediatric Infectious Disease, Riley Hospital for Children, Indiana University School of Medicine, Indianapolis, Indiana

MARKUS PÄÄKKÖNEN, MD, PhD
Clinical Researcher, Department of Orthopaedics and Traumatology, Turku University Hospital, University of Turku, Turku, Finland

HEIKKI PELTOLA, MD, PhD
Professor, Department of Pediatrics, Children's Hospital, Helsinki University Central Hospital, University of Helsinki, Helsinki, Finland

MICHAEL E. PICHICHERO, MD
Director, Center for Infectious Diseases and Immunology, Rochester General Hospital Research Institute, Rochester General Hospital, Rochester, New York

SWETHA G. PINNINTI, MD
Fellow, Division of Pediatric Infectious Diseases, The University of Alabama at Birmingham, Birmingham, Alabama

MARK R. SCHLEISS, MD
Professor and Director, Division of Pediatric Infectious Diseases and Immunology, American Legion and Auxiliary Heart Research Foundation Chair in Pediatrics, Associate Head for Research, Department of Pediatrics, Center for Infectious Diseases and Microbiology Translational Research, University of Minnesota Medical School, Minneapolis, Minnesota

PAUL W. SPEARMAN, MD
Nahmias-Schinazi Professor and Chief, Division of Pediatric Infectious Diseases, Vice Chair for Research, Emory Department of Pediatrics, Chief Research Officer, Children's Healthcare of Atlanta, Emory University, Atlanta, Georgia

BARBARA J. STOLL, MD
George W. Brumley, Jr. Professor and Chair of the Department of Pediatrics, Medical Director of Children's Healthcare of Atlanta at Egleston, President of the Emory-Children's Center, Atlanta, Georgia

ELIZABETH C. SWANSON, DO
Fellow, Division of Pediatric Infectious Diseases and Immunology, Department of Pediatrics, Center for Infectious Diseases and Microbiology Translational Research, University of Minnesota Medical School, Minneapolis, Minnesota

JILL E. WEATHERHEAD, MD
Departments of Medicine and Pediatrics, National School of Tropical Medicine, Baylor College of Medicine, Houston, Texas

LAILA WOC-COLBURN, MD
Department of Medicine, National School of Tropical Medicine, Baylor College of Medicine, Houston, Texas

CHARLES R. WOODS, MD, MS
Professor of Pediatrics and Vice Chair for Faculty Development, Department of Pediatrics, University of Louisville School of Medicine, Louisville, Kentucky

Contents

PEDIATRIC CLINICS OF NORTH AMERICA

FORTHCOMING ISSUES

June 2013
Pediatric Critical Care Medicine
Derek Wheeler, MD, *Editor*

August 2013
Pediatric Otolaryngology
Harold S. Pine, MD, *Editor*

October 2013
Pediatric Emergencies
Richard Lichenstein, MD, *Editor*

RECENT ISSUES

February 2012
Breastfeeding Updates for the Pediatrician
Ardythe L. Morrow, PhD, and
Caroline J. Chantry, MD, *Editors*

December 2012
Safety and Reliability in Pediatrics
Brian R. Jacobs, MD, and
Max J. Coppes, MD, *Editors*

October 2012
Neonatal and Pediatric Clinical Pharmacology
John N. van den Anker, MD,
Max J. Coppes, MD, and
Gideon Koren, MD, *Editors*

RELATED INTEREST

Infectious Disease Clinics of North America December 2012 (Volume 26:4)
Care of the Patient with Hepatitis C Virus Infection
Barbara H. McGovern, MD, *Editor*

Preface

Pediatric Infectious Diseases

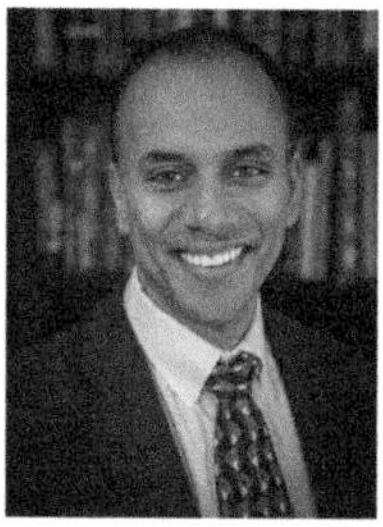

Chandy C. John, MD, MS
Editor

I'm delighted to introduce this issue of the *Pediatric Clinics of North America*, which highlights "Advances in Evaluation, Diagnosis, and Treatment of Pediatric Infectious Diseases." The 11 articles in this issue cover common childhood infections, such as otitis media and community-acquired pneumonia, and infections that inspire questions because they are less common, such as parasitic and travel-related infections. I'm grateful to the authors for providing succinct, up-to-date, and highly clinically relevant articles. Reading through them, I felt that I had just been given an expert tutorial on the latest in pediatric infectious diseases—as indeed I had!

Because pediatrics starts with the neonate, the first 3 articles address key neonatal infections. Drs Beth Swanson and Mark Schleiss start with an article summarizing the latest findings on congenital cytomegalovirus (CMV) infection, the most common cause of acquired hearing loss in children. They outline advances in diagnosis and treatment and provide a simple algorithm for evaluation of the child with suspected CMV and assessment of whether a child with known CMV infection requires ganciclovir treatment. Dr Schleiss, who has been at the forefront of CMV vaccine development, also gives a brief update on the current state of CMV vaccines. Drs Swetha Pinninti and David Kimberlin follow with an article on neonatal herpes simplex virus (HSV) infection, highlighting advances in this area and providing guidelines for evaluation and treatment of mothers with genital HSV infection and infants born to these mothers. Data from Dr Kimberlin's 2011 *New England Journal of Medicine* article provide the rationale and criteria for follow-up treatment of children with neonatal HSV infection with oral acyclovir, after initial intravenous acyclovir treatment. Drs Andres Camacho-Gonzales, Paul Spearman, and Barbara Stoll review the latest information on diagnosis and treatment of neonatal sepsis. The authors provide insight on which of the many diagnostic markers currently being studied may become clinically useful and discuss the risks for development of antibiotic-resistant bacteria in neonatal intensive care units.

Pediatr Clin N Am 60 (2013) xv–xvii
http://dx.doi.org/10.1016/j.pcl.2013.01.001
0031-3955/13/$ – see front matter

The next section focuses on common childhood infections. Dr Michael Pichichero leads off this section with an update on acute otitis media. Dr Pichichero, who has studied and published on otitis media for decades, carefully delineates the criteria for a diagnosis of acute otitis media and compares this condition (and its prognosis) with otitis media with effusion. Dr Pichichero notes that tympanocentesis aspirates from children in Rochester, New York in 2011 showed a predominance of nontypable *Haemophilus influenzae* and *Moraxella catarrhalis*, most of which were β-lactamase–producing organisms. The shift to these organisms may reflect effectiveness of the current 13-valent pneumococcal conjugate vaccine. Dr Pichichero notes that, in areas where *H influenzae* and *M catarrhalis* predominate as causes of acute otitis media, amoxicillin-clavulanate may be a more appropriate first choice for treatment than amoxicillin. Dr Itzhak Brook then discusses the evaluation, diagnosis, and treatment of acute and chronic sinusitis. Dr Brook's research on the contribution of anaerobic organisms to chronic sinusitis transformed our understanding of that condition, and his concise and informative article on acute and chronic sinusitis provides an excellent update on these common yet sometimes difficult-to-diagnose conditions in children. Drs Markus Pääkkönen and Heikki Peltola's article on bone and joint infections outlines their pioneering studies of these infections. In these studies, they demonstrated that for uncomplicated osteomyelitis and septic arthritis, short courses of intravenous therapy, followed by high-dose oral therapy, are as effective as the traditional longer courses of intravenous therapy. Their review provides a new, evidence-based approach to the evaluation and therapy of acute osteomyelitis and septic arthritis. Dr Pui-Ying Iroh Tam then provides a succinct evidence-based review of community-acquired pneumonia in children, outlining current standards for evaluation and diagnosis of pneumonia, and highlighting areas of controversy in treatment of pneumonia in children.

The section on tick-borne and parasitic infections in children starts with a review by Dr Charles Woods, an expert in many areas of clinical pediatric infectious disease research, on Rocky Mountain spotted fever. Dr Woods discusses new findings in the evaluation and diagnosis of Rocky Mountain spotted fever, including the utility of a PCR-based diagnosis. Drs Meagan Barry, Jill Weatherhead, Peter Hotez, and Laila Woc-Colborn review parasitic infections endemic to the United States. Parasitic infections in the US are more common than is often realized, so the article provides a much-needed synthesis of information on the current approach to diagnosis, evaluation, and treatment of these infections, delivered by experts from the new National School of Tropical Medicine at the Baylor College of Medicine.

The final section focuses on infections in immigrant and traveling children. Nearly ten thousand children are adopted every year from other countries to the United States. Dr Judith Eckerle and I review the infectious problems common to these children, which are quite different from those of children born in the United States. Our recommendations come from the current literature and from our clinical experience at the University of Minnesota International Adoption Clinic, the first and still busiest international adoption clinic in the United States. Travel by parents and children to countries in Asia, South America, and Africa is increasing, making travel-related infection an important topic for the pediatrician. The comprehensive overview of travel-related infections in children by Drs Thomas Fox, John Manaloor, and John Christenson provides up-to-date information on how to prepare children for international travel and how to evaluate the ill child returning from international travel.

Together, these articles provide an excellent and current overview of common infections in children, from the neonate to the traveling or immigrant child. They are highly relevant to the practice of clinical pediatrics and should stand as valuable reference articles for years to come. I hope you enjoy reading them as much as I did and find them useful to your clinical practice.

Chandy C. John, MD, MS
Division of Global Pediatrics and
Division of Pediatric Infectious Diseases
Department of Pediatrics
University of Minnesota Medical School
717 Delaware Street SE, Room 366
Minneapolis, MN 55414, USA

E-mail address:
ccj@umn.edu

Congenital Cytomegalovirus Infection

New Prospects for Prevention and Therapy

Elizabeth C. Swanson, DO, Mark R. Schleiss, MD*

KEYWORDS

• Congenital cytomegalovirus (CMV) infection • Antiviral therapy • Newborn screening
• Sensorineural hearing loss • CMV vaccines

KEY POINTS

- In the developed world, cytomegalovirus (CMV) is the most common congenital viral infection, with an overall birth prevalence of approximately 0.6%.
- Approximately 10% of congenitally infected infants have signs and symptoms of disease at birth, and these symptomatic infants have a substantial risk of subsequent neurologic sequelae. These include sensorineural hearing loss, mental retardation, microcephaly, development delay, seizure disorders, and cerebral palsy.
- The public health impact of congenital CMV infection is underestimated and underrecognized by both the lay public and health care providers.
- Antiviral therapy for children with symptomatic central nervous system congenital CMV infection is effective at reducing the risk of long-term disabilities and should be offered to families with affected newborns.
- An effective preconceptual vaccine against CMV could, by preventing congenital infection, protect against long-term neurologic sequelae and other disabilities. A variety of active and passive immunization strategies are in clinical trials and are likely to be licensed in the next few years. Until a vaccine is licensed, preventive strategies aimed at reducing transmission should be emphasized and public awareness increased, particularly among women of childbearing age.

INTRODUCTION

Cytomegalovirus (CMV) is a ubiquitous herpesvirus spread by close interpersonal contact through saliva, blood, genital secretions, urine, or breast milk that infects up to 90% of the US population by the eighth decade of life and establishes lifelong latency in monocytes and granulocytes.[1–3] Maternal transmission to the fetus of a new or

---

Support: Support from NIH HD068229 and HD038416 is acknowledged.
Division of Pediatric Infectious Diseases and Immunology, Department of Pediatrics, Center for Infectious Diseases and Microbiology Translational Research, University of Minnesota Medical School, 2001 6th Street Southeast, Minneapolis, MN 55455, USA
* Corresponding author.
E-mail address: schleiss@umn.edu

Pediatr Clin N Am 60 (2013) 335–349
http://dx.doi.org/10.1016/j.pcl.2012.12.008 pediatric.theclinics.com
0031-3955/13/$ – see front matter

reactivated latent infection may occur at any gestation, leading to congenital CMV. About 20,000 to 40,000 infants per year in the United States are born with congenital CMV infection, with a corresponding incidence of 0.6% to 0.7% of all deliveries of the developed world, making CMV the most common of the congenital viral infections.[4–7] CMV is mostly asymptomatic or mildly symptomatic when acquired as a primary infection in infants, children, and adults; however, it can be devastating to immunocompromised hosts, including infected newborns, and results in more long-term neurodevelopmental morbidity than any other perinatally acquired infection. The most frequently observed neurodevelopmental sequela is sensorineural hearing loss (SNHL): indeed, congenital CMV infection is estimated to be the leading non-hereditary cause of SNHL.[8,9]

Despite its frequency and disabling consequences, congenital CMV is less known to the general population than other conditions with lower prevalence, such as Down syndrome, fetal alcohol syndrome, and spina bifida. This lack of awareness is problematic given that currently the only way to prevent fetal infection is through careful hygienic practices, such as hand washing and avoidance of potential sources of CMV. This review summarizes the current state of knowledge regarding the epidemiology, pathogenesis, diagnosis, treatment, and prognosis of congenital CMV infection. New and emerging strategies for prevention and therapy are emphasized, including vaccines currently in clinical trials. Key principles of management, including appropriate use of consultants, are summarized. Finally, potential resources for parents raising a child with symptomatic congenital CMV infection are provided.

EPIDEMIOLOGY

Cytomegalovirus is a ubiquitous infection and most individuals are eventually exposed to this agent. There is no seasonality to infection. Patient populations with an increased incidence of primary infection include breastfeeding infants, toddlers and care providers in group daycare, and sexually active adolescents.[10–16] CMV infections are generally asymptomatic in immunocompetent individuals, but may produce a heterophile-negative mononucleosis syndrome in approximately 10% of primary infections in older children and adults.[17] CMV seroprevalence demonstrates striking geographic and racial variation and tends to be highest in South America, Africa, and Asia and lowest in Western Europe and the United States. Seroprevalence is higher among nonwhites and among individuals of lower socioeconomic status.[18,19] The factors responsible for geographic and racial variation in seroprevalence remain incompletely understood.

The biggest risk factor for CMV transmission in women of reproductive age is exposure to urine and saliva of young children, and mothers of children who are shedding CMV are 10 times more likely to seroconvert than women in other comparison groups.[12,20,21] Children in group daycare represent a particularly important reservoir of CMV. It is postulated that maternal CMV infection could be prevented during pregnancy through education and behavioral changes. However, many women have not heard of CMV; obstetricians may not discuss CMV prevention with their patients, and these opportunities are missed.[20] A lack of public knowledge of CMV is a major barrier to disease control. A recent study using a national mail survey showed that awareness of CMV was very low.[20] Only 7% of men and 13% of women had heard of congenital CMV. Awareness of other congenital infections, such as rubella and toxoplasmosis, was slightly greater despite their lesser prevalence. This lack of awareness is particularly troubling given that CMV is fairly easy to inactivate through simple hand-washing interventions.[22]

CONGENITAL AND PERINATAL CMV INFECTIONS: CLINICAL PRESENTATION

CMV infection may be acquired in an infant via congenital, intrapartum, or postnatal routes. Infection of the newborn may occur secondary to exposure to CMV-infected cervical secretions during vaginal delivery or via ingestion of CMV-infected breast milk, but these types of infections rarely result in significant symptoms or sequelae in term babies.[23] Postnatal acquisition of CMV by breast-feeding has little significance, is not associated with long-term disability, and rarely causes clinical signs of illness in term infants. In contrast, low-birth-weight premature infants are at significant risk for CMV disease following acquisition of infection via breast milk. CMV also can cause disease in a premature infant when acquired by transfusion. Premature infants may demonstrate worsening respiratory status, neutropenia, or septic appearance (with apnea, bradycardia, pallor, and bowel distention) at the onset of infection, regardless of whether the virus was acquired postnatally from human milk or transfusions.[24,25] For premature infants acquiring infection postnatally, CMV's ability to cause long-term sequelae independent from prematurity remains unclear, although minor effects on motor development have been suggested.[25–27] A recent study suggested that postnatal CMV infection of preterm infants did not result in an increased risk of SNHL.[28]

Congenital CMV occurs transplacentally and may result in symptomatic or asymptomatic infection in the neonate. The likelihood of fetal transmission and symptomatic disease is much greater during primary versus nonprimary maternal CMV infection. It is estimated that 1% to 4% of CMV-seronegative mothers will become infected during pregnancy, and 30% to 40% of these infected women will transmit the virus to the fetus. Nonprimary maternal CMV infections can also result in fetal transmission. These infections may represent reactivated latent infection or reinfection with a new strain in seropositive women. Currently it is estimated that 10% to 30% of women with preconception immunity become reinfected, and 1% to 3% will transmit to the fetus.[5,6,19,29,30] Symptoms of disease in the newborn and long-term neurodevelopmental sequelae can occur after transmission in the setting of primary or recurrent infection. Symptoms occur in 11% to –12.7% of all neonates with congenital CMV according to 2 recent meta-analyses.[4,5] Clinical findings include intrauterine growth restriction, hydrops, generalized petechiae, purpura, thrombocytopenia, jaundice, hepatosplenomegaly, pneumonitis, microcephaly, periventricular calcifications, seizures, chorioretinitis, sensorineural hearing loss, bone abnormalities, abnormal dentition, and hypocalcified enamel. **Table 1** summarizes the frequencies of these findings as noted in a review of 106 infants with symptomatic congenital CMV infection, as well as the most common associated laboratory abnormalities.[31]

The differential diagnosis of congenital CMV includes other congenital viral infections, toxoplasmosis, and syphilis, given that many of the presenting symptoms are nonspecific. For example, rubella may also present with petechiae, bony defects, and sensorineural hearing loss.[32] Neonatal enteroviral infections, particularly infections with the recently described parechoviruses, can be associated with fetal brain injury and long-term sequalae.[33] Neonatal HSV infection may present with seizures; parvovirus B19 may present with hepatomegaly and anemia; and lymphocytic choriomeningitis virus may present with microcephaly, chorioretinitis, and intracranial calcifications.[34]

Long-term sequelae occur following both symptomatic and asymptomatic congenital infections, with the more frequent and severe sequelae occurring in symptomatic infants. It has been estimated that 40% to 58% of infants who are symptomatic at birth go on to develop sequelae,[4] and these may include sensorineural hearing loss, vision loss, mental retardation, seizure disorder, cerebral palsy, visual deficits,

Table 1
Clinical and laboratory abnormalities in symptomatic congenital CMV infection

Finding	Frequency (%)
Petechiae	76
Neurologic, one or more of the following:	68
Microcephaly	53
Lethargy/hopotonia	27
Poor suck	19
Seizures	7
Jaundice	67
Hepatosplenomegaly	60
Small for gestational age (weight <10 percentile)	50
Prematurity (<38 wk gestation)	34
Elevated ALT (>80 units/L)	83
Thrombocytopenia:	
$<100 \times 10^3/mm^3$	77
$<50 \times 10^3/mm^3$	53
Conjugated hyperbilirubinemia:	
Direct bilirubin >2 mg/dL	81
Direct bilirubin >4 mg/dL	69
Hemolysis	51
Increased CSF protein (>120 mg/dL)	46

Data from Boppana SB, Pass RF, Britt WJ, et al. Symptomatic congenital cytomegalovirus infection: neonatal morbidity and mortality. Pediatr Infect Dis J 1992;11:93.

or developmental delay.[31,35,36] Approximately 13.5% of the asymptomatic neonates may still go on to develop neurodevelopment injury, which most commonly manifests as hearing loss.[4] Hearing loss is most common when CMV infection occurs in the first or second trimester.[37,38] Sensorineural hearing loss following symptomatic or asymptomatic congenital infection is often progressive, can be unilateral or bilateral, and may be absent at birth, only to become clinically manifest later in childhood.[39–43] About 21% of all hearing loss at birth and 25% of hearing loss at 4 years of age is attributable to congenital CMV infection; therefore, these children require regular hearing evaluations and early intervention.[44]

DIAGNOSTIC EVALUATION

There is no universal screening for CMV in mothers or newborns. Pregnant mothers can be diagnosed by seroconversion from immunoglobin G (IgG) -negative to IgG-positive status, or by positive immunoglobin M (IgM) if confirmed with low-avidity IgG (IgM may remain positive for 6–9 months after the end of acute phase infection).[30] Fetal infection is diagnosed by positive viral culture or polymerase chain reaction (PCR) from amniotic fluid. Diagnosis in the neonate is made by viral detection in body fluids via PCR, culture, or antigen testing (pp65 antigen) within the first 3 weeks of life.[45] The finding of CMV antibodies or viral DNA after this point makes congenital versus postnatally acquired infection difficult to distinguish. Antibody titers cannot reliably make the diagnosis as maternal CMV IgG crosses the placenta, and neonates mount weak IgM responses. The preferred specimens are saliva and urine as newborns shed high levels of the virus from these fluids. Saliva samples may be more easily obtained and have been shown to be as reliable as urine samples in diagnosing CMV, so some propose that saliva PCR should be considered the investigation of choice.[46–48]

For the primary care clinician, having an appropriate index of suspicion is key. In addition to the signs, symptoms, and laboratory abnormalities noted in **Table 1**, CMV diagnostic studies should also be considered in infants with more subtle potential manifestations of illness, such as mild growth retardation, or a failed newborn hearing screen. Once the diagnosis is confirmed, further laboratory tests, imaging, and eye and hearing assessments are indicated. Complete blood count and liver function tests may reveal pancytopenia and hepatitis, and coagulation studies may be abnormal in the setting of hepatitis. Renal function is checked as a baseline before beginning treatment with ganciclovir (see later discussion). A range of seizure disorders, including infantile spasm, have been described, and ongoing consultation with a pediatric neurologist may be necessary.[49] Neuroimaging is an important component of management. Available techniques for neuroimaging assessment include cerebral ultrasound, computed tomography, and magnetic resonance imaging (MRI) for suspected or proven congenital infection. Cranial ultrasound is a good screening tool, with subsequent MRI being recommended for definitive evaluation, particularly for infants with abnormal ultrasound examination, microcephaly, or neurological findings (**Fig. 1**).[50,51] A recent review elegantly summarized the pattern of neurodevelopmental injury as a function of timing of acquisition of brain infection in utero.[51] This review noted that lesions occurring prior to 18 weeks gestational age commonly include lissencephaly with thin cerebral cortex, cerebellar hypoplasia, ventriculomegaly, periventricular calcification, and delay in myelination. At 18 to 24 weeks, migrational abnormalities may occur, including polymicrogyria, schizencephaly, and periventricular cysts. Third trimester infections may be associated with central nervous system (CNS) lesions that may include delayed myelination, dysmyelination, calcification, and white matter disease. Ophthalmologic assessment should be performed on all infants with congenital CMV infection. Ophthalmologic signs are seen in a large percentage of symptomatic infants and include chorioretinitis, optic atrophy, and cortical visual impairment.[52] Strabismus is also a common long-term ophthalmologic complication.[53] Audiologic assessment should be performed on all infants with

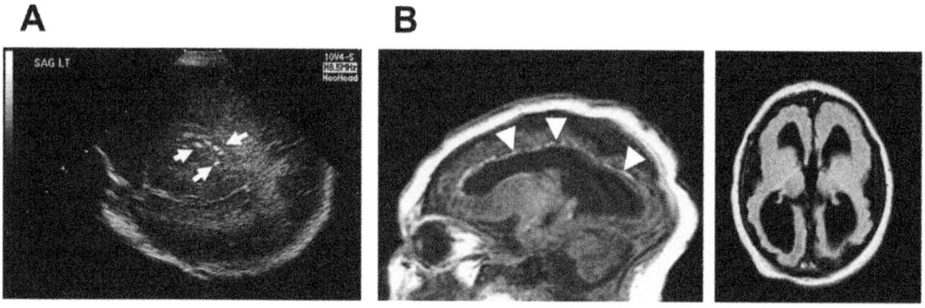

Fig. 1. (*A*) Head ultrasound (sagittal view) from a newborn infant with symptomatic congenital CMV infection. Intracranial and periventricular calcifications are noted (*arrows*). This infant went on to have severe bilateral SNHL and other developmental disabilities. (*B*) Brain MRI of infant with congenital CMV infection. Fetal CMV infection was first identified in utero and immune globulin therapy commenced. Sagittal (*left panel*) and axial (*right panel*) views are demonstrated. T1-Weighted, 1.5-T images demonstrate ventriculomegaly, periventricular calcifications, marked loss of brain volume with reduced white matter, pachygyria, and lissencephaly on the surface, and very thin cortex. Sagittal view demonstrates calcifications most clearly (*arrowheads*). This infant went on to manifest a seizure disorder and moderate bilateral SNHL.

congenital CMV infection; as noted, SNHL may be absent at birth, and progressive in nature, and frequent evaluations are required throughout childhood to evaluate for the possibility of hearing deterioration.[39] At a minimum, audiologic assessment should be performed every 6 months for the first 3 years of life and annually thereafter. For children with severe-to-profound hearing loss caused by congenital CMV, cochlear implantation is a successful intervention.[54,55] Hypoplasia and hypocalcification of tooth enamel are common in children with congenital CMV infection,[56] and regular dental visits are an important component of the long-term care of these infants. Children with evidence of cerebral palsy may require consultative care from a clinician expert in the management of this disorder. Several suggested diagnostic studies and potential specialty referrals are noted in **Box 1**; however, it should be noted that the range of management issues for any given child may be quite variable, and not all children with congenital CMV will require all of these services.

Box 1
Potential diagnostic studies and subspecialty consultations in the management of congenital CMV infection

Potential diagnostic studies

- Diagnostic virology
- PCR and/or culture of infant urine, blood, and saliva
- Specimens must be obtained before day 21 of life to confirm congenital infection (vs postnatal acquisition)
- Neurodiagnostic imaging
- Head ultrasound, good screening examination in neonatal period
- MRI of brain more definitive for symptomatic/affected infants
- Ophthalmologic evaluation
- Audiologic evaluation
- Newborn hearing screening in nursery
- Definitive auditory-evoked response on follow-up evaluation
- Complete blood count, platelet counts, transaminases, bilirubin for symptomatic infants
- Electroencephalography if seizures clinically evident or suspected

Potential consultants

- Audiology
- Otolaryngology
- Pediatric infectious disease
- Neurology
- Physical medicine/rehabilitation
- Orthopedics
- Developmental pediatrics
- Pediatric ophthalmology
- Pediatric dentistry

Not all children with congenital CMV will require all of these studies. The need for specific studies will be guided by the clinical picture in the individual child.

TREATMENT

Treatment of congenital CMV infection with antivirals should be instituted in infants with evidence of CNS involvement, including SNHL, and should be considered in infants with serious end-organ disease (hepatitis, pneumonia, thrombocytopenia). The cornerstone of antiviral therapy is ganciclovir, which was the first compound licensed specifically for treatment of CMV infections. Ganciclovir is a synthetic acyclic nucleoside analogue, structurally similar to guanine. Its structure is similar to that of acyclovir, and, like acyclovir, it requires phosphorylation for antiviral activity. Following phosphorylation by a viral protein known as pUL97, cellular enzymes phosphorylate the monophosphate form to diphosphate and triphosphate metabolites; the ganciclovir triphosphate metabolite then exerts its antiviral effect in the CMV-infected cell. The first reports of the use of ganciclovir therapy for congenital CMV infection date to the late 1980s.[57] In subsequent reports,[58,59] ganciclovir has been shown to be generally safe and well-tolerated when used in newborns and has appeared to be useful in the management of severe, focal, end-organ disease in infants. No sustained effect on CMV shedding at mucosal sites can be expected: once therapy is completed, infants resume the excretion of CMV in their urine and saliva.

In addition to its role in the management of severe CMV end-organ disease, it has become increasingly clear that ganciclovir also provides long-term neurodevelopmental benefit for some infants with congenital CMV infection. These benefits were demonstrated in a phase III randomized double-blind study of parenteral ganciclovir in neonates with symptomatic congenital CMV infection.[60] This study indicated that 84% of 25 ganciclovir recipients either had improved hearing or maintained normal hearing between baseline and 6 months. In contrast, only 59% of 17 control patients had improved or stable hearing ($P = .06$). Results were even more encouraging when the study and control groups were compared for subsequent maintenance of normal hearing. None (0%) of 25 ganciclovir-treated infants had worsening in hearing between baseline and 6-month follow-up, compared with 7 (41%) of 17 control patients ($P<.01$). The study further examined whether a therapeutic benefit was noted after 12 months of follow-up. Among 43 patients who had a brainstem-evoked response study at both baseline and 1 year or beyond, 5 (21%) of 24 ganciclovir recipients had worsening of hearing versus 13 (68%) of 19 control patients ($P<.01$). A subsequent report compared long-term neurodevelopmental outcomes in infants treated with ganciclovir therapy and untreated infants, using the Denver Developmental Screening Test.[61] This study indicated that infants receiving intravenous ganciclovir therapy had fewer developmental delays at 6 and 12 months compared with untreated infants.

Based on these data as well as the data regarding ganciclovir treatment and hearing outcomes, 6 weeks of intravenous ganciclovir therapy is recommended in the management of babies with symptomatic congenital CMV disease involving the CNS (**Fig. 2**). Treatment should be initiated within the first month of life. Infants need to be monitored closely for toxicity, especially neutropenia, which may be observed in up to 60% of infants on long-term therapy.[62] Care must be taken, and dosage adjustments made, when treating infants with impaired renal function.[63] Treatment of infants with ganciclovir should be approached with realistic expectations and should be undertaken with the assistance of an expert familiar with the use of this medication in infants. The risk of toxicity needs to be explained to parents, and it must be stressed that ganciclovir will not reverse established CNS injury. If neutropenia occurs on therapy, human granulocyte colony-stimulating factor therapy can be administered and is usually effective in restoring an adequate neutrophil count, such that therapy may be continued. Ganciclovir or valganciclovir (if the infant is

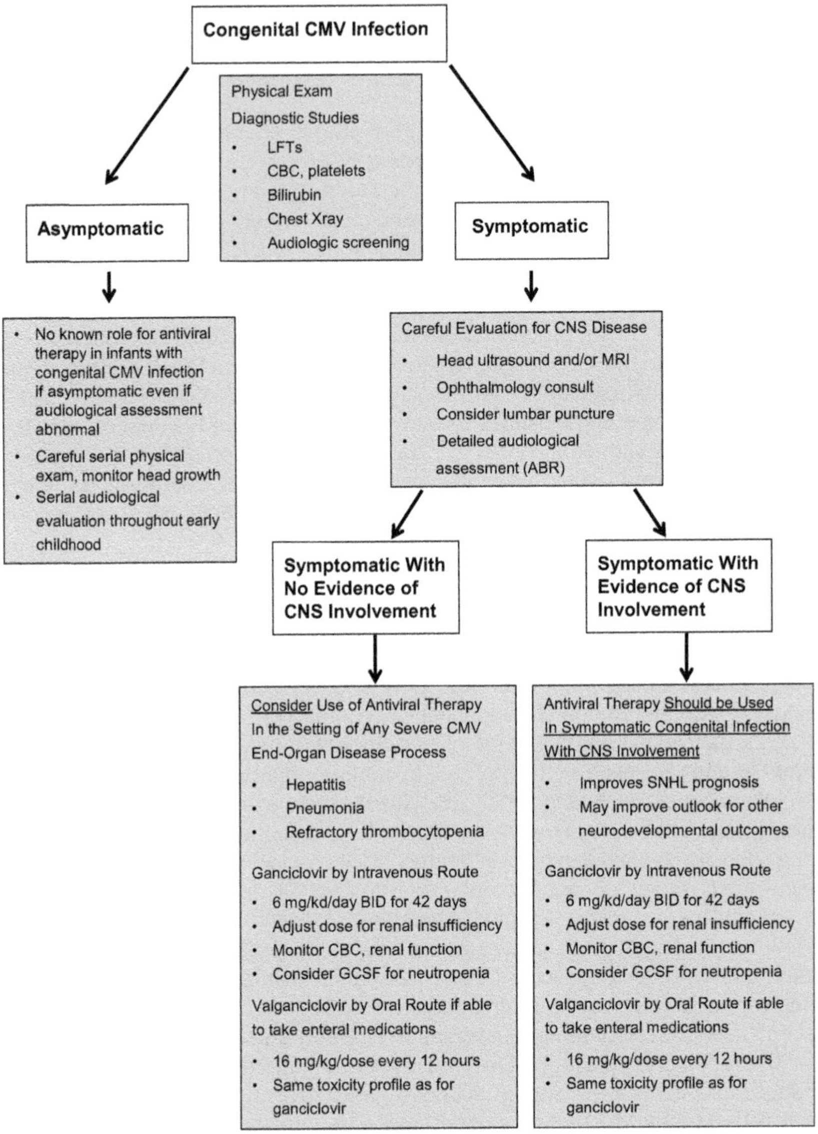

Fig. 2. Management strategies for congenital CMV infection. Congenital CMV infection may be either asymptomatic or symptomatic at birth. Asymptomatic congenital infection is rarely recognized (because there is seldom any clinical impetus to evaluate an asymptomatic newborn), but may be diagnosed as an incidental finding, or because of concern regarding a primary maternal infection during pregnancy. It is possible that more asymptomatic congenital infections will be recognized in the future because of ongoing programs evaluating the potential value of performing universal CMV screening on all newborns.[46] Such infants require frequent audiologic screening, but are not known to benefit from antiviral therapy. Infants with symptomatic congenital CMV infection should be evaluated for CNS involvement (by ophthalmologic evaluation, CNS imaging studies, audiologic evaluation, and, when feasible, lumbar puncture). If CNS involvement is noted, 6 weeks of therapy with ganciclovir is known to improve hearing and possibly neurodevelopmental outcomes. Oral valganciclovir is an alternative. Infants with symptomatic infection without CNS involvement are not known to benefit from antiviral therapy. ABR, auditory-evoked response; CBC, complete blood count; GCSF, granulocyte colony-stimulating factor; LFT, liver function tests.

able to take an orally administered medication, see later discussion) may also be considered in neonates with symptomatic end-organ disease other than CNS disease (hepatitis, pneumonia, thrombocytopenia), but the efficacy of treatment of non-CNS symptomatic congenital CMV infection has not been assessed in any large multicenter studies (see **Fig. 2**).

An alternative to intravenous ganciclovir for neonates who are candidates for oral medication is the use of its oral prodrug, valganciclovir. This approach is attractive insofar as it obviates the need for placement of a central venous catheter for 6 weeks of intravenous therapy. Valganciclovir is very well absorbed following oral administration. It is rapidly metabolized following oral dosing into ganciclovir. A suspension formulation is licensed and available, and although not licensed for the treatment of congenital CMV, its use can be considered as an alternative to intravenous therapy. Studies in neonates have demonstrated stable drug levels following oral dosing.[63,64] Currently, data from a clinical trial of 6 weeks versus 6 months of valganciclovir performed by the Collaborative Antiviral Study Group are being analyzed toward the goal of determining whether long-term therapy confers additional neurodevelopmental benefits to infants.[62] Although anecdotal reports from uncontrolled studies suggest that long-term oral therapy is well tolerated and possibly effective,[65,66] there is insufficient evidence at this point to recommend a long-term (6 months) course of therapy for infants with congenital CMV infection. Similarly, it remains unclear if treatment initiated beyond the neonatal period provides any benefit with respect to neurodevelopmental outcomes, although additional studies of this question are warranted.

Consensus guidelines for antiviral management of congenital CMV have not been formulated in the United States, although some recommended guidelines from Europe have been published with proposed treatment algorithms (see **Fig. 2**).[48,67] Other antiviral agents are available for CMV infection, including drugs such as foscarnet and cidofovir,[68] but there is little experience with the use of these agents in infants, and at the current time their usefulness is limited to exceptional circumstances, such as the emergence of antiviral resistance to ganciclovir and/or in the treatment of immunocompromised infants with serious CMV end-organ disease.[69]

PROSPECTS FOR PREVENTION: ACTIVE AND PASSIVE IMMUNIZATION

Development of a CMV vaccine is the most promising strategy for addressing the problem of congenital CMV. An effective vaccine could, by preventing neurologic sequelae and other disabilities, provide a newborn with a lifetime of benefit. A report from the Institute of Medicine of the National Academy of Sciences placed CMV in its highest priority category for vaccine development, concluding that a vaccine would be strongly cost-saving.[70] Several CMV vaccines are currently being evaluated in several clinical trials. A live-attenuated strain of CMV, the Towne strain, has been evaluated as a potential vaccine in a number of studies, including several studies in immunocompromised solid organ transplant patients at risk for CMV disease.[71–73] Although the Towne vaccine has elicited humoral and cellular immune responses in these studies and demonstrated an effect on CMV disease, its potential as a vaccine against congenital CMV infection was called into question in a study of young women with children attending group daycare. In this study, the Towne vaccine showed no reduction in the rate of infection of Towne-vaccinated mothers compared with placebo-inoculated mothers.[74] An approach to improve the immunogenicity of a live virus CMV vaccine has recently been undertaken by engineering recombinant "chimeras" of the attenuated Towne strain and the less attenuated, low-passage Toledo strain, and these vaccines are also in clinical trials.[75] In addition to live virus vaccines, purified protein and DNA subunit vaccines are also in clinical trials.[76] These vaccines focus on the virally encoded proteins that are the key targets of both the humoral and the cellular immune response to CMV. A vaccine based on the immunodominant CMV envelope glycoprotein, gB, was recently studied in adolescent and young adult women, with the primary endpoint reported in this study being time to primary CMV infection. Primary CMV infection was confirmed in 8% in the vaccine group, compared with 14% in the placebo group, an overall efficacy of 50%.[77] Additional evidence of the efficacy of the gB subunit vaccine was demonstrated in a placebo-controlled phase II study in solid organ transplant recipients.[78] It is hoped that ongoing and future clinical trials will lead to the licensure of a CMV vaccine in the not-too-distant future.

In addition to active immunization strategies, passive immunization, based on administration of anti-CMV immune globulin to women at risk of transmitting CMV to the fetus, is currently an intensely active area of clinical research. In a study of pregnant women with a primary CMV infection, whose amniotic fluid contained either CMV or CMV DNA, subjects were offered intravenous CMV hyperimmune globulin (HIG), in 2 different dose regimens, a "therapy" regimen or a "prevention" regimen.[79] In the therapy group, only 1 in 31 women gave birth to an infant with CMV disease (defined as an infant who was symptomatic at birth and handicapped at 2 or more years of age) compared with 7 of 14 women in an untreated control group. Similar benefits were noted in the prevention group. The administration of HIG to women in the primary infection group was associated with significant reductions in placental pathologic abnormalities, and with regression of cerebral structural abnormalities in some infants.[80,81] Another retrospective, observational study of HIG reported a trend toward reduced intrauterine transmission of CMV.[82] The use of HIG during pregnancy has also been reported to be associated with improved neurodevelopmental outcomes in infants in the first year of life.[83] Randomized controlled trials of HIG are warranted in high-risk pregnancies to validate the protective effect of passive immunization.

SUMMARY

Congenital CMV infection is common and underrecognized. Pediatricians and primary care physicians should be familiar with maternal risk factors and clinical clues in newborns that might suggest the diagnosis of congenital infection. Increased public awareness is needed, particularly among women of childbearing age. Therapeutic options are available, both for women who have transmitted CMV to the developing fetus and for symptomatic newborns. Children with congenital CMV infection are at risk for adverse neurodevelopmental outcomes, particularly SNHL. The pediatrician plays an essential role in the long-term anticipatory management of children with congenital CMV infection. Progress toward development of a CMV vaccine has accelerated. Eventual licensure of a vaccine coupled with increased recognition of the importance of this common and disabling disease will make inroads into reducing the impact of this virus on the health and well-being of children. Parents of children with congenital CMV have formed support groups and created Web sites for fostering knowledge and awareness (eg, www.buckbuck.org; www.congenitalcmvfoundation.org; www.averysjourney.com; www.stopcmv.org) and these organizations can be a useful source of information for parents and clinicians alike who are seeking answers regarding this major public health problem.

REFERENCES

1. Staras SA, Dollard SC, Radford KW, et al. Seroprevalence of cytomegalovirus infection in the United States, 1988-1994. Clin Infect Dis 2006;43(9):1143–51.

2. Kondo K, Xu J, Mocarski ES. Human cytomegalovirus latent gene expression in granulocyte-macrophage progenitors in culture and in seropositive individuals. Proc Natl Acad Sci U S A 1996;93(20):11137–42.
3. Hargett D, Shenk TE. Experimental human cytomegalovirus latency in CD14+ monocytes. Proc Natl Acad Sci U S A 2010;107(46):20039–44.
4. Dollard SC, Grosse SD, Ross DS. New estimates of the prevalence of neurological and sensory sequelae and mortality associated with congenital cytomegalovirus infection. Rev Med Virol 2007;17(5):355–63.
5. Kenneson A, Cannon MJ. Review and meta-analysis of the epidemiology of congenital cytomegalovirus (CMV) infection. Rev Med Virol 2007;17(4):253–76.
6. Nyholm JL, Schleiss MR. Prevention of maternal cytomegalovirus infection: current status and future prospects. Int J Womens Health 2010;2:23–35.
7. Leung AK, Sauve RS, Davies HD. Congenital cytomegalovirus infection. J Natl Med Assoc 2003;95(3):213–8.
8. Nance WE, Lim BG, Dodson KM. Importance of congenital cytomegalovirus infections as a cause for pre-lingual hearing loss. J Clin Virol 2006;35(2):221–5.
9. Fowler KB, Boppana SB. Congenital cytomegalovirus (CMV) infection and hearing deficit. J Clin Virol 2006;35(2):226–31.
10. Stagno S, Reynolds DW, Pass RF, et al. Breast milk and the risk of cytomegalovirus infection. N Engl J Med 1980;302(19):1073–6.
11. Pass RF, Hutto C, Ricks R, et al. Increased rate of cytomegalovirus infection among parents of children attending day-care centers. N Engl J Med 1986;314(22):1414–8.
12. Hyde TB, Schmid DS, Cannon MJ. Cytomegalovirus seroconversion rates and risk factors: implications for congenital CMV. Rev Med Virol 2010;20(5):311–26.
13. Marshall BC, Adler SP. The frequency of pregnancy and exposure to cytomegalovirus infections among women with a young child in day care. Am J Obstet Gynecol 2009;200(2):163.e1–5.
14. Sohn YM, Oh MK, Balcarek KB, et al. Cytomegalovirus infection in sexually active adolescents. J Infect Dis 1991;163(3):460–3.
15. Stadler LP, Bernstein DI, Callahan ST, et al. Seroprevalence of cytomegalovirus (CMV) and risk factors for infection in adolescent males. Clin Infect Dis 2010;51(10):e76–81.
16. Staras SA, Flanders WD, Dollard SC, et al. Influence of sexual activity on cytomegalovirus seroprevalence in the United States, 1988-1994. Sex Transm Dis 2008;35(5):472–9.
17. Horwitz CA, Henle W, Henle G, et al. Clinical and laboratory evaluation of cytomegalovirus-induced mononucleosis in previously healthy individuals. Report of 82 cases. Medicine (Baltimore) 1986;65(2):124–34.
18. Bate SL, Dollard SC, Cannon MJ. Cytomegalovirus seroprevalence in the United States: the national health and nutrition examination surveys, 1988-2004. Clin Infect Dis 2010;50(11):1439–47.
19. Cannon MJ, Schmid DS, Hyde TB. Review of cytomegalovirus seroprevalence and demographic characteristics associated with infection. Rev Med Virol 2010;20(4):202–13.
20. Cannon MJ, Westbrook K, Levis D, et al. Awareness of and behaviors related to child-to-mother transmission of cytomegalovirus. Prev Med 2012;54(5):351–7.
21. Revello MG, Campanini G, Piralla A, et al. Molecular epidemiology of primary human cytomegalovirus infection in pregnant women and their families. J Med Virol 2008;80(8):1415–25.
22. Cannon MJ, Davis KF. Washing our hands of the congenital cytomegalovirus disease epidemic. BMC Public Health 2005;5:70.

23. Schleiss MR. Acquisition of human cytomegalovirus infection in infants via breast milk: natural immunization or cause for concern? Rev Med Virol 2006;16(2):73–82.
24. Buxmann H, Miljak A, Fischer D, et al. Incidence and clinical outcome of cytomegalovirus transmission via breast milk in preterm infants </=31 weeks. Acta Paediatr 2009;98(2):270–6.
25. Kurath S, Halwachs-Baumann G, Muller W, et al. Transmission of cytomegalovirus via breast milk to the prematurely born infant: a systematic review. Clin Microbiol Infect 2010;16(8):1172–8.
26. Hamprecht K, Maschmann J, Jahn G, et al. Cytomegalovirus transmission to preterm infants during lactation. J Clin Virol 2008;41(3):198–205.
27. Bryant P, Morley C, Garland S, et al. Cytomegalovirus transmission from breast milk in premature babies: does it matter? Arch Dis Child Fetal Neonatal Ed 2002;87(2):F75–7.
28. Nijman J, van Zanten BG, de Waard AK, et al. Hearing in preterm infants with postnatally acquired cytomegalovirus infection. Pediatr Infect Dis J 2012;31:1082–4.
29. Boppana SB, Rivera LB, Fowler KB, et al. Intrauterine transmission of cytomegalovirus to infants of women with preconceptional immunity. N Engl J Med 2001; 344(18):1366–71.
30. Stagno S, Pass RF, Cloud G, et al. Primary cytomegalovirus infection in pregnancy. Incidence, transmission to fetus, and clinical outcome. JAMA 1986;256(14): 1904–8.
31. Boppana SB, Pass RF, Britt WJ, et al. Symptomatic congenital cytomegalovirus infection: neonatal morbidity and mortality. Pediatr Infect Dis J 1992;11(2):93–9.
32. Freij BJ, South MA, Sever JL. Maternal rubella and the congenital rubella syndrome. Clin Perinatol 1988;15(2):247–57.
33. Verboon-Maciolek MA, Krediet TG, Gerards LJ, et al. Severe neonatal parechovirus infection and similarity with enterovirus infection. Pediatr Infect Dis J 2008; 27(3):241–5.
34. Bale JF Jr, Murph JR. Congenital infections and the nervous system. Pediatr Clin North Am 1992;39(4):669–90.
35. Conboy TJ, Pass RF, Stagno S, et al. Early clinical manifestations and intellectual outcome in children with symptomatic congenital cytomegalovirus infection. J Pediatr 1987;111(3):343–8.
36. Pass RF, Stagno S, Myers GJ, et al. Outcome of symptomatic congenital cytomegalovirus infection: results of long-term longitudinal follow-up. Pediatrics 1980;66(5):758–62.
37. Foulon I, Naessens A, Foulon W, et al. Hearing loss in children with congenital cytomegalovirus infection in relation to the maternal trimester in which the maternal primary infection occurred. Pediatrics 2008;122(6):e1123–7.
38. Pass RF, Fowler KB, Boppana SB, et al. Congenital cytomegalovirus infection following first trimester maternal infection: symptoms at birth and outcome. J Clin Virol 2006;35(2):216–20.
39. Dahle AJ, Fowler KB, Wright JD, et al. Longitudinal investigation of hearing disorders in children with congenital cytomegalovirus. J Am Acad Audiol 2000;11(5): 283–90.
40. Fowler KB, Dahle AJ, Boppana SB, et al. Newborn hearing screening: will children with hearing loss caused by congenital cytomegalovirus infection be missed? J Pediatr 1999;135(1):60–4.
41. Dollard SC, Schleiss MR, Grosse SD. Public health and laboratory considerations regarding newborn screening for congenital cytomegalovirus. J Inherit Metab Dis 2010;33(Suppl 2):S249–54.

42. Grosse SD, Ross DS, Dollard SC. Congenital cytomegalovirus (CMV) infection as a cause of permanent bilateral hearing loss: a quantitative assessment. J Clin Virol 2008;41(2):57–62.
43. Foulon I, Naessens A, Foulon W, et al. A 10-year prospective study of sensorineural hearing loss in children with congenital cytomegalovirus infection. J Pediatr 2008;153(1):84–8.
44. Morton CC, Nance WE. Newborn hearing screening–a silent revolution. N Engl J Med 2006;354(20):2151–64.
45. Bhatia P, Narang A, Minz RW. Neonatal cytomegalovirus infection: diagnostic modalities available for early disease detection. Indian J Pediatr 2010;77(1):77–9.
46. Boppana SB, Ross SA, Shimamura M, et al. Saliva polymerase-chain-reaction assay for cytomegalovirus screening in newborns. N Engl J Med 2011;364(22):2111–8.
47. Yamamoto AY, Mussi-Pinhata MM, Marin LJ, et al. Is saliva as reliable as urine for detection of cytomegalovirus DNA for neonatal screening of congenital CMV infection? J Clin Virol 2006;36(3):228–30.
48. Kadambari S, Williams EJ, Luck S, et al. Evidence based management guidelines for the detection and treatment of congenital CMV. Early Hum Dev 2011;87(11):723–8.
49. Cheeran MC, Lokensgard JR, Schleiss MR. Neuropathogenesis of congenital cytomegalovirus infection: disease mechanisms and prospects for intervention. Clin Microbiol Rev 2009;22(1):99–126 [table of contents].
50. Lanari M, Capretti MG, Lazzarotto T. Neuroimaging examination of newborns in vertically acquired infections. J Matern Fetal Neonatal Med 2011;24(Suppl 1):117–9.
51. Lanari M, Capretti MG, Lazzarotto T, et al. Neuroimaging in CMV congenital infected neonates: how and when. Early Hum Dev 2012;88(Suppl 2):S3–5.
52. Ghekiere S, Allegaert K, Cossey V, et al. Ophthalmological findings in congenital cytomegalovirus infection: when to screen, when to treat? J Pediatr Ophthalmol Strabismus 2012;49(5):274–82.
53. Coats DK, Demmler GJ, Paysse EA, et al. Ophthalmologic findings in children with congenital cytomegalovirus infection. J AAPOS 2000;4(2):110–6.
54. Shin JJ, Keamy DG Jr, Steinberg EA. Medical and surgical interventions for hearing loss associated with congenital cytomegalovirus: a systematic review. Otolaryngol Head Neck Surg 2011;144(5):662–75.
55. Lee DJ, Lustig L, Sampson M, et al. Effects of cytomegalovirus (CMV) related deafness on pediatric cochlear implant outcomes. Otolaryngol Head Neck Surg 2005;133(6):900–5.
56. Stagno S, Pass RF, Thomas JP, et al. Defects of tooth structure in congenital cytomegalovirus infection. Pediatrics 1982;69(5):646–8.
57. Fan-Havard P, Nahata MC, Brady MT. Ganciclovir–a review of pharmacology, therapeutic efficacy and potential use for treatment of congenital cytomegalovirus infections. J Clin Pharm Ther 1989;14(5):329–40.
58. Vallejo JG, Englund JA, Garcia-Prats JA, et al. Ganciclovir treatment of steroid-associated cytomegalovirus disease in a congenitally infected neonate. Pediatr Infect Dis J 1994;13(3):239–41.
59. Nigro G, Scholz H, Bartmann U. Ganciclovir therapy for symptomatic congenital cytomegalovirus infection in infants: a two-regimen experience. J Pediatr 1994;124(2):318–22.
60. Kimberlin DW, Lin CY, Sanchez PJ, et al. Effect of ganciclovir therapy on hearing in symptomatic congenital cytomegalovirus disease involving the central nervous system: a randomized, controlled trial. J Pediatr 2003;143(1):16–25.

61. Oliver SE, Cloud GA, Sanchez PJ, et al. Neurodevelopmental outcomes following ganciclovir therapy in symptomatic congenital cytomegalovirus infections involving the central nervous system. J Clin Virol 2009;46(Suppl 4):S22–6.
62. Nassetta L, Kimberlin D, Whitley R. Treatment of congenital cytomegalovirus infection: implications for future therapeutic strategies. J Antimicrob Chemother 2009;63(5):862–7.
63. Marshall BC, Koch WC. Antivirals for cytomegalovirus infection in neonates and infants: focus on pharmacokinetics, formulations, dosing, and adverse events. Paediatr Drugs 2009;11(5):309–21.
64. Stronati M, Lombardi G, Garofoli F, et al. Pharmacokinetics, pharmacodynamics and clinical use of valganciclovir in newborns with symptomatic congenital Cytomegalovirus infection. Curr Drug Metab 2012;14(2):208–15.
65. Amir J, Wolf DG, Levy I. Treatment of symptomatic congenital cytomegalovirus infection with intravenous ganciclovir followed by long-term oral valganciclovir. Eur J Pediatr 2010;169(9):1061–7.
66. del Rosal T, Baquero-Artigao F, Blazquez D, et al. Treatment of symptomatic congenital cytomegalovirus infection beyond the neonatal period. J Clin Virol 2012;55(1):72–4.
67. Coll O, Benoist G, Ville Y, et al. Guidelines on CMV congenital infection. J Perinat Med 2009;37(5):433–45.
68. Razonable RR. Strategies for managing cytomegalovirus in transplant recipients. Expert Opin Pharmacother 2010;11(12):1983–97.
69. Blackman SC, Lurain NS, Witte DP, et al. Emergence and compartmentalization of fatal multi-drug-resistant cytomegalovirus infection in a patient with autosomal-recessive severe combined immune deficiency. J Pediatr Hematol Oncol 2004;26(9):601–5.
70. Arvin AM, Fast P, Myers M, et al. Vaccine development to prevent cytomegalovirus disease: report from the National Vaccine Advisory Committee. Clin Infect Dis 2004;39(2):233–9.
71. Plotkin SA, Smiley ML, Friedman HM, et al. Towne-vaccine-induced prevention of cytomegalovirus disease after renal transplants. Lancet 1984;1(8376):528–30.
72. Plotkin SA, Smiley ML, Friedman HM, et al. Prevention of cytomegalovirus disease by Towne strain live attenuated vaccine. Birth Defects Orig Artic Ser 1984;20(1):271–87.
73. Plotkin SA, Starr SE, Friedman HM, et al. Effect of Towne live virus vaccine on cytomegalovirus disease after renal transplant. A controlled trial. Ann Intern Med 1991;114(7):525–31.
74. Adler SP, Starr SE, Plotkin SA, et al. Immunity induced by primary human cytomegalovirus infection protects against secondary infection among women of childbearing age. J Infect Dis 1995;171(1):26–32.
75. Heineman TC, Schleiss M, Bernstein DI, et al. A phase 1 study of 4 live, recombinant human cytomegalovirus Towne/Toledo chimeric vaccines. J Infect Dis 2006;193(10):1350–60.
76. Sung H, Schleiss MR. Update on the current status of cytomegalovirus vaccines. Expert Rev Vaccines 2010;9(11):1303–14.
77. Pass RF, Zhang C, Evans A, et al. Vaccine prevention of maternal cytomegalovirus infection. N Engl J Med 2009;360(12):1191–9.
78. Griffiths PD, Stanton A, McCarrell E, et al. Cytomegalovirus glycoprotein-B vaccine with MF59 adjuvant in transplant recipients: a phase 2 randomised placebo-controlled trial. Lancet 2011;377(9773):1256–63.
79. Nigro G, Adler SP, La Torre R, et al. Passive immunization during pregnancy for congenital cytomegalovirus infection. N Engl J Med 2005;353(13):1350–62.

80. La Torre R, Nigro G, Mazzocco M, et al. Placental enlargement in women with primary maternal cytomegalovirus infection is associated with fetal and neonatal disease. Clin Infect Dis 2006;43(8):994–1000.
81. Nigro G, Torre RL, Pentimalli H, et al. Regression of fetal cerebral abnormalities by primary cytomegalovirus infection following hyperimmunoglobulin therapy. Prenat Diagn 2008;28(6):512–7.
82. Buxmann H, Stackelberg OM, Schlosser RL, et al. Use of cytomegalovirus hyperimmunoglobulin for prevention of congenital cytomegalovirus disease: a retrospective analysis. J Perinat Med 2012;40(4):439–46.
83. Visentin S, Manara R, Milanese L, et al. Early primary cytomegalovirus infection in pregnancy: maternal hyperimmunoglobulin therapy improves outcomes among infants at 1 year of age. Clin Infect Dis 2012;55(4):497–503.

Neonatal Herpes Simplex Virus Infections

Swetha G. Pinninti, MD[a], David W. Kimberlin, MD[b,*]

KEYWORDS

• Neonatal herpes • Acyclovir • Polymerase chain reaction • Antiviral therapy

KEY POINTS

- Neonatal herpes simplex virus (HSV) infection can be difficult to differentiate from other causes of neonatal sepsis.
- The three major forms of neonatal HSV infection are disseminated disease (25% of cases); central nervous system (CNS) disease (30%); and skin, eye, and mouth disease (45%).
- The use of high-dose acyclovir for neonatal HSV disease has dramatically reduced mortality and morbidity from this disease.
- Disseminated HSV disease has a higher mortality rate (29%) than CNS disease (4%), but a lower frequency of disabilities 1 year after disease (disseminated, 17%; CNS, 69%).
- Neonates with HSV disease should receive oral acyclovir suppressive therapy for 6 months after completion of intravenous acyclovir treatment.
- New guidelines provide an evidence-based approach to evaluation and treatment of neonates born to women with active genital herpetic lesions.

VIRAL STRUCTURE

Herpes simplex viruses (HSV)-1 and -2 belong to alphaherpesviridae and are large, enveloped virions with an icosahedral nucleocapsid arranged around a linear, double-stranded DNA core. There is considerable cross-reactivity between HSV-1 and -2 glycoproteins, which mediate attachment to and penetration into cells and evoke host immune responses. Antigenic specificity is provided by glycoprotein gG, with the antibody response allowing for distinction between HSV-1 and -2.

Funding Sources: Dr Pinninti: None. Dr Kimberlin: NIH, Cellex, GSK (All monies go directly to the University).
Conflict of Interest: None.
This work was supported under contract with the Division of Microbiology and Infectious Diseases of the National Institute of Allergy and Infectious Diseases (N01-AI-30025, N01-AI-65306, N01-AI-15113, N01-AI-62554).
[a] Division of Pediatric Infectious Diseases, The University of Alabama at Birmingham, 1600 Seventh Avenue South, CHB 308, Birmingham, AL 35233, USA; [b] Division of Pediatric Infectious Diseases, The University of Alabama at Birmingham, 1600 Seventh Avenue South, CHB 303, Birmingham, AL 35233, USA
* Corresponding author.
E-mail address: dkimberlin@peds.uab.edu

Pediatr Clin N Am 60 (2013) 351–365
http://dx.doi.org/10.1016/j.pcl.2012.12.005 **pediatric.theclinics.com**
0031-3955/13/$ – see front matter

MATERNAL GENITAL HERPES

Terminology

Primary infection refers to acquisition of HSV-1 or -2 without prior exposure to either virus and hence no preformed antibodies. Nonprimary infection refers to acquisition of HSV-2 in an individual with prior HSV-1 antibodies and vice versa.

Reactivation is isolation of same type of virus from genital lesions as pre-existing type-specific antibodies. Symptomatic shedding refers to presence of lesions characteristic of genital herpes and detection of HSV-1 or -2 from the lesions by culture or polymerase chain reaction (PCR). Subclinical shedding refers to isolation of HSV-1 or -2 from genital mucosa by culture or PCR in the absence of lesions.

Epidemiology of Genital Infections During Pregnancy

Genital herpes infections are caused by HSV-1 or -2 and most infections are asymptomatic. HSV-2 seroprevalence among pregnant women is estimated to be 20% to 30% with approximately 10% of HSV-2 seronegative women living with a seropositive partner and hence at risk for acquisition of genital herpes during pregnancy.[1,2] Among discordant couples, women seronegative for HSV-1 and -2 have an estimated 3.7% chance for seroconversion, whereas the risk for women already seropositive for HSV-1 to seroconvert to HSV-2 is estimated to be 1.7%.[3] Similar to nonpregnant women, two-thirds of women who acquire genital HSV infection during pregnancy are either asymptomatic or have nonspecific symptoms. Among women with history of genital herpes acquired before pregnancy, 75% have at least one recurrence during pregnancy and 14% have prodromal symptoms or lesions at the time of delivery.[4,5] For neonatal transmission, women must be shedding the virus symptomatically or asymptomatically around the time of delivery. It has been shown that 0.2% to 0.39%[6] of all pregnant women shed HSV in the genital tract around the time of delivery irrespective of prior history of HSV, and this incidence of shedding increases to 0.77% to 1.4% among women with prior history of recurrent genital herpes.[7,8]

Distinguishing primary and nonprimary first-episode genital herpes episodes during pregnancy is based on information obtained from combination of genital culture or PCR data and serology. The risk of transmission of HSV to the neonate remains significantly higher with primary maternal infections acquired closer to the time of delivery compared with recurrent infections (50%–60% with primary infections vs <3% for recurrent infections), most likely caused by decreased transplacentally acquired antibody levels in the neonate and exposure in the birth canal to increased quantities of virus for longer duration.[9] Fortunately, most genital herpes infections during pregnancy are recurrent and are associated with a lower risk of transmission to the neonate.

NEONATAL HERPES

Epidemiology

HSV infection of the neonate is an uncommon occurrence with an estimated rate of approximately 1 in 3200 deliveries.[10] Neonatal HSV infections occur far less frequently compared with other serious neonatal infections overall. With approximately 4 million deliveries per year in the United States, an estimated 1500 cases of neonatal HSV disease occur annually in the United States.[11] When compared with other reportable congenital infections, such as syphilis, toxoplasmosis, and rubella, the overall incidence of neonatal HSV disease is higher yet the disease still does not require mandatory reporting.[12]

Factors Influencing Transmission of HSV to Neonate

Factors that influence transmission of HSV to neonate include the following:

1. Type of maternal infection (primary vs secondary)[6,10,13]
2. Maternal antibody status[10,14,15]
3. Mode of delivery (vaginal vs cesarean section)[10]
4. Duration of rupture of membranes[10,13]
5. Integrity of cutaneous barrier (use of fetal scalp electrodes and other instrumentation)[10]
6. Type of HSV (HSV-1 vs -2)[10]

The risk of neonatal acquisition of HSV is significantly higher with first-episode primary and first-episode nonprimary maternal infections when compared with recurrent genital infections. Brown and colleagues[10] evaluated approximately 40,000 pregnant women to assess the effect of maternal serologic status and cesarean section on transmission of HSV to the neonate. Of the approximately 40,000 women in the study who had cultures obtained from the external genitalia, approximately 31,000 women had serologic results available. Of these, 121 women were identified who were asymptomatically shedding virus at the time of delivery and who had serologic analysis. The risk of neonatal transmission was identified as 57% with first-episode primary infection compared with 25% with first-episode nonprimary infection and 2% with recurrent genital HSV infections. This study, for the first time, also documented the protective effect of cesarean section in preventing neonatal HSV. Other statistically significant risk factors in this large study for transmission of HSV to neonate were isolation of HSV-1 from genital lesions when compared with HSV-2 and use of invasive monitoring techniques, such as fetal scalp electrodes.

In a smaller study of approximately 7000 women at risk of acquiring HSV during pregnancy, Brown and colleagues[3] documented a maternal seroconversion rate of 3.2% and noted that HSV seroconversion completed before labor was not associated with increased neonatal morbidity but infections acquired close to labor were associated with increased incidence of neonatal HSV and worse morbidity.

Cesarean delivery has been proved to be effective in preventing the transmission of HSV to the neonate.[16] It is important, however, to note that neonatal HSV cases have occurred despite cesarean delivery before rupture of membranes.[2,17] Evidence also exists for prolonged rupture of membranes[13] and disruption of mucocutaenous barrier by the use of fetal scalp electrodes and other instrumentation to affect the acquisition of neonatal HSV disease.[10,18]

Prematurity as a risk factor for acquisition of neonatal HSV is not well studied. Although there is a larger proportion of premature infants with neonatal HSV compared with the general population and neonatal HSV infections in this population is associated with significant mortality and morbidity,[19] it is not well known if genital herpes leads to prematurity or prematurity increases the risk of acquiring neonatal HSV.[20]

Although it has been shown that the chances of acquisition of HSV-1 are decreased in women seropositive for HSV-2, transmission of HSV-1 to the neonate has been documented to be high irrespective of primary or recurrent infection when compared with HSV-2 transmission patterns.[10]

Neonatal HSV Disease Classification and Clinical Presentation

Neonatal HSV is acquired during one of three time periods: (1) in utero (5%); (2) peripartum (85%); or (3) postnatal (10%). HSV infection acquired in the intrauterine, peripartum, or postnatal period is classified into the following types and is predictive of mortality and morbidity (**Table 1**)[21–25]: disseminated disease; central nervous system (CNS) disease; and skin, eye, or mouth (SEM) disease.

Intrauterine infection

In utero infection with HSV is a rare entity but is unlikely to be missed because of presentation at birth and extent of involvement. It occurs in approximately 1 in 300,000 deliveries.[26] Affected infants present with a triad of clinical findings[27–29]: cutaneous (scarring, rash, aplasia cutis, hyperpigmentation or hypopigmentation); ophthalmologic (microphthalmia, chorioretinitis, optic atrophy); and neurologic (intracranial calcifications, microcephaly, encephalomalacia).

Disseminated disease

In the preantiviral era, disseminated HSV infections accounted for one-half to two-thirds of all children with neonatal HSV disease. Since the development and use of antiviral therapy, disseminated disease has decreased to approximately 25% of all neonatal herpes[2] and usually presents around day 10 to 12 of life. Two-thirds of infants with disseminated disease also have concurrent encephalitis. Disseminated disease involves multiple organs, including CNS, lungs, liver, adrenal, and SEM. Although presence of a vesicular rash greatly facilitates identification of neonates with HSV disease, 20% of infants with disseminated disease never develop a vesicular rash.[2,25,30] These patients usually present with viral sepsis, including respiratory failure, hepatic failure, and disseminated intravascular coagulation. Death from disseminated disease is usually caused by severe coagulopathy and extensive hepatic and pulmonary involvement.

CNS disease

Almost one-third of cases of neonatal herpes disease present as encephalitis and are categorized as CNS disease with or without skin involvement[2] and tend to present later than the other two entities at 16 to 19 days of life.[25] Clinical manifestations include

Table 1
Clinical presentations of neonatal HSV disease

Clinical Characteristic	Disseminated Disease	CNS Disease	SEM Disease
Mode of acquisition	Peripartum/postpartum	Peripartum/postpartum	Peripartum/postpartum
Frequency	25%	30%	45%
Sites of involvement	CNS, liver, lung, adrenal, skin, eye, mucus membranes	Central nervous system with or without skin involvement	Skin, eye, mucus membranes
Presentation	Encephalitis, respiratory failure, hepatic failure, disseminated intravascular coagulation ± rash	Seizures, lethargy, irritability, poor feeding, temperature instability ± rash	± vesicular rash
Mortality	29%	4%	—
Normal development 1 y after treatment without subsequent antiviral suppressive therapy	83%	31%	100%

focal or generalized seizures, lethargy, irritability, poor feeding, temperature instability, and bulging fontanelle. A total of 60% to 70% of infants with CNS disease have skin lesions at some point during the course of the illness.[25] In the absence of skin lesions, the clinical presentation is indistinguishable from other causes of viral or bacterial sepsis. Mortality in these neonates is usually caused by devastating brain destruction with acute neurologic and autonomic dysfunction. Unlike herpes simplex encephalitis beyond the neonatal period, where there is a higher predilection for the temporal lobe to be involved, neonatal HSV often involves multiples areas of the brain.

SEM disease

Infection limited to SEM has historically accounted for 20% of cases of neonatal herpes disease but has increased to approximately 45% with the introduction of antiviral therapy.[2] Eighty percent of neonates with SEM disease have a vesicular rash on physical examination and usually present to medical attention around day 10 to 12 of life.[25]

Differential Diagnosis

Several other infectious and non-infectious conditions mimic neonatal HSV disease. Bacterial pathogens include group B *Streptococcus*, *Listeria monocytogenes*, *Staphylococcus aureus*, *Escherichia coli*, and other gram-negative bacteria. Viral exanthematous infections that are confused for neonatal HSV include varicella-zoster virus infection, enteroviral sepsis, and symptomatic cytomegalovirus infection. Noninfectious cutaneous disorders should be considered and include erythema toxicum, incontinentia pigmenti, and Bednar's aphthae.

EVALUATION OF THE NEONATE WITH SUSPECTED HSV INFECTION

Viral Culture

Isolation of HSV by culture remains the definitive method of diagnosing neonatal HSV infection (**Box 1**). Conjunctivae, nasopharynx, mouth, and anus (surface cultures) are swabbed and transported in appropriate transport media on ice to a diagnostic virology laboratory for inoculation into cell culture systems that are monitored for cytopathic effects.[30] Typing of an isolate may be performed by one of several techniques for prognostic purposes. Others sites from which HSV can be cultured include cerebrospinal fluid (CSF) and blood. Of sites routinely cultured for HSV, skin and eye or conjunctival cultures provide the greatest yield.[25]

Polymerase Chain Reaction

The application of PCR to CSF samples has revolutionized the diagnosis of CNS neonatal herpes disease.[31–35] However, performance of PCR is highly dependent on the manner the CSF sample is collected, stored, and transported to the laboratory.[36] The overall sensitivities of CSF PCR in neonatal HSV disease have ranged from 75% to 100%, with overall specificities ranging from 71% to 100%.[33,34,37] The results of the PCR should always be interpreted, taking into consideration the clinical presentation of the neonate. A negative PCR result from the CSF does not rule out neonatal HSV disease, because the test may be negative in very early stages of the infection as a result of low viral load or the sensitivity of the test being used. In comparison, blood PCR in neonatal HSV has been evaluated to a lesser extent and in smaller cohorts.[34,35,38]

Serologic Testing

Serologic diagnosis of neonatal HSV is not very helpful and is not usually recommended because of transplacentally acquired maternal IgG, which confounds the assessment of neonatal antibody levels during acute infection. Serial antibody assessment

Box 1
Evaluation and treatment of neonatal HSV disease

1. Specimens to obtain before initiating anti-viral therapy
   a. CSF – Indices, bacterial culture, HSV DNA PCR
   b. Surface cultures ± PCR
   c. Base of vesicle or suspicious lesions culture ± PCR
   d. Whole Blood – PCR
   e. Whole Blood – Alanine aminotransferase (ALT)
2. Treatment of Neonatal HSV
   a. Intravenous Acyclovir
   b. Dose – 60 mg/kg/day divided in 3 doses
3. Duration of Treatment:
   a. SEM Disease – 14 days
   b. CNS Disease – Minimum 21 days[a]
   c. Disseminated Disease – 21 days
4. Antiviral Suppressive Therapy after Treatment (SEM, CNS and Disseminated Disease):
   a. Oral acyclovir 300 mg/m2/dose, three times a day for 6 months
   b. Monitor absolute neutrophil count while on therapy

[a] In neonates with positive CSF HSV PCR at the end of therapy, antiviral therapy should be continued until PCR negativity is achieved.

From Pickering L, Baker C, Kimberlin D, et al. Herpes Simplex. In: Pickering L, editor. Red book. Report of the Committee on Infectious Diseases. 29th edition. Elk Grove Village (IL): American Academy of Pediatrics; 2012. p. 398–408; with permission.

may be useful in specific circumstances where a mother with primary genital HSV late in gestation transfers very little antibody to the neonate. Overall, serologic studies play no role in the diagnosis of neonatal HSV infection and are not currently recommended for diagnostic purposes.

Specimens to Obtain Before Starting Antiviral Therapy

Before initiation of empiric parenteral antiviral therapy, the following specimens should be collected to aid in the diagnosis of neonatal HSV disease or to determine if antiviral therapy may be discontinued if HSV has been excluded[30]:

1. CSF for indices, bacterial culture, and HSV DNA PCR
2. Swab for viral culture from the base of vesicles, suspicious areas, and mucous membrane lesions for viral culture; PCR may be performed in addition to cultures, if desired
3. Swab from mouth, conjunctiva, nasopharynx, and rectum (surface cultures) for viral culture; PCR may be performed in addition to cultures, if desired
4. Whole blood for HSV DNA PCR
5. Blood to determine alanine aminotransferase (ALT)

TREATMENT OF NEONATAL HSV

The earliest antiviral agents effective against HSV included 5-iodo-2′-doexyuridine and 1-β-D-arabinofuranosylcytosine, but were found to be too toxic for human use.

Vidarabine, licensed for use in the United States in 1977, was the first antiviral for which the therapeutic efficacy outweighed toxicity for use in cases of life-threatening HSV disease. Because of toxicity associated with administration of intravenous vidarabine, its use was restricted by the Food and Drug Administration to life-threatening HSV and varicella-zoster virus infections.[21] In the 1980s, a landmark study comparing the efficacy of intravenous vidarabine with lower-dose acyclovir (30 mg/kg/d administered three times a day for 10 days) for neonatal herpes disease[22] found a lack of therapeutic superiority of the lower-dose acyclovir over vidarabine. Acyclovir was soon the treatment of choice because of its safety profile and ease of administration. Subsequently, a higher dose of acyclovir (60 mg/kg/d divided in three doses for 14–21 days) has been shown to remarkably improve mortality associated with neonatal HSV disease.[24]

The current recommendations are to treat all neonates with HSV disease parenterally with acyclovir given at 60 mg/kg/d divided every 8 hours.[24,30] The dosing interval may need to be increased in premature infants depending on their renal clearance.[39] Duration of treatment is 14 days for infants with SEM disease and 21 days for neonates with CNS and disseminated disease presentations.[30] All neonates with CNS involvement should have repeat CSF PCR performed on CSF at the end of therapy to document a negative CSF PCR result and for CSF indices. HSV DNA detected in CSF after completion of acyclovir therapy has been associated with poorer outcomes.[33] In those rare neonates with positive CSF PCR at the end of therapy, antiviral therapy should be continued until PCR negativity is achieved.[25,30,33] Because the significance of blood DNA PCR positivity remains largely unknown, serial measurement of blood DNA PCR for assessing response to therapy is not recommended at this time.[30] Although a retrospective study that compared the prevalence of neonatal HSV disease with bacterial meningitis among infants admitted through the emergency department for sepsis evaluation revealed that the incidence for both entities was similar, the number of infants with neonatal herpes included in the study was too small to draw any definite conclusions about empiric antiviral coverage for all infants undergoing sepsis evaluation in the first month.[40] Experts in the field differ regarding opinion about empiric coverage for such infants.[41,42]

Prognosis

Mortality

In the preantiviral era, 85% of neonates with disseminated disease and 50% of neonates with CNS disease died by 1 year of age.[21] Currently, with the use of the higher dose of acyclovir (60 mg/kg/d divided in three doses for 21 days), 1-year mortality has been reduced to 29% for disseminated disease and 4% for CNS disease.[24] Risk factors associated with higher mortality include lethargy and severe hepatitis in neonates with disseminated disease and lethargy and seizures in infants with CNS disease.[25]

Morbidity

In the preantiviral era, 50% of survivors with disseminated disease and 33% of neonates with CNS disease developed normally at 12 months of age.[21] After the initiation of high-dose acyclovir, 83% of neonates with disseminated disease and 31% with CNS disease develop normally at 12 months of age.[21,24] Seizures before or at the time of initiation of antiviral therapy has been associated with increased risk of morbidity in neonates with disseminated and CNS disease.[24]

Morbidity after SEM disease has dramatically improved after initiation of antiviral therapy. In the preantiviral era, 38% of the infants with SEM disease developed developmental disabilities at the age of 12 months, and after introduction of vidarabine and lower-dose acyclovir the percentages dropped to 12% and 2%, respectively.[22] None of the infants with SEM disease in the high-dose acyclovir study developed developmental disabilities at 12 months age.[24]

Antiviral Suppressive Therapy After Treatment

The outcome of neonatal herpes depends on the extent of disease. Approximately 20% of survivors with disseminated disease have neurologic sequelae compared with 70% of neonates with CNS disease.[24] A phase III, placebo-controlled trial performed by the National Institute of Allergy and Infectious Diseases Collaborative Antiviral Study Group showed good evidence for use of acyclovir-suppressive therapy for 6 months after completion of standard therapy for neonatal HSV disease. Infants with CNS disease stratified to the treatment arm were found to have better neurodevelopmental outcomes compared with the placebo group, and infants with SEM disease were found to have less frequent recurrence of skin lesions while receiving suppressive therapy.[43] Although almost half of infants enrolled in an earlier small phase I/II trial were found to have increased incidence of neutropenia,[44] the phase III trial of acyclovir-suppressive therapy found similar rates of neutropenia in the treatment and placebo arms of the study,[43] although the *p*-value approached statistical significance. The current recommendation for antiviral-suppressive therapy after completion of treatment of neonatal herpes disease is to treat with oral acyclovir at 300 mg/m^2/dose, three times a day for 6 months. Absolute neutrophil counts should be monitored at 2 and 4 weeks and monthly thereafter after initiation of suppressive therapy.[30] Orally administered acyclovir, however, has low bioavailability and requires frequent dosing. Recently, pharmacokinetic and safety profile of an extemporaneously compounded valacyclovir oral suspension in pediatric patients 1 month to 11 years was assessed. Clearance of acyclovir after administration of valacyclovir was found to be prolonged in infants younger than 3 months compared with older age groups,[45] and at this time valacyclovir should not be used for prolonged antiviral suppression after neonatal HSV disease.

Approach to an Infant Exposed to HSV During Maternal Primary or Recurrent Genital HSV Infection

Recommendations for the management of infants exposed to HSV in the intrapartum period until recently were based on expert opinion and did not take into consideration the change in epidemiology of genital HSV (primary vs recurrent infections and HSV-1 vs -2 infections in women). The most recent Clinical Report endorsed by the American Academy of Pediatrics provides evidence-based guidance on the management of neonates born to women with active genital herpetic lesions (**Box 2**).[46]

The recommendations take into consideration maternal serologic status, presence of genital lesions at the time of delivery, and route of delivery. The recommendations are applicable only to institutions that have access to PCR facilities and require neonatal and obstetric clinicians involved to work very closely with laboratory personnel for timely access to laboratory results. Moreover, the guidelines are only applicable to care of infants exposed to HSV from maternal genital lesions present at the time of delivery and not to situations of asymptomatic shedding.

Testing of women in labor

All women with genital lesions characteristic of HSV at the time of delivery should have viral culture and PCR sent off from the lesions. Further characterization of type as HSV-1 or -2 is required for correlation with serology to determine status of maternal infection (primary vs recurrent).

Box 2
Management of infants born to women with genital lesions at delivery

1. Determine maternal serologic and virologic status
   a. Send viral culture and PCR for HSV from genital lesions at delivery
   b. Characterize type of HSV (HSV-1 vs -2)
   c. Determine maternal HSV serology
   d. Determine status of maternal infection at delivery (primary vs recurrent infection)
2. Infants born to women with lesions at delivery with genital herpes before pregnancy
   a. Determine status of maternal infection at delivery (primary vs recurrent infection)
   b. Obtain surface cultures and blood DNA PCR from neonate for viral culture ± PCR at 24 hours
   c. Obtain CSF for HSV PCR and serum ALT level if previously mentioned tests positive
   d. Neonatal HSV infection: treat pre-emptively with intravenous acyclovir for 10 days
   e. Neonatal HSV disease: treat with intravenous acyclovir for 21 days (CNS/disseminated disease) or 14 days (SEM disease)
3. Infants born to women with genital lesions at delivery without genital herpes before pregnancy
   a. Determine status of maternal infection at delivery (primary vs recurrent infection)
   b. Obtain surface cultures, blood DNA PCR, serum ALT, and CSF for HSV PCR from neonate for viral culture ± PCR at 24 hours
   c. Initiate treatment with intravenous acyclovir
   d. Maternal recurrent infection and neonate asymptomatic: discontinue acyclovir
   e. Maternal first episode primary or nonprimary maternal infection and neonate asymptomatic: treat pre-emptively with acyclovir for 10 days
   f. Neonatal HSV infection: treat pre-emptively with acyclovir for 10 days
   g. Neonatal HSV disease: treat with intravenous acyclovir for 21 days (CNS/disseminated disease) or 14 days (SEM disease)

Management of newborns born to women with lesions at delivery and a history of genital herpes before pregnancy

For women with a history of genital herpes before pregnancy, the likelihood of lesions present at delivery being recurrent is high and the risk of transmission to the infant is low (<3%). At approximately 24 hours after delivery, surface cultures (conjunctiva, mouth, nasopharynx, rectum, and scalp electrode site when present) and blood DNA PCR should be obtained for viral culture and PCR. It is not required to start acyclovir therapy in these neonates because of lesser risk for acquisition of neonatal HSV. Waiting for 24 hours after delivery before collection of samples is recommended to differentiate contamination of neonatal skin by maternal secretions during the birth process versus true HSV infection of the baby. It is acceptable to discharge these infants who continue to be clinically well at 48 hours with instructions to caregivers for very close monitoring and immediate medical attention with development of any findings concerning for neonatal HSV.

If the surface and blood virologic studies are negative at 5 days, further evaluation of the infant is recommended only with the development of any signs suggestive of neonatal HSV in the subsequent 6 weeks. If the surface and blood virologic studies are positive, suggesting HSV infection, a full evaluation (CSF for indices and HSV PCR, serum ALT level) is recommended to determine presence and extent of HSV disease. Under these circumstances, therapy with intravenous acyclovir should be initiated in these infants as soon as possible.

If the results of the evaluation are negative (normal CSF indices and negative CSF HSV PCR, normal ALT measurement), suggestive of neonatal HSV infection, preemptive treatment for 10 days with parenteral acyclovir should be administered to prevent the progression of HSV infection to HSV disease. If the evaluation is suggestive of neonatal HSV disease (abnormal CSF indices with HSV CSF PCR positive or elevated serum ALT), treatment with acyclovir should be continued for 21 days for CNS or disseminated neonatal HSV disease as discussed previously, followed by oral suppressive therapy with acyclovir for 6 months.

Management of newborns born to women with lesions at delivery and no history of genital herpes before pregnancy

In women without a history of genital herpes before pregnancy, the presence of genital lesions at labor could represent primary infection (>50% risk of transmission to neonate); nonprimary infection (25% risk of transmission to neonate); or recurrent infection (<3% risk of transmission). The information obtained from viral culture and PCR of these lesions and maternal serologic status obtained at delivery should guide the clinician in determining the type of maternal infection and risk for transmission to the neonate and guide approach to management of neonate.

At approximately 24 hours after birth, surface cultures (eye, mouth, nasopharynx, and rectum) and blood for HSV DNA PCR should be obtained from the neonate. Because of the higher risk of transmission of HSV to neonates in these circumstances, CSF for determination of indices and HSV PCR and serum for ALT level should be obtained simultaneously, as should initiation of treatment with intravenous acyclovir.

If the maternal serology and virologic studies are more suggestive of a recurrent infection and the infant remains asymptomatic with no evidence of HSV infection or disease (negative result on surface cultures, blood DNA PCR, CSF PCR, and normal ALT level), discontinuation of parenteral acyclovir with instructions for close monitoring and re-evaluation with the development of any new signs is recommended.

If the maternal studies are suggestive of a primary or nonprimary genital infection and the neonate remains asymptomatic and lacks evidence of HSV infection or disease, treatment with 10 days of parenteral acyclovir is recommended (preemptive therapy).

With maternal recurrent or nonprimary infections involving infants with evidence of HSV infection or HSV disease, the guidelines are similar to those outlined in the approach to an infant born to a mother with history of genital herpes before pregnancy: 10 days of parenteral acyclovir for HSV infection (preemptive therapy), 14 days of parenteral acyclovir for neonatal SEM disease, and 21 days of parenteral acyclovir therapy for CNS or disseminated disease with documentation of negative CSF HSV PCR before stopping parenteral acyclovir therapy followed by 6 months of oral acyclovir-suppressive therapy as discussed previously.

STRATEGIES FOR PREVENTION OF NEONATAL HERPES

Cesarean Delivery

Delivery of the infant by cesarean section in women with active genital lesions can reduce the infant's risk of acquiring HSV[10,13] and is recommended when genital lesions or prodromal symptoms are present at the time of delivery,[16] although it does not completely eliminate the risk of neonatal HSV. Cesarean delivery is more likely to be effective if performed before rupture of membranes, but in situations where rupture of membranes has occurred and genital lesions are observed on physical examination cesarean delivery is recommended to minimize exposure of the neonate to HSV.[16] Physicians involved in the care of neonates should be aware that delivery by cesarean section does not entirely prevent transmission of HSV to the neonate. Transmission of HSV has been documented in circumstances where cesarean section was performed before rupture of membranes.[2,17] Cesarean section is not currently recommended for women with a prior history of genital herpes and no active lesions or prodromal symptoms at the time of delivery.[16,47] Protocols as outlined previously should be followed for care of neonates exposed to maternal genital lesions suggestive of HSV infection.

Antiviral Suppressive Therapy

In women with active recurrent genital herpes, antiviral suppressive therapy with acyclovir/valacyclovir initiated at 36 weeks of gestation has been associated with decreased genital lesions at the time of delivery and decreased viral detection by culture or PCR with a reduced need for cesarean section. Use of such suppressive therapy is an increasing practice among obstetricians and is recommended by the American College of Obstetricians and Gynecologists,[16] even though subclinical viral shedding is not entirely suppressed. The use of such a practice in preventing neonatal HSV disease is not well studied. The Acyclovir in Pregnancy Registry, which recorded the outcomes of pregnancy in which in utero exposure to acyclovir or valacyclovir occurred, observed no adverse fetal outcomes or birth defects in fetuses exposed to these drugs.[48] The number of neonates in the registry was too small to draw any conclusions regarding efficacy or safety to the neonate from the use of such suppressive therapy during pregnancy.

A recent multicenter case series reported eight cases of infants with neonatal HSV disease acquired from mothers despite receiving antiviral suppressive therapies beyond 36 weeks of gestation.[29] Overall, although maternal antiviral suppressive therapy decreases the incidence of genital recurrences at labor, the extent to which these drugs prevent neonatal acquisition remains unknown and requires further research.

HSV Vaccine

Several attempts to develop a vaccine for genital herpes have been futile. An earlier HSV-2 gD subunit vaccine adjuvanted with alum was found to be effective in preventing HSV-1 or -2 genital herpes (~75% vaccine efficacy) and HSV-2 infection. However, efficacy was limited only to women who were HSV-1 and -2 seronegative before vaccination. There was no reported efficacy in men or women who were HSV-1 seropositive before vaccination.[49] Most recently, the results of a randomized, double-blind trial testing the efficacy of the same HSV-2 gD subunit vaccine involving women seronegative for HSV-1 and -2 were reported. The vaccine was found to have an efficacy of 58% for preventing HSV-1 genital herpes but lacked efficacy for preventing HSV-2 genital herpes.[50] Currently, no vaccine has proved to be effective for preventing acquisition of HSV-1 or -2.

Prevention of Maternal HSV Acquisition During Pregnancy

Various strategies have been recommended to prevent maternal acquisition during pregnancy but none have been tested in large-scale trials.[12,51] The first approach is to screen all women with an IgG-based assay at 24 to 28 weeks of gestation. Women identified to be seropositive but unaware of a prior infection would benefit from education regarding significance of this finding and identification of recurrent lesions and prodromal symptoms, particularly at the time of labor. Women found to be seronegative or seropositive to either HSV-1 or -2 should be counseled to avoid oral-genital and genital-genital contact, respectively. This strategy does not take into account the serostatus or exposure risk to the sexual partner.

The second approach recommends screening all couples for HSV serology at 14 to 18 weeks and appropriate counseling based on serology results for both partners. This approach might not be applicable in situations where a single partner cannot be identified or the partner changes during the course of pregnancy.

The third approach is to advise all pregnant women to abstain from all forms of sexual contact during the third trimester of pregnancy. The final approach might particularly be applicable in situations where serologic testing is either unavailable or is economically not feasible.

The feasibility of these approaches has not been tested in any studies and the applicability and cost-effectiveness of such interventions requires further study. The American College of Obstetricians and Gynecologists currently does not recommend routine screening of asymptomatic women for HSV during pregnancy.[16]

Prevention of Postnatal Acquisition

Although most neonatal HSV infections are acquired in the peripartum period, 10% of cases are acquired in the postpartum period by exposure to the virus from open lesions of caretakers. There have also been reports of neonatal HSV infections after Jewish ritual circumcision involving orogenital contact[52] and it is important for physicians involved in the care of children to educate parents about the risks involved in such practices. Although it is recommended that infected household contacts and family members avoid contact with a newborn, it is prudent for infected healthcare personnel with active herpetic whitlow lesions to not be responsible for direct care of neonates.[30]

REFERENCES

1. Kulhanjian JA, Soroush V, Au DS, et al. Identification of women at unsuspected risk of primary infection with herpes simplex virus type 2 during pregnancy. N Engl J Med 1992;326(14):916–20.
2. Whitley RJ, Corey L, Arvin A, et al. Changing presentation of herpes simplex virus infection in neonates. J Infect Dis 1988;158(1):109–16.
3. Brown ZA, Selke S, Zeh J, et al. The acquisition of herpes simplex virus during pregnancy. N Engl J Med 1997;337(8):509–15.
4. Sheffield JS, Hill JB, Hollier LM, et al. Valacyclovir prophylaxis to prevent recurrent herpes at delivery: a randomized clinical trial. Obstet Gynecol 2006;108(1):141–7.
5. Watts DH, Brown ZA, Money D, et al. A double-blind, randomized, placebo-controlled trial of acyclovir in late pregnancy for the reduction of herpes simplex virus shedding and cesarean delivery. Am J Obstet Gynecol 2003;188(3):836–43.
6. Brown ZA, Benedetti J, Ashley R, et al. Neonatal herpes simplex virus infection in relation to asymptomatic maternal infection at the time of labor. N Engl J Med 1991;324(18):1247–52.
7. Arvin AM, Hensleigh PA, Prober CG, et al. Failure of antepartum maternal cultures to predict the infant's risk of exposure to herpes simplex virus at delivery. N Engl J Med 1986;315(13):796–800.
8. Vontver LA, Hickok DE, Brown Z, et al. Recurrent genital herpes simplex virus infection in pregnancy: infant outcome and frequency of asymptomatic recurrences. Am J Obstet Gynecol 1982;143(1):75–84.

9. Sullender WM, Yasukawa LL, Schwartz M, et al. Type-specific antibodies to herpes simplex virus type 2 (HSV-2) glycoprotein G in pregnant women, infants exposed to maternal HSV-2 infection at delivery, and infants with neonatal herpes. J Infect Dis 1988;157(1):164–71.
10. Brown ZA, Wald A, Morrow RA, et al. Effect of serologic status and cesarean delivery on transmission rates of herpes simplex virus from mother to infant. JAMA 2003;289(2):203–9.
11. Kimberlin DW. Neonatal herpes simplex infection. Clin Microbiol Rev 2004;17(1): 1–13.
12. Corey L, Wald A. Maternal and neonatal herpes simplex virus infections. N Engl J Med 2009;361(14):1376–85.
13. Nahmias AJ, Josey WE, Naib ZM, et al. Perinatal risk associated with maternal genital herpes simplex virus infection. Am J Obstet Gynecol 1971;110(6):825–37.
14. Prober CG, Sullender WM, Yasukawa LL, et al. Low risk of herpes simplex virus infections in neonates exposed to the virus at the time of vaginal delivery to mothers with recurrent genital herpes simplex virus infections. N Engl J Med 1987;316(5):240–4.
15. Yeager AS, Arvin AM. Reasons for the absence of a history of recurrent genital infections in mothers of neonates infected with herpes simplex virus. Pediatrics 1984;73(2):188–93.
16. ACOG Practice Bulletin. Clinical management guidelines for obstetrician-gynecologists. No. 82 June 2007. Management of herpes in pregnancy. Obstet Gynecol 2007;109(6):1489–98.
17. Peng J, Krause PJ, Kresch M. Neonatal herpes simplex virus infection after cesarean section with intact amniotic membranes. J Perinatol 1996;16(5):397–9.
18. Kaye EM, Dooling EC. Neonatal herpes simplex meningoencephalitis associated with fetal monitor scalp electrodes. Neurology 1981;31(8):1045–7.
19. O'Riordan DP, Golden WC, Aucott SW. Herpes simplex virus infections in preterm infants. Pediatrics 2006;118(6):e1612–20.
20. Overall JC. Herpes simplex virus infection of the fetus and newborn. Pediatr Ann 1994;23(3):131–6.
21. Whitley RJ, Nahmias AJ, Soong SJ, et al. Vidarabine therapy of neonatal herpes simplex virus infection. Pediatrics 1980;66(4):495–501.
22. Whitley R, Arvin A, Prober C, et al. A controlled trial comparing vidarabine with acyclovir in neonatal herpes simplex virus infection. Infectious Diseases Collaborative Antiviral Study Group. N Engl J Med 1991;324(7):444–9.
23. Whitley R, Arvin A, Prober C, et al. Predictors of morbidity and mortality in neonates with herpes simplex virus infections. The National Institute of Allergy and Infectious Diseases Collaborative Antiviral Study Group. N Engl J Med 1991;324(7):450–4.
24. Kimberlin DW, Lin CY, Jacobs RF, et al. Safety and efficacy of high-dose intravenous acyclovir in the management of neonatal herpes simplex virus infections. Pediatrics 2001;108(2):230–8.
25. Kimberlin DW, Lin CY, Jacobs RF, et al. Natural history of neonatal herpes simplex virus infections in the acyclovir era. Pediatrics 2001;108(2):223–9.
26. Baldwin S, Whitley RJ. Intrauterine herpes simplex virus infection. Teratology 1989;39(1):1–10.
27. Hutto C, Arvin A, Jacobs R, et al. Intrauterine herpes simplex virus infections. J Pediatr 1987;110(1):97–101.
28. Monif GR, Kellner KR, Donnelly WH. Congenital herpes simplex type II infection. Am J Obstet Gynecol 1985;152(8):1000–2.

29. Pinninti SG, Angara R, Feja KN, et al. Neonatal herpes disease following maternal antenatal antiviral suppressive therapy: a multicenter case series. J Pediatr 2012; 161(1):134–138.e1–3.
30. Pickering L, Baker C, Kimberlin D, et al. Herpes Simplex. In: Pickering L, editor. Red book. Report of the Committee on Infectious Diseases. 29th edition. Elk Grove Village (IL): American Academy of Pediatrics; 2012. p. 398–408.
31. Barbi M, Binda S, Primache V, et al. Use of Guthrie cards for the early diagnosis of neonatal herpes simplex virus disease. Pediatr Infect Dis J 1998;17(3):251–2.
32. Diamond C, Mohan K, Hobson A, et al. Viremia in neonatal herpes simplex virus infections. Pediatr Infect Dis J 1999;18(6):487–9.
33. Kimberlin DW, Lakeman FD, Arvin AM, et al. Application of the polymerase chain reaction to the diagnosis and management of neonatal herpes simplex virus disease. National Institute of Allergy and Infectious Diseases Collaborative Antiviral Study Group. J Infect Dis 1996;174(6):1162–7.
34. Kimura H, Futamura M, Kito H, et al. Detection of viral DNA in neonatal herpes simplex virus infections: frequent and prolonged presence in serum and cerebrospinal fluid. J Infect Dis 1991;164(2):289–93.
35. Malm G, Forsgren M. Neonatal herpes simplex virus infections: HSV DNA in cerebrospinal fluid and serum. Arch Dis Child Fetal Neonatal Ed 1999;81(1):F24–9.
36. Atkins JT. HSV PCR for CNS infections: pearls and pitfalls. Pediatr Infect Dis J 1999;18(9):823–4.
37. Troendle-Atkins J, Demmler GJ, Buffone GJ. Rapid diagnosis of herpes simplex virus encephalitis by using the polymerase chain reaction. J Pediatr 1993;123(3): 376–80.
38. Lewensohn-Fuchs I, Osterwall P, Forsgren M, et al. Detection of herpes simplex virus DNA in dried blood spots making a retrospective diagnosis possible. J Clin Virol 2003;26(1):39–48.
39. Englund JA, Fletcher CV, Balfour HH. Acyclovir therapy in neonates. J Pediatr 1991;119:129–35.
40. Caviness AC, Demmler GJ, Almendarez Y, et al. The prevalence of neonatal herpes simplex virus infection compared with serious bacterial illness in hospitalized neonates. J Pediatr 2008;153(2):164–9.
41. Kimberlin DW. When should you initiate acyclovir therapy in a neonate? J Pediatr 2008;153(2):155–6.
42. Long SS. In defense of empiric acyclovir therapy in certain neonates. J Pediatr 2008;153(2):157–8.
43. Kimberlin DW, Whitley RJ, Wan W, et al. Oral acyclovir suppression and neurodevelopment after neonatal herpes. N Engl J Med 2011;365(14):1284–92.
44. Kimberlin D, Powell D, Gruber W, et al. Administration of oral acyclovir suppressive therapy after neonatal herpes simplex virus disease limited to the skin, eyes and mouth: results of a phase I/II trial. Pediatr Infect Dis J 1996;15(3): 247–54.
45. Kimberlin DW, Jacobs RF, Weller S, et al. Pharmacokinetics and safety of extemporaneously compounded valacyclovir oral suspension in pediatric patients from 1 month through 11 years of age. Clin Infect Dis 2010;50(2):221–8.
46. Kimberlin DW, Brady MT, Byington MT, et al. American Academy of Pediatrics Committee on Infectious Diseases, in conjunction with COFN and ACOG: Policy Statement - Guidance on management of neonates born to women with active genital herpes lesions. in press.
47. Roberts SW, Cox SM, Dax J, et al. Genital herpes during pregnancy: no lesions, no cesarean. Obstet Gynecol 1995;85(2):261–4.

48. Stone KM, Reiff-Eldridge R, White AD, et al. Pregnancy outcomes following systemic prenatal acyclovir exposure: conclusions from the international acyclovir pregnancy registry, 1984-1999. Birth Defects Res A Clin Mol Teratol 2004;70(4): 201–7.
49. Stanberry LR, Spruance SL, Cunningham AL, et al. Glycoprotein-D-adjuvant vaccine to prevent genital herpes. N Engl J Med 2002;347(21):1652–61.
50. Belshe RB, Leone PA, Bernstein DI, et al. Efficacy results of a trial of a herpes simplex vaccine. N Engl J Med 2012;366(1):34–43.
51. Brown ZA, Gardella C, Wald A, et al. Genital herpes complicating pregnancy. Obstet Gynecol 2005;106(4):845–56.
52. Centers for Disease Control and Prevention (CDC). Neonatal herpes simplex virus infection following Jewish ritual circumcisions that included direct orogenital suction—New York City, 2000-2011. MMWR Morb Mortal Wkly Rep 2012;61: 405–9.

Neonatal Infectious Diseases

Evaluation of Neonatal Sepsis

Andres Camacho-Gonzalez, MD, MSc[a,*], Paul W. Spearman, MD[a], Barbara J. Stoll, MD[b]

KEYWORDS

- Neonatal sepsis • Immature immunity • Early and late onset disease
- Biologic markers • Treatment

KEY POINTS

- The adoption of Centers for Disease Control and Prevention guidelines for intrapartum antibiotic prophylaxis to reduce vertical transmission of Group B streptococcus (GBS) resulted in an 80% decrease in neonatal GBS sepsis.
- Nonetheless, GBS and *Escherichia coli* remain the most common causes of early-onset sepsis in neonates.
- Coagulase-negative staphylococci are now the most common cause of late-onset neonatal sepsis, particularly in low birth weight infants.
- Among commonly used biomarkers, limited studies suggest that serial C-reactive protein levels and serial assessment of immature:total neutrophil counts provide the best negative predictive value for neonatal sepsis.
- No biomarker to date provides a good positive predictive value for neonatal sepsis.
- Newer biomarkers and broad-based and real-time polymerase chain reaction have demonstrated promise in the early detection of neonatal sepsis, but further study is required to determine if they will be useful in clinical practice.
- Among recent interventions to prevent neonatal sepsis, the use of fluconazole prophylaxis in very low birth weight infants is the only intervention that has shown repeated efficacy in multiple trials.
- Other interventions to prevent neonatal sepsis, such as antistaphylococcal monoclonal antibodies and lactoferrin administration, show early promise but require larger studies to determine real-world efficacy.

[a] Division of Pediatric Infectious Diseases, Emory Department of Pediatrics, Children's Healthcare of Atlanta, Emory University, 2015 Uppergate Drive, Suite 500, Atlanta, GA 30322, USA; [b] Department of Pediatrics, Children's Healthcare of Atlanta at Egleston, Emory-Children's Center, 2015 Uppergate Drive, Suite 200, Atlanta, GA 30322, USA
* Corresponding author.
E-mail address: acamac2@emory.edu

Pediatr Clin N Am 60 (2013) 367–389
http://dx.doi.org/10.1016/j.pcl.2012.12.003 pediatric.theclinics.com
0031-3955/13/$ – see front matter

EPIDEMIOLOGY OF NEONATAL SEPSIS

Neonatal sepsis remains a feared and serious complication, especially among very low birth weight (VLBW) preterm infants. Neonatal sepsis is divided into early-onset and late-onset sepsis, based on timing of infection and presumed mode of transmission. Early-onset sepsis (EOS) is defined by onset in the first week of life, with some studies limiting EOS to infections occurring in the first 72 hours that are caused by maternal intrapartum transmission of invasive organisms. Late-onset sepsis (LOS) is usually defined as infection occurring after 1 week and is attributed to pathogens acquired postnatally. Risk factors for neonatal sepsis include maternal factors, neonatal host factors, and virulence of infecting organism (**Table 1**).

In the United States, widespread acceptance of intrapartum antibiotic prophylaxis (IAP) to reduce vertical transmission of Group B Streptococcal (GBS) infections in high-risk women has resulted in a significant decline in rates of EOS GBS infection.[1] Overall, it is not believed that IAP has resulted in a change in pathogens associated with EOS; however, some studies among VLBW preterm infants have shown an increase in EOS caused by *Escherichia coli*.[2] A recent study done by the Eunice Kennedy Shriver National Institute of Child Health and Human Development (NICHD) Neonatal Research Network (NRN) estimated the overall incidence of EOS to be 0.98 cases per 1000 live births, with increasing rates in premature infants.[3] Studies with stratification of disease burden by gestational age and race have shown that black preterm neonates have a significantly higher incidence of neonatal sepsis as compared with the rest of the population, accounting for 5.14 cases per 1000 births with a case fatality rate of 24.4%.[4]

Despite efforts to detect GBS colonization during pregnancy and provide appropriate GBS prophylaxis to colonized mothers, not all cases of early-onset GBS are prevented and GBS continues to be the most common cause of EOS in term neonates. Sepsis caused by *E coli* has increased in recent years, mainly affecting preterm newborns weighing less than 2500 g at birth, and is considered the most common cause of EOS in this weight group. *E coli* is frequently associated with severe

Table 1
Risk factors for the development of neonatal sepsis

Source	Risk Factor
Early-onset neonatal sepsis	Maternal Group B streptococcal colonization Chrorioamnionitis Premature rupture of membranes Prolonged rupture of membranes (>18 h) Maternal urinary tract infection Multiple pregnancies Preterm delivery (<37 wk)
Late-onset neonatal sepsis	Breakage of the natural barriers (skin and mucosa) Prolonged indwelling catheter use Invasive procedures (eg, endotracheal intubation) Necrotizing enterocolitis Prolonged use of antibiotics H_2-receptor blocker or proton pump inhibitor use
Neonatal[a]	Prematurity • Decreased passage of maternal immunoglobulin and specific antibodies • Immature function of immune system

[a] Increases the risk for both early-onset and late-onset neonatal sepsis.

infections and meningitis and it has become the leading cause of sepsis-related mortality among VLBW infants (24.5%).[4] Together, GBS and *E coli* account for about 70% of cases of EOS in the neonatal period.[5,6]

Rates of LOS are most common in preterm low birth weight infants. Studies from the NICHD NRN report that approximately 21% of VLBW infants weighing less than 1500 g, developed 1 or more episode of blood culture–confirmed LOS, with rates inversely related to gestational age (GA) (58% at 22 weeks GA and 20% at 28 weeks GA).[7,8] Intrapartum antibiotic prophylaxis has not had an impact on rates of LOS.[1,9] VLBW preterm infants are at particular risk for LOS in part because of prolonged hospitalization and prolonged use of indwelling catheters, endotracheal tubes, and other invasive procedures. Several studies have documented rates of LOS from 1.87 to 5.42, with decreasing rates as birth weight increases.[6,7] Coagulase-negative staphylococci (CoNS) have emerged as the most commonly isolated pathogens among VLBW infants with LOS.

DEVELOPMENT OF THE IMMUNE SYSTEM AND INCREASED RISK OF NEONATES TO INFECTIONS

The development of the immune system entails a number of changes that occur during the first years of life. Neonates, especially preterm infants, are relatively immunocompromised because of immaturity of the immune system, as well as decreased placental passage of maternal antibodies. Here we highlight some of the components of the neonatal immune system that are immature and contribute to increased susceptibility to serious bacterial, fungal, and viral infections.

Innate Immune System

The innate immune system produces an immediate immunologic response and is capable of doing this without previous exposure to a specific pathogen. Recognition of pathogens occurs by identification of conserved biologic regions known as pathogen-associated molecular patterns (PAMPs). Recognition receptors, such as TOLL-like receptors, NOD-like receptors and RIG-like receptors, identify and respond to PAMPs with the production of cytokines and proinflammatory responses that activate the adaptive immune system.[10] Studies comparing neonatal and adult innate immune functions show that neonatal cells have a decreased ability to produce inflammatory cytokines, especially tumor necrosis factor (TNF) and interleukin (IL)-6.[11] In addition, they induce IL-10 production, which in itself is capable of inhibiting synthesis of proinflammatory cytokines.[12] Neutrophil and dendritic cell functions are also reduced; neutrophils show a decreased expression of adhesion molecules, as well as a decreased response to chemotactic factors,[13,14] and dendritic cells have a decreased capacity of producing IL-12 and interferon (IFN) gamma. The overall reduction in cytokine production in neonates also results in decreased activation of natural killer cells.[15] Impairment of the innate immune system leads to an increased susceptibility to bacterial and viral infection in this population.

Adaptive Immune System

The adaptive branch of the immune system is designed to eliminate specific pathogens. In newborns, the adaptive immune system slowly increases its function toward an adultlike response, minimizing the otherwise overwhelming inflammatory response that would occur when infants transition from a sterile to a colonized environment.[16] Decreased cytotoxic function (strong T-helper 2 polarization with decreased IFN-gamma production), lack of isotype switching, and overall immaturity and decreased memory (because of limited pathogen exposure at time of birth), reduce the neonate's ability to respond effectively to infections.[17–20] For example, the reduction of cell-mediated immunity increases the risks of infections caused by intracellular pathogens, such as *Listeria*, *Salmonella*, herpes simplex virus (HSV), cytomegalovirus, and enteroviruses.

Transplacental passage of maternal immunoglobulin G (IgG) is inversely related to gestational age and limits the functional ability of the neonate to respond to certain pathogens.[21,22] Minimal IgG is transported to the fetus in the first trimester, whereas fetal IgG rises in the second trimester from approximately 10% at 17 to 22 weeks' gestation to 50% at 28 to 32 weeks' gestation.[23,24] Thus, preterm infants lack adequate humoral protection against a number of infant pathogens, whereas term infants will often be protected against most vaccine-preventable neonatal infections through transplacental passage from the mother's serum. Histologic studies have also demonstrated that the marginal zone of the spleen is not fully developed until 2 years of age, increasing the infant's susceptibility to encapsulated bacterial infections (*Streptococcus pneumoniae*, *Haemophilus influenzae*, *Neisseria meningitidis*).[25] Finally, transfer of IgA, IgG, cytokines, and antibacterial peptides present in human milk may be compromised, especially in premature babies. The lack of secretory IgA decreases the ability of the neonate to respond to environmental pathogens.[26]

Complement

Complement levels increase with increasing gestational age, but are only about 50% of adult levels at term. Reduced complement levels are associated with deficient opsonization and impaired bacterial killing. Although both pathways seem to be capable of being activated, there may be variations in their activation level. In addition, profound C9 deficiency has been observed in neonates, reducing the ability to form bacteriolytic C5b-9 (m), which will increase the risk of acquiring severe invasive bacterial infections.[27,28]

ETIOLOGIC AGENTS IN NEONATAL SEPSIS

The etiologic agents associated with neonatal sepsis in the United States have changed over time.[5] In this section, we review current data on organisms associated with early-onset and late-onset neonatal sepsis (**Table 2**).

EARLY-ONSET SEPSIS

Group B-streptococcus

Despite widespread use of IAP to prevent vertical transmission of invasive GBS disease, missed opportunities for prevention exist and GBS remains the most common

Table 2
Organisms associated with early-onset and late-onset neonatal sepsis

Early-Onset Sepsis	Late-Onset Sepsis
Group B *Streptococcus*	Coagulase-negative *Staphylococcus*
Escherichia coli	*Staphylococcus aureus*
Listeria monocytogenes	Enterococci
Other streptococci: *Streptococcus pyogenes*, viridans group streptococci, *Streptococcus pneumoniae*	Multidrug-resistant gram-negative rods (*E coli, Klebsiella, Pseudomonas, Enterobacter, Citrobacter, Serratia*)
Enterococci	*Candida*
Nontypable *Haemophilus influenzae*	

organism associated with EOS in the United States. According to the Centers for Disease Control and Prevention (CDC), rates of early-onset invasive GBS disease have declined by 80% since the CDC prevention guidelines were first published.[9] GBS are gram-positive encapsulated bacteria for which 10 different serotypes have been identified; serotype III strains are responsible for most of disease (54%).[29] GBS commonly colonize the gastrointestinal (GI) and genital tracts, with rates up to 20% in the adult population.[30] Transmission occurs late in pregnancy or during labor and delivery, and the likelihood of disease, as well as the severity, has been associated with the density of recto-vaginal carriage.[31,32] GBS possess different virulence factors that determine its ability to cause invasive disease: (1) capsular polysaccharide, which helps evade phagocytosis; (2) pili, which allows adherence of GBS to the host's epithelial cells as well as transepithelial migration; and (3) C5a peptidase, which inhibits human C5a, a neutrophil chemoattractant produced during complement activation. Among infected newborns, clinical manifestations develop very early after delivery and most infants will have signs of respiratory distress and cardiovascular instability. Infants with early-onset GBS are at increased risk for meningitis. Rapid deterioration of the clinical status is expected unless prompt antibiotic management is started. Risk of death is inversely related to gestational age, with mortality of 20% to 30% among infected infants of less than 33 weeks' gestation, compared with a mortality of 2% to 3% in full-term infants.[1,33]

Escherichia coli

E coli, a gram-negative rod that commonly colonizes the maternal urogenital and GI tracts, is considered the second most common cause of neonatal sepsis in term infants and the most common cause in VLBW neonates with rates of 5.09 per 1000 live births.[3,34,35] The antigenic structure of *E coli* is represented by multiple antigens (O), (K), and (H), which in combination account for the genetic diversity of the bacteria. Strains with the K1 antigen have been associated with the development of neonatal sepsis and meningitis, as well as with increased risk of mortality when compared with K1-negative strains.[36] Some studies suggest a more aggressive presentation for infants infected with *E coli*, with a higher risk of thrombocytopenia and death in the first days of life.[3] Several US studies have shown high rates of ampicillin resistance in *E coli* strains that infect newborns. Although some studies have shown an association between intrapartum antibiotic exposure and ampicillin-resistant *E coli*, ampicillin resistance has increased throughout the community and a direct link between intrapartum use of ampicillin and the higher likelihood of resistance has not been established.[3,37–39]

Listeria monocytogenes

Listeria is a facultative anaerobic, gram-positive bacterium found in soil, decaying vegetation, fecal flora, and raw unprocessed food.[40] Multiple virulence factors allow *Listeria* to escape the immune system, including listeriolysin, which helps the organism avoid the oxidative stress of phagolysosomes, allowing intracellular replication. *Listeria* proteins ActA, phospholipase C, and lecithinase allow polymerization of actin and lysis of phagosomal membranes, enabling cell-to-cell transmission.[41,42] Pregnant women have 17% higher risk of *Listeria* infection than nonpregnant women, and infection has been associated with spontaneous abortions and stillbirths. Early neonatal infections have a similar clinical presentation, as EO GBS infections, with respiratory distress, sepsis, and meningitis. In severe cases, patients may present with a granulomatous rash (small patches with erythematous base), known as granulomatosis infantisepticum. Most cases of neonatal *Listeria* are caused by serotypes 1, 2, and 4, with the latter serotype responsible for almost all cases of meningitis.[43] Suspicion for *Listeria* sepsis should be increased in ill infants of mothers who have consumed raw milk, unpasteurized cheeses, or other unprocessed food products that have been contaminated with the organism.[44,45]

Other Bacterial Etiologic Agents Seen in EOS

Other less common but important pathogens associated with EOS include other streptococci (*Streptococcus pyogenes*, viridans group streptococci, *S pneumoniae*), enterococci, staphylococci, and nontypable *H influenzae*. *S pyogenes* (group A Streptococcus [GAS]) was once the predominant organism responsible for neonatal sepsis. Although overall incidence has decreased significantly, severe cases of EO GAS continue to be reported. A recent literature review identified 38 cases of neonatal GAS sepsis (24 with EOS). Patients were most likely to present with pneumonia and empyema (42%) or toxic shock syndrome (17%); 70% of the isolates were M1 serotype and they were all susceptible to penicillin. Mortality was estimated to be 38% among patients with EOS.[46] The presentation of pneumococcus, groups C and G streptococci, and viridans streptococci neonatal sepsis is very similar to GBS infection, and transmission seems to be secondary to bacterial colonization of the maternal genital tract.[47–51] Enterococcal EOS is usually mild compared with LOS and is characterized by either a mild respiratory illness or diarrhea without a focal infection. *Enterococcus faecalis* is more frequently isolated than *Enterococcus faecium,* and most of the isolates remain ampicillin susceptible.[52] Although nontypable *H influenzae* frequently colonizes the maternal genital tract, neonatal infection is relatively rare, but with high mortality rates, especially in preterm neonates.[3,53] Hershckowitz and colleagues[54] reported a cluster of 9 cases with 3 deaths; similar high mortality rates were reported in a series by Takala and colleagues.[55]

LOS

The increased survival of preterm low birth weight infants, particularly those who are VLBW, with need for prolonged hospitalization and use of invasive procedures and devices, especially long-term intravascular catheters, results in ongoing risk of infection. LOS is largely caused by organisms acquired from the environment after birth. The following section reviews the most common organisms associated with LOS (see **Table 2**).

CoNS and Staphylococcus aureus

CoNS has emerged as the single most commonly isolated pathogen among VLBW infants with LOS and is associated with 22% to 55% of LOS infections among VLBW infants.[56,57] *S aureus* is associated with 4% to 8%.[7,58] *Staphylococcus* commonly colonizes the human skin and mucous membranes and is capable of adhering to plastic surfaces with the subsequent formation of biofilms. These biofilms protect the bacteria from antibiotic penetration and can produce substances that will help them evade the immune system. Although CoNS infections are usually secondary to *Staphylococcus epidermidis,* other strains such as *Staphylococcus capitis*, *Staphylococcus haemolyticus,* and *Staphylococcus hominis* have also been reported.[59] Methicillin-resistant *S aureus* (MRSA) has been isolated in 28% of staphylococcal infections in preterm neonates with no significant differences between MRSA and methicillin-susceptible organisms in terms of morbidity, mortality, and length of hospital stay. Overall, 25% of infants infected with MRSA die, with no significant difference in death rates between infants infected with MRSA or methicillin-susceptible *S aureus*.[58]

Gram-negative Organisms

Gram-negative organisms are associated with about one-third of cases of LOS, but 40% to 69% of deaths due to sepsis in this age group. Transmission occurs from the hands of health care workers, colonization of the GI tract, contamination of total parenteral nutrition or formulas, and bladder catheterization devices.[60,61] The most common gram-negative organisms isolated include *E coli*, *Klebsiella*, *Pseudomonas*, *Enterobacter*, *Citrobacter*, and *Serratia*.[62] In some case series, *Klebsiella* is recognized as the most common gram-negative agent associated with LOS, ranging from 20% to 31% of cases.[63,64] Infections caused by *Pseudomonas* have been associated with the highest mortality.[65] *Citrobacter* is uniquely associated with brain abscesses, but dissemination can occur to other organs. Its ability to survive intracellularly has been linked to the capacity of creating chronic central nervous system (CNS) infections and abscesses.[66,67]

Candida Infections

Infections caused by *Candida* species are the third leading cause of LOS in premature infants. Risk factors of infection include low birth weight, use of broad-spectrum antibiotics, male gender, and lack of enteral feedings.[68] *Candida albicans* and *Candida parapsilosis* are the species most commonly associated with disease in neonates.[69,70] Poor outcomes, including higher mortality rates and neurodevelopmental impairment, have been associated with the ability of the organisms to express virulence traits, such as adherence factors and cytotoxic substances.[71] *Candida* easily grows in blood culture media, but its isolation may require larger volumes of blood than normally obtained in neonates and therefore multiple cultures may be necessary to document infection and clearance. Among those with a positive cerebrospinal fluid (CSF) culture, as many as 50% will have a negative blood culture; the discordance of blood and CSF cultures underscores the need for a lumbar puncture (LP).[68] Prompt removal of contaminated catheters is also recommended based on the ability of *Candida* species to create biofilms, as well as better survival rates and neurodevelopmental outcomes in patients who had early removal and clearance of the infection.[68]

HSV

HSV is a potentially devastating cause of late-onset neonatal infection. HSV should be included in the differential diagnosis and treatment strategy of newborns who present with signs and symptoms of sepsis, especially after the first few days of life. For a detailed discussion on neonatal HSV infection, refer to the article by Kimberlin and colleagues, elsewhere in this issue.

CLINICAL MANIFESTATIONS

Both EOS and LOS have nonspecific clinical manifestations (**Table 3**). The importance of a lumbar puncture in neonates with suspected sepsis and without specific CNS clinical manifestations is underscored by studies showing growth of CSF cultures despite negative blood cultures, especially in VLBW infants.[72]

DIAGNOSTIC METHODS

Early diagnosis of neonatal sepsis is challenging because clinical characteristics are nonspecific and difficult to differentiate from those of noninfectious etiologies, and because the repertoire of ancillary laboratory tests is limited and not always reliable. Blood culture remains the gold standard for diagnosis of neonatal sepsis, but the

Table 3
Clinical manifestations in patients with early-onset and late-onset neonatal sepsis

Sepsis/Meningitis	Temperature instability Respiratory distress Apnea Jaundice & feeding intolerance Bulging fontanel Seizures
Other	Skin lesions: may occur in disseminated staphylococcal, *Listeria,* and *Candida* infections Joint and bone: may be the preceding event

rate of positivity is low, influenced by factors such as intrapartum antimicrobial administration and limitations in blood volume per culture that can be obtained in neonates.[73,74] Here we review the standard evaluation of neonatal sepsis, followed by a discussion of recent data on inflammatory markers and diagnostic methods in neonatal sepsis.

General Evaluation of Neonatal Sepsis

A neonate with signs and symptoms of sepsis (see **Table 3**) requires prompt evaluation and initiation of antibiotic therapy. Blood, CSF (as clinical condition allows), and urine cultures (useful only after the third day of life) should be obtained.[72,75,76] Chest radiograph is indicated in patients having respiratory symptoms. If disseminated herpes is suspected (herpetic skin lesions, elevated hepatic transaminases, maternal peripartum herpes infection), surface cultures from conjunctiva, mouth, skin, and anus, as well as herpes DNA polymerase chain reaction (PCR) from CSF and blood should also be ordered.[77,78] Ancillary tests, such as complete blood count (CBC) and C-reactive protein (CRP), should not preclude a sepsis evaluation in a neonate, because they can be normal (see the following sections).[79] If positive, however, they can be useful in supporting the diagnosis and determining length of therapy. Careful maternal and exposure history targeted toward identifying potential risk factors (see **Table 1**), as well as a complete physical examination, including skin and catheter insertion sites, should be obtained.

Complete Blood Cell Count

Contrary to older children and adults, the white blood cell (WBC) count does not accurately predict infection in neonates. A recent multicenter review of CBCs and blood cultures in neonates admitted to 293 neonatal intensive care units (NICUs) in the United States, showed that low WBC and absolute neutrophil counts, as well as high immature-to-total neutrophil ratio (I:T ratio) were associated with increasing odds of infection (odds ratios 5.38, 6.84, and 7.90, respectively); however, the test sensitivities for detection of sepsis were low.[80] Studies looking at serial values of WBC counts and I:T ratios have shown better outcomes. Murphy and Weiner,[81] in a single-center historical cohort study, showed that 2 serial normal I:T ratios and a negative blood culture in the first 24 hours of life had a negative predictive value (NPV) of 100% (95% confidence interval [CI]: 99.905%–100%), but the specificity and positive predictive value were 51.0% and 8.8% respectively. CBC values need to be interpreted cautiously and in conjunction with other clinical and laboratory parameters.

CRP

CRP was first described in the 1930s and since then multiple studies have shown elevation of the CRP in several infectious and noninfectious etiologies that share a common background of inflammation or tissue injury.[82] In neonates, serial measurements of the CRP in the first 24 to 48 hours of symptoms increases the sensitivity of the test, with suggestion that normal CRP values during this period have a 99% negative predicted value for determination of infection.[83,84] In contrast, elevated levels of CRP may be more difficult to interpret, especially for diagnosis of EOS, because factors such as premature rupture of membranes (PROM), maternal fever, pregnancy-induced hypertension, prenatal steroid use, and fetal distress may also cause elevation of the CRP.[85,86] Additionally, studies have suggested a physiologic variation of the CRP during the first few days of life limiting the use of single values.[86] Gestational age influences CRP kinetics, with preterm infants having a lower and shorter CRP response compared with healthy term infants.[87,88] Studies suggest that CRP is best used as part of a group of ancillary diagnostic tests to help determine if an infant has infection, rather than as a single test.

Procalcitonin

Tissue release of procalcitonin (PCT) increases with infection, making it a potential marker for early detection of sepsis. PCT differs from CRP, in that PCT levels increase more rapidly and may be more useful for detection of EOS. Auriti and colleagues,[89] in a multicenter, prospective observational study of 762 neonates, showed a significant increase in the median value of PCT level in neonates with sepsis compared with those without sepsis (3.58 vs 0.49 ng/mL; $P<.001$), In addition, a cutoff value of 2.4 ng/mL was suggested as the most accurate level for differentiation of sepsis in neonates regardless of gestational age, with a sensitivity of 62% and a specificity of 84%. A meta-analysis of 16 studies (1959 neonates), showed that PCT had a pooled sensitivity and specificity of 81% and 79% respectively.[90] Although these are promising results, further studies are needed to clarify the use of PCT in clinical practice.

Mannose-Binding Lectin

Mannose-binding lectin (MBL) is a plasma protein, primarily produced by the liver, with an important role in the innate immune defense. MBL activates the lectin pathway of the complement system, increasing opsonization and enhancing phagocytosis.[91] Genetic polymorphisms in the MBL gene have been associated with an increased risk of sepsis. In a recent study in which MBL levels were measured in 93 neonates, development of sepsis was associated with lower levels of MBL and with the presence of BB genotype in exon 1 of the MBL gene. MBL remains a research tool with further studies needed to confirm diagnostic utility.[92]

Cytokine Profile

Multiple cytokines have been studied for diagnosis of neonatal sepsis including IL-6, IL-8, IL-10, and TNF-alpha. IL-6 and IL-8 increase very rapidly with bacterial invasion, but they promptly normalize in serum levels (within the first 24 hours), limiting their ability to be used as clinical markers. TNF-alpha has not shown to have high sensitivity, but the ratio of IL-10 and TNF-alpha has been used for diagnosis of LOS in VLBW neonates with some success.[93,94] Evaluating a combination of cytokine profiles may increase the likelihood of identifying infection more than single measurements.

Neutrophil CD64 and Neutrophil/Monocyte CD11B

The specific markers, neutrophil CD64 and neutrophil/monocyte CD11B, are cell surface antigens whose production increases after activation of leukocytes by bacteria and therefore can potentially be used for diagnosis of neonatal sepsis. Their upregulation precedes that of CRP, suggesting potential use in EOS. A recent study by Genel and colleagues[95] showed that CD64 had a sensitivity and specificity to accurately identify neonatal sepsis of 81% and 77% respectively, with an NPV of 75%. Similarly, CD11b had a sensitivity and specificity of 66% and 71%. Cost and processing time may be barriers to use of these markers in clinical practice.

Molecular Techniques for Early Detection of Neonatal Sepsis

Important advances have been made in molecular diagnostics, and studies of real-time PCR and a broad range of conventional PCR assays suggest improved sensitivity and specificity for sepsis diagnosis. A meta-analysis done by Pammi[96] found that sensitivity and specificity of real-time PCR was 0.96 (95% CI for sensitivity: 0.65–1.00 and 95% CI for specificity: 0.92–0.98). Similarly, broad-range PCR had a sensitivity of 0.95 (95% CI 0.84–0.98) and specificity of 0.98 (0.95–1.0); however, neither test achieved the minimum limits of sensitivity or specificity set up by the study and results were insufficient to replace blood cultures for diagnosis of neonatal sepsis. Currently these techniques should be seen as adjunctive methods in the diagnosis of neonatal sepsis, with limitations that include the inability to provide information about antibiotic susceptibility, as well as significant cost of implementation in clinical practice. An exception to this is the use of HSV PCR for the diagnosis of HSV encephalitis, which is the gold standard test for this condition. The role of HSV PCR from the blood in diagnosing disseminated HSV infection is less clear.

Genomics and Proteomics

Exciting alternatives for detection of neonatal sepsis include the use of genomics and proteomics for identification of host response biomarkers. Genomics targets genes that are upregulated with infection and proteomics analyzes the structure, function, and interactions of proteins produced by a particular gene. Early studies in neonates have suggested potential utility in these techniques for identification of sepsis and necrotizing enterocolitis. A score based on proapolipoprotein CII (Pro-apoC2) and a des-arginine variant of serum amyloid, was used to withhold antibiotics in 45% of patients with suspected infection and to discontinue antibiotics in 16%.[93,97] Studies are needed for validation of this score, as well as for detection of other potential biomarkers.

TREATMENT

Prevention and Infection Control Practices

Prevention of neonatal sepsis is the goal, through implementation of what is known and development of new prevention strategies. Maternal prenatal care continues to be important for prevention of EO GBS sepsis with identification of maternal carriage of GBS through universal screening for all pregnant women. Early recognition of chorioamnionitis, with appropriate antimicrobial therapy for the mother, decreases maternal fetal transmission. The recent CDC GBS prevention guidelines emphasize the need for universal maternal GBS screening at 35 to 37 weeks of gestation and includes chromogenic agar and nucleic amplification tests as newer diagnostic techniques that can be used to increase the yield of GBS identification. The guidelines also clarify the definition of adequate intrapartum prophylaxis as the use of penicillin, ampicillin, or cefazolin at least 4 hours before delivery (**Table 4**). Clindamycin and vancomycin, which can be used in penicillin-allergic patients, are not considered effective prophylaxis therapy.[9] Other potential prevention strategies include rapid GBS testing during labor and a safe and effective GBS vaccine. Diagnostic tests during labor will identify colonized women who either had a negative screen at 35 to 37 weeks or were not screened before labor. Further studies are needed to improve sensitivity and specificity of rapid tests.[98]

Efforts to reduce hospital-acquired late-onset infections require much closer attention to appropriate hand washing, infection control, and proper techniques for placement and management of central catheters. Recently, the American Academy of Pediatrics published guidelines for the prevention of health care–associated infections in the NICU. These guidelines emphasize the need for 100% compliance with appropriate hand-washing techniques and recommend use of alcohol-based products for hand hygiene. Catheter bundles that include guidelines for insertion and management of central lines have been shown to reduce risk of central line–associated bloodstream infection.[99–102] The use of heparin for prevention of line infections has been successful in single-center randomized studies, but has not been confirmed in larger multicenter studies; therefore, its routine use is not recommended.[103,104] Daily check lists that document continued need for central lines to reduce duration of line use and a goal of zero central line–associated infections should be the responsibility of the whole health care team.[99]

Prevention Strategies

A variety of interventions to decrease rates of neonatal sepsis have been studied, including postnatal use of lactoferrin, antistaphylococcal monoclonal antibodies, intravenous immunoglobulin (IVIG), granulocyte-macrophage colony-stimulating factors, probiotics, glutamine, and fluconazole prophylaxis for invasive candida infection (**Table 5**).

IVIG

Delay in the synthesis of immunoglobulin and a decrease in transplacental antibody transfer in neonates suggested that the use of IVIG could be a potential strategy for prevention of neonatal sepsis. In 1994, a randomized controlled trial in 2416 infants failed to show a decreased incidence of nosocomial infections, morbidity/mortality, and duration of hospital stay among VLBW infants.[105] A follow-up meta-analysis of 10 trials showed that mortality was reduced with the use of IVIG in suspected (relative risk [RR] 0.58, 95% CI 0.38–0.89) and proven infection (RR 0.55, 95% CI 0.31–0.98), but the investigators caution about their conclusions based on concerns about individual study quality.[106] Recently, the International Neonatal Immunotherapy Study randomized 3493 infants with suspected or proven sepsis to receive either 2 doses of polyvalent IgG immune globulin or placebo 48 hours apart. Their primary outcome

Table 4
Recommended intrapartum antibiotic prophylaxis for Group B *Streptococcus*–positive women

Antibiotic	Dose
Penicillin G	5 million units IV as an initial dose followed by 2.5 million units every 4 h until delivery
Ampicillin	2 g IV as an initial dose, followed by 1 g IV every 4 h until delivery
Cefazolin	2 g IV as an initial dose, followed by 1 g IV every 8 h until delivery

Abbreviation: IV, intravenous.

Table 5
Evidence of strategies for prevention of neonatal sepsis

Prevention Strategy	Notes
Lactoferrin	Small studies show reduction of both fungal and bacterial infection; large studies needed.
Intravenous immunoglobulin	No proven efficacy for prevention of neonatal sepsis.
Antistaphylococcal monoclonal antibodies	Monoclonal antibodies against capsular polysaccharide and clumping Factor A have shown no effect in prevention of sepsis. Antilipoteichoic acid antibodies may have an effect but further randomized controlled studies are required.
Probiotics	No proven efficacy for neonatal sepsis. Useful as prevention of necrotizing enterocolitis.
GM-CSF/G-CSF	No proven efficacy of neonatal sepsis.
Glutamine	No proven efficacy of neonatal sepsis.
Fluconazole	Efficacious in prevention of *Candida* sepsis in VLBW infants.

Abbreviations: G-CSF, granulocyte colony-stimulating factor; GM-CSF, granulocyte-macrophage colony-stimulating factor; VLBW, very low birth weight.

was rate of death or major disability at the age of 2 years. There was no difference in the primary outcome between the 2 groups (RR 1.00, 95% CI 0.92–1.08).[107]

Antistaphylococcal monoclonal antibodies

Because of the burden of staphylococcal infections in neonatal sepsis, different antistaphylococcal monoclonal antibodies had been developed. These include antibodies against the capsular polysaccharide antigen, antibodies against microbial surface components that recognize adhesive matrix molecules, antibodies to clumping factor A, and anti-lipoteichoic acid (LTA) antibodies.[108–110] Initial animal studies, as well as phase I and II trials in humans, showed that capsular-directed antibodies and anti-clumping factor A were well tolerated and had the potential to reduce staphylococcal sepsis[111,112]; however, a meta-analysis showed that their efficacy in decreasing staphylococcal infections was limited and recommended against their use.[113] Recently, Weisman and colleagues[110] showed safety and tolerance of pagibaximab (anti-LTA antibody) at doses of 60 and 90 mg/kg in VLBW infants, with those receiving 90 mg/kg per dose showing no staphylococcal sepsis. Although these are exciting results, randomized controlled studies are needed to further confirm these findings.

Granulocyte/Granulocyte-macrophage colony-stimulating factors

Granulocyte-macrophage colony-stimulating factor (GM-CSF) increases T-Helper 1 immune responses and enhances bactericidal activity by stimulating neutrophils and monocytes. Animal studies have shown that both GM-CSF and granulocyte colony-stimulating factor (G-CSF), given before bacterial inoculation, decrease mortality. A single blinded multicenter study looking at the use of GM-CSF and the development of sepsis showed that although the absolute neutrophil count on the treatment arm increased significantly faster (P = .002), there was no difference in sepsis-free survival to day 14 from study entry (risk difference −8%, 95% CI −18% to 3%).[114] A meta-analysis that included 4 small studies had similar results (RR 0.89, 95% CI 0.43–1.86).[96]

Glutamine

Based on promising adult studies, glutamine supplementation has been suggested as a potential intervention to reduce neonatal sepsis. A randomized double-blinded study from the NICHD NRN among 1433 extremely low birth weight infants showed no difference in mortality and late-onset sepsis outcomes (RR 1.07, 95% CI 0.97–1.17; $P = .18$).[115] Similar results were obtained in a meta-analysis of 5 trials that included 2240 neonates looking at the effects of glutamine in the incidence of culture-proven invasive infection (RR 1.01, 95% CI 0.91–1.13).[116] Glutamine supplementation is not currently recommended as a strategy to decrease or prevent neonatal sepsis.

Probiotics

Evidence continues to grow regarding the use of probiotics to prevent necrotizing enterocolitis,[117,118] but data on use of probiotics for prevention of neonatal sepsis are limited and contradictory. A major problem with the use of probiotics is the lack of standardization and federal regulation. If probiotics are considered food additives, no formal evaluation is required and a wide of variety of products are available. Some investigators have stressed the need for review and approval by the Food and Drug Administration, especially if probiotics are to be used in at-risk VLBW infants. Although small studies have indicated potential benefits of probiotics in decreasing neonatal sepsis, a recent meta-analysis (RR 0.90, 95% CI 0.76–1.07) and a systematic review (RR 0.98, 95% CI 0.81–1.18) found no evidence that probiotics decreased sepsis in preterm VLBW infants.[117,119]

Lactoferrin

Lactoferrin is a glycoprotein present in human milk that contains immunomodulatory properties by increasing cytokine production in the gut and associated lymphoid tissue, as well as by showing antibioticlike activities against gram-negative and gram-positive bacteria. A recent multicenter randomized study in 472 VLBW neonates demonstrated decreased bacterial and fungal LOS among newborns treated with lactoferrin (5.9% in lactoferrin group vs 17.3% in controls, $P = .002$).[120] Further studies are needed to confirm these findings and to evaluate optimal dosage as well as short-term and long-term safety.

Fluconazole prophylaxis

Studies have documented that fluconazole prophylaxis among high-risk VLBW infants is effective in reducing the number of severe infections. Kaufman and colleagues[121] found a 22% decrease in risk of fungal colonization among infants weighing less than 1000 g who were on fluconazole prophylaxis. In addition, they found no fungal invasive infections in those who received fluconazole compared with 20% in the placebo group. Similar results were obtained by the Italian Task Force in 322 neonates who were randomized to receive fluconazole or placebo.[122] The success in decreasing the incidence of fungal infections in the neonatal units has not been translated into decreased mortality; however, all prospective studies of fluconazole prophylaxis have consistently revealed decreasing mortality trends.[121–124] In addition, Healy and colleagues,[125] in a retrospective 4-year study looking at the incidence of invasive candidiasis, showed that there were no attributable deaths among patients who received fluconazole prophylaxis compared with 21% of those who did not. Current recommendations advocate for the use of fluconazole prophylaxis in infants with birth weights of less than 1000 g in neonatal units with high rates of invasive candidiasis.[126] Recently, Kaufman and colleagues[123] reported an 8-year to 10-year follow-up study evaluating the long-term and neurodevelopmental outcomes of fluconazole prophylaxis. They found no significant neurodevelopmental impairment or difference in head circumference growth and cholestasis in patients on prophylaxis when compared with placebo. A larger study is needed to verify these findings. Another important aspect of fluconazole prophylactic use has been the concern regarding emergence of fluconazole-resistant strains; however, studies have failed to show such an association, and a significant increase in fluconazole-resistant *Candida* species has not yet occurred.[125]

Judicious Use of Antibiotics

Appropriate use of antibiotics is important to save lives and reduce complications. Indiscriminate use increases risk of multidrug-resistant organisms and other complications, including disseminated candida infections and necrotizing enterocolitis.[127,128] Reports of vancomycin-resistant enterococcus, beta lactamase–producing organisms (*E coli, Klebsiella, Enterobacter*), and highly resistant *Acinetobacter*, *Burkholderia*, *Chryseobacterium meningosepticum,* and *Serratia* are increasing in the neonatal population, calling for a judicious use of antibiotics.[129–134] A study looking at antibiotic prescribing practices in 4 NICUs found that approximately 28% of the established antibiotic courses and 24% of antibiotic days were inappropriate for the prescribing indication. The most common cause of inappropriate use was excessive continuation of antibiotics, rather than inappropriate initiation, followed by inability to target the specific pathogen once isolated.[135] General principles for antibiotic use, as well as effective antibiotic stewardship programs, may help decrease misuse of antibiotics in the NICU (**Table 6**). Such programs require developing antibiotic guidelines and education initiatives, accompanied by preprescription approval and postprescription review (ie, modification of empiric antibiotic regimen, dose optimization, therapeutic monitoring, oral antimicrobial conversion, and drug-drug interactions). Close involvement and communication among an infectious disease specialist, neonatologist, clinical pharmacist, and infection control and microbiology personnel are essential for the success of the program.[136] Efforts to document and measure the success of stewardship programs are important as well as generating nonpunitive feedback on antibiotic prescription practices. The NICU has specific characteristics in antibiotic prescription practices, as multiple providers may be involved in the decision of initiating, continuing, or discontinuing antibiotics; adapting programs to such characteristics is important.[137] Recently, the CDC launched the *Get Smart for Health Care* campaign, which focuses on improving antibiotic use in inpatient/outpatient health care facilities and offers tools for implementation and improvement of stewardship efforts (http://www.cdc.gov/getsmart/healthcare).

Ampicillin and gentamicin continue to be the preferred antibiotics for empiric treatment of suspected early-onset neonatal sepsis. Increasing ampicillin-resistant *E coli* in some centers has led to increased use of third-generation cephalosporins as part of the empiric treatment; however, studies have shown a potential association with

Table 6
Principles for antibiotic use

Empiric initiation of antibiotics	Use only when bacterial infections are likely and discontinue empiric treatment when they have not been identified.
Switch antibiotics based on susceptibility patterns	Change the antibiotic agents to those with the narrowest spectrum.
Define duration of antibiotic therapy	Establish a final duration of antibiotic management based on the disease process.

Table 7
Duration of antibiotic therapy in neonatal sepsis based on clinical presentation

Clinical Presentation	Duration of Antibiotic Therapy
Early-onset sepsis without meningitis	10 d
Late-onset sepsis without meningitis	10–14 d
Meningitis: early-onset or late-onset sepsis	14–21 d[a]

[a] Gram-negative rod meningitis: will require at least 21 days of therapy.

increased mortality and the development of multidrug-resistant organisms associated with this practice. In addition, cephalosporins are not active against *Listeria* and enterococcus. In LOS, coverage with vancomycin should be considered, especially in hospitalized VLBW infants at risk for CoNS infection.

Definitive therapy should be chosen based on antibiotic susceptibilities. Combination therapy for gram-negative organisms is not required for patients without meningitis, and for patients with an inducible B-lactamase–producing organism (*Serratia*, indol-positive *Proteus*, *Citrobacter,* and *Enterobacter*), the use of a carbapenem should be considered. The duration of therapy is based on the disease process (**Table 7**).

Amphotericin and fluconazole continue to be the antifungal drugs of choice for treatment of neonatal candidiasis. Local susceptibility patterns should be followed if *Candida glabrata*, *Candida krusei,* or *Candida lusitaniae* are isolated, as susceptibility of these species to both fluconazole and amphotericin may be decreased. *C krusei* is intrinsically fluconazole resistant, and may have reduced susceptibility to amphotericin, whereas *C lusitanaie* is among the few *Candida* species to show full in vitro resistance to amphotericin in some isolates. *Candida tropicalis* and *Candida parapsilosis* are frequently resistant to fluconazole, although resistance rates vary by area, but they are usually susceptible to amphotericin. The experience with the use of echinocandins (micafungin, caspofungin, anidulafungin) in neonates continues to increase, but their use is not yet approved in this population, and their poor CNS penetration is also a concern.[138] Micafungin is the echinocandin that has been studied the most in the neonatal population and these studies show that higher doses may be required, especially for better CNS penetration.[139–141]

SUMMARY

Neonatal sepsis continues to be a significant cause of morbidity and mortality in term and preterm infants. Although GBS and *E coli* are the most common pathogens associated with EOS, and CoNS are the most frequently isolated agents in newborns with LOS, other organisms, as well as multidrug-resistant pathogens, need to be considered. Development of accurate novel early diagnostic markers will allow clinicians to better assess the risk of infection and need for antibiotic therapy. Adherence to infection-control policies, including attention to strict hand hygiene, antibiotic stewardship, and catheter management, are required to decrease the number of infections in hospitalized neonates.

REFERENCES

1. Verani JR, McGee L, Schrag SJ. Prevention of perinatal group B streptococcal disease—revised guidelines from CDC, 2010. MMWR Recomm Rep 2010;59:1–36.

2. Stoll BJ, Hansen N, Fanaroff AA, et al. Changes in pathogens causing early-onset sepsis in very-low-birth-weight infants. N Engl J Med 2002;347:240–7.
3. Stoll BJ, Hansen NI, Sanchez PJ, et al. Early onset neonatal sepsis: the burden of group B Streptococcal and *E. coli* disease continues. Pediatrics 2011;127:817–26.
4. Weston EJ, Pondo T, Lewis MM, et al. The burden of invasive early-onset neonatal sepsis in the United States, 2005-2008. Pediatr Infect Dis J 2011;30:937–41.
5. Bizzarro MJ, Raskind C, Baltimore RS, et al. Seventy-five years of neonatal sepsis at Yale: 1928-2003. Pediatrics 2005;116:595–602.
6. Vergnano S, Menson E, Kennea N, et al. Neonatal infections in England: the NeonIN surveillance network. Arch Dis Child Fetal Neonatal Ed 2011;96:F9–14.
7. Stoll BJ, Hansen N, Fanaroff AA, et al. Late-onset sepsis in very low birth weight neonates: the experience of the NICHD Neonatal Research Network. Pediatrics 2002;110:285–91.
8. Stoll BJ, Hansen NI, Bell EF, et al. Neonatal outcomes of extremely preterm infants from the NICHD Neonatal Research Network. Pediatrics 2010;126:443–56.
9. Baker CJ, Byington CL, Polin RA. Policy statement—Recommendations for the prevention of perinatal group B streptococcal (GBS) disease. Pediatrics 2011;128:611–6.
10. Kumar S, Ingle H, Prasad DV, et al. Recognition of bacterial infection by innate immune sensors. Crit Rev Microbiol 2012. [Epub ahead of print].
11. Kollmann TR, Crabtree J, Rein-Weston A, et al. Neonatal innate TLR-mediated responses are distinct from those of adults. J Immunol 2009;183:7150–60.
12. Belderbos ME, Levy O, Stalpers F, et al. Neonatal plasma polarizes TLR4-mediated cytokine responses towards low IL-12p70 and high IL-10 production via distinct factors. PLoS One 2012;7:e33419.
13. Carr R. Neutrophil production and function in newborn infants. Br J Haematol 2000;110:18–28.
14. Levy O. Innate immunity of the newborn: basic mechanisms and clinical correlates. Nat Rev Immunol 2007;7:379–90.
15. Guilmot A, Hermann E, Braud VM, et al. Natural killer cell responses to infections in early life. J Innate Immun 2011;3:280–8.
16. Schelonka RL, Maheshwari A, Carlo WA, et al. T cell cytokines and the risk of blood stream infection in extremely low birth weight infants. Cytokine 2011;53:249–55.
17. Tolar J, Hippen KL, Blazar BR. Immune regulatory cells in umbilical cord blood: T regulatory cells and mesenchymal stromal cells. Br J Haematol 2009;147:200–6.
18. Risdon G, Gaddy J, Horie M, et al. Alloantigen priming induces a state of unresponsiveness in human umbilical cord blood T cells. Proc Natl Acad Sci U S A 1995;92:2413–7.
19. Takahashi N, Kato H, Imanishi K, et al. Change of specific T cells in an emerging neonatal infectious disease induced by a bacterial superantigen. Microbiol Immunol 2009;53:524–30.
20. Sautois B, Fillet G, Beguin Y. Comparative cytokine production by in vitro stimulated mononucleated cells from cord blood and adult blood. Exp Hematol 1997;25:103–8.
21. Palmeira P, Quinello C, Silveira-Lessa AL, et al. IgG placental transfer in healthy and pathological pregnancies. Clin Dev Immunol 2012;2012:985646.

22. van den Berg JP, Westerbeek EA, van der Klis FR, et al. Transplacental transport of IgG antibodies to preterm infants: a review of the literature. Early Hum Dev 2011;87:67–72.
23. Malek A. Ex vivo human placenta models: transport of immunoglobulin G and its subclasses. Vaccine 2003;21:3362–4.
24. Malek A, Sager R, Kuhn P, et al. Evolution of maternofetal transport of immunoglobulins during human pregnancy. Am J Reprod Immunol 1996;36:248–55.
25. Zandvoort A, Timens W. The dual function of the splenic marginal zone: essential for initiation of anti-TI-2 responses but also vital in the general first-line defense against blood-borne antigens. Clin Exp Immunol 2002;130:4–11.
26. Brandtzaeg P. The mucosal immune system and its integration with the mammary glands. J Pediatr 2010;156:S8–15.
27. Hogasen AK, Overlie I, Hansen TW, et al. The analysis of the complement activation product SC5 b-9 is applicable in neonates in spite of their profound C9 deficiency. J Perinat Med 2000;28:39–48.
28. Suzuki-Nishimura T, Uchida MK. Binding of spin-labeled fatty acids and lysophospholipids to hydrophobic region of calmodulin. J Biochem 1991;110:333–8.
29. Imperi M, Gherardi G, Berardi A, et al. Invasive neonatal GBS infections from an area-based surveillance study in Italy. Clin Microbiol Infect 2011;17:1834–9.
30. Tomlinson MW, Schmidt NM, Rourke JW Jr, et al. Rectovaginal *Staphylococcus aureus* colonization: is it a neonatal threat? Am J Perinatol 2011;28:673–6.
31. Yancey MK, Duff P, Kubilis P, et al. Risk factors for neonatal sepsis. Obstet Gynecol 1996;87:188–94.
32. Regan JA, Klebanoff MA, Nugent RP, et al. Colonization with group B streptococci in pregnancy and adverse outcome. VIP Study Group. Am J Obstet Gynecol 1996;174:1354–60.
33. Schrag SJ, Zywicki S, Farley MM, et al. Group B streptococcal disease in the era of intrapartum antibiotic prophylaxis. N Engl J Med 2000;342:15–20.
34. Tsai CH, Chen YY, Wang KG, et al. Characteristics of early-onset neonatal sepsis caused by *Escherichia coli*. Taiwan J Obstet Gynecol 2012;51:26–30.
35. Bizzarro MJ, Dembry LM, Baltimore RS, et al. Changing patterns in neonatal *Escherichia coli* sepsis and ampicillin resistance in the era of intrapartum antibiotic prophylaxis. Pediatrics 2008;121:689–96.
36. Kaczmarek A, Budzynska A, Gospodarek E. Prevalence of genes encoding virulence factors among *Escherichia coli* with K1 antigen and non-K1 *E. coli* strains. J Med Microbiol 2012;61(Pt 10):1360–5.
37. Schrag SJ, Hadler JL, Arnold KE, et al. Risk factors for invasive, early-onset *Escherichia coli* infections in the era of widespread intrapartum antibiotic use. Pediatrics 2006;118:570–6.
38. Al-Hasan MN, Lahr BD, Eckel-Passow JE, et al. Antimicrobial resistance trends of *Escherichia coli* bloodstream isolates: a population-based study, 1998-2007. J Antimicrob Chemother 2009;64:169–74.
39. Puopolo KM, Eichenwald EC. No change in the incidence of ampicillin-resistant, neonatal, early-onset sepsis over 18 years. Pediatrics 2010;125:e1031–8.
40. Versalovic J. Manual of clinical microbiology. 10th edition. Washington, DC: ASM Press; 2012.
41. Shetron-Rama LM, Marquis H, Bouwer HG, et al. Intracellular induction of *Listeria monocytogenes* actA expression. Infect Immun 2002;70:1087–96.
42. Moors MA, Levitt B, Youngman P, et al. Expression of listeriolysin O and ActA by intracellular and extracellular *Listeria monocytogenes*. Infect Immun 1999;67:131–9.

43. Smith B, Kemp M, Ethelberg S, et al. *Listeria monocytogenes*: maternal-foetal infections in Denmark 1994-2005. Scand J Infect Dis 2009;41:21–5.
44. CDC. From the Centers for Disease Control. Foodborne listeriosis—United States, 1988-1990. JAMA 1992;267:2446–8.
45. Schlech WF 3rd. Foodborne listeriosis. Clin Infect Dis 2000;31:770–5.
46. Miyairi I, Berlingieri D, Protic J, et al. Neonatal invasive group A streptococcal disease: case report and review of the literature. Pediatr Infect Dis J 2004;23: 161–5.
47. Prommalikit O, Mekmullica J, Pancharoen C, et al. Invasive pneumococcal infection in neonates: 3 case reports. J Med Assoc Thai 2010;93(Suppl 5):S46–8.
48. Malhotra A, Hunt RW, Doherty RR. *Streptococcus pneumoniae* sepsis in the newborn. J Paediatr Child Health 2012;48:E79–83.
49. Gomez M, Alter S, Kumar ML, et al. Neonatal *Streptococcus pneumoniae* infection: case reports and review of the literature. Pediatr Infect Dis J 1999;18:1014–8.
50. Appelbaum PC, Friedman Z, Fairbrother PF, et al. Neonatal sepsis due to group G streptococci. Acta Paediatr Scand 1980;69:559–62.
51. West PW, Al-Sawan R, Foster HA, et al. Speciation of presumptive viridans streptococci from early onset neonatal sepsis. J Med Microbiol 1998;47:923–8.
52. Dobson SR, Baker CJ. Enterococcal sepsis in neonates: features by age at onset and occurrence of focal infection. Pediatrics 1990;85:165–71.
53. Ault KA. Vaginal flora as the source for neonatal early onset *Haemophilus influenzae* sepsis. Pediatr Infect Dis J 1994;13:243.
54. Hershckowitz S, Elisha MB, Fleisher-Sheffer V, et al. A cluster of early neonatal sepsis and pneumonia caused by nontypable *Haemophilus influenzae*. Pediatr Infect Dis J 2004;23:1061–2.
55. Takala AK, Pekkanen E, Eskola J. Neonatal *Haemophilus influenzae* infections. Arch Dis Child 1991;66:437–40.
56. Didier C, Streicher MP, Chognot D, et al. Late-onset neonatal infections: incidences and pathogens in the era of antenatal antibiotics. Eur J Pediatr 2012; 171:681–7.
57. Lim WH, Lien R, Huang YC, et al. Prevalence and pathogen distribution of neonatal sepsis among very-low-birth-weight infants. Pediatr Neonatol 2012; 53:228–34.
58. Shane AL, Hansen NI, Stoll BJ, et al. Methicillin-resistant and susceptible *Staphylococcus aureus* bacteremia and meningitis in preterm infants. Pediatrics 2012;129:e914–22.
59. de Silva GD, Kantzanou M, Justice A, et al. The ica operon and biofilm production in coagulase-negative Staphylococci associated with carriage and disease in a neonatal intensive care unit. J Clin Microbiol 2002;40:382–8.
60. Drudy D, Mullane NR, Quinn T, et al. *Enterobacter sakazakii*: an emerging pathogen in powdered infant formula. Clin Infect Dis 2006;42:996–1002.
61. Tresoldi AT, Padoveze MC, Trabasso P, et al. *Enterobacter cloacae* sepsis outbreak in a newborn unit caused by contaminated total parenteral nutrition solution. Am J Infect Control 2000;28:258–61.
62. Cohen-Wolkowiez M, Moran C, Benjamin DK, et al. Early and late onset sepsis in late preterm infants. Pediatr Infect Dis J 2009;28:1052–6.
63. Bell Y, Barton M, Thame M, et al. Neonatal sepsis in Jamaican neonates. Ann Trop Paediatr 2005;25:293–6.
64. Leibovitz E, Flidel-Rimon O, Juster-Reicher A, et al. Sepsis at a neonatal intensive care unit: a four-year retrospective study (1989-1992). Isr J Med Sci 1997; 33:734–8.

65. Townsend S, Hurrell E, Forsythe S. Virulence studies of *Enterobacter sakazakii* isolates associated with a neonatal intensive care unit outbreak. BMC Microbiol 2008;8:64.
66. Etuwewe O, Kulshrestha R, Sangra M, et al. Brain abscesses due to *Citrobacter koseri* in a pair of twins. Pediatr Infect Dis J 2009;28:1035.
67. Townsend SM, Pollack HA, Gonzalez-Gomez I, et al. *Citrobacter koseri* brain abscess in the neonatal rat: survival and replication within human and rat macrophages. Infect Immun 2003;71:5871–80.
68. Benjamin DK Jr, Stoll BJ, Fanaroff AA, et al. Neonatal candidiasis among extremely low birth weight infants: risk factors, mortality rates, and neurodevelopmental outcomes at 18 to 22 months. Pediatrics 2006;117:84–92.
69. Neu N, Malik M, Lunding A, et al. Epidemiology of candidemia at a children's hospital, 2002 to 2006. Pediatr Infect Dis J 2009;28:806–9.
70. Chitnis AS, Magill SS, Edwards JR, et al. Trends in Candida central line-associated bloodstream infections among NICUs, 1999-2009. Pediatrics 2012; 130:e46–52.
71. Bliss JM, Wong AY, Bhak G, et al. Candida virulence properties and adverse clinical outcomes in neonatal candidiasis. J Pediatr 2012;161:441–447.e2.
72. Stoll BJ, Hansen N, Fanaroff AA, et al. To tap or not to tap: high likelihood of meningitis without sepsis among very low birth weight infants. Pediatrics 2004;113:1181–6.
73. Jawaheer G, Neal TJ, Shaw NJ. Blood culture volume and detection of coagulase negative staphylococcal septicaemia in neonates. Arch Dis Child Fetal Neonatal Ed 1997;76:F57–8.
74. Neal PR, Kleiman MB, Reynolds JK, et al. Volume of blood submitted for culture from neonates. J Clin Microbiol 1986;24:353–6.
75. Visser VE, Hall RT. Urine culture in the evaluation of suspected neonatal sepsis. J Pediatr 1979;94:635–8.
76. Wiswell TE, Baumgart S, Gannon CM, et al. No lumbar puncture in the evaluation for early neonatal sepsis: will meningitis be missed? Pediatrics 1995;95:803–6.
77. Lakeman FD, Whitley RJ. Diagnosis of herpes simplex encephalitis: application of polymerase chain reaction to cerebrospinal fluid from brain-biopsied patients and correlation with disease. National Institute of Allergy and Infectious Diseases Collaborative Antiviral Study Group. J Infect Dis 1995;171:857–63.
78. Simko JP, Caliendo AM, Hogle K, et al. Differences in laboratory findings for cerebrospinal fluid specimens obtained from patients with meningitis or encephalitis due to herpes simplex virus (HSV) documented by detection of HSV DNA. Clin Infect Dis 2002;35:414–9.
79. Christensen RD, Rothstein G, Hill HR, et al. Fatal early onset group B streptococcal sepsis with normal leukocyte counts. Pediatr Infect Dis 1985;4:242–5.
80. Hornik CP, Benjamin DK, Becker KC, et al. Use of the complete blood cell count in early-onset neonatal sepsis. Pediatr Infect Dis J 2012;31:799–802.
81. Murphy K, Weiner J. Use of leukocyte counts in evaluation of early-onset neonatal sepsis. Pediatr Infect Dis J 2012;31:16–9.
82. Tillett WS, Francis T. Serological reactions in pneumonia with a non-protein somatic fraction of pneumococcus. J Exp Med 1930;52:561–71.
83. Hengst JM. The role of C-reactive protein in the evaluation and management of infants with suspected sepsis. Adv Neonatal Care 2003;3:3–13.
84. Philip AG, Mills PC. Use of C-reactive protein in minimizing antibiotic exposure: experience with infants initially admitted to a well-baby nursery. Pediatrics 2000; 106:E4.

85. Chiesa C, Signore F, Assumma M, et al. Serial measurements of C-reactive protein and interleukin-6 in the immediate postnatal period: reference intervals and analysis of maternal and perinatal confounders. Clin Chem 2001;47:1016–22.
86. Forest JC, Lariviere F, Dolce P, et al. C-reactive protein as biochemical indicator of bacterial infection in neonates. Clin Biochem 1986;19:192–4.
87. Chiesa C, Natale F, Pascone R, et al. C reactive protein and procalcitonin: reference intervals for preterm and term newborns during the early neonatal period. Clin Chim Acta 2011;412:1053–9.
88. Hofer N, Muller W, Resch B. Non-infectious conditions and gestational age influence C-reactive protein values in newborns during the first 3 days of life. Clin Chem Lab Med 2011;49:297–302.
89. Auriti C, Fiscarelli E, Ronchetti MP, et al. Procalcitonin in detecting neonatal nosocomial sepsis. Arch Dis Child Fetal Neonatal Ed 2012;97:F368–70.
90. Vouloumanou EK, Plessa E, Karageorgopoulos DE, et al. Serum procalcitonin as a diagnostic marker for neonatal sepsis: a systematic review and meta-analysis. Intensive Care Med 2011;37:747–62.
91. Neth O, Jack DL, Dodds AW, et al. Mannose-binding lectin binds to a range of clinically relevant microorganisms and promotes complement deposition. Infect Immun 2000;68:688–93.
92. Ozkan H, Koksal N, Cetinkaya M, et al. Serum mannose-binding lectin (MBL) gene polymorphism and low MBL levels are associated with neonatal sepsis and pneumonia. J Perinatol 2012;32:210–7.
93. Ng PC, Li K, Wong RP, et al. Proinflammatory and anti-inflammatory cytokine responses in preterm infants with systemic infections. Arch Dis Child Fetal Neonatal Ed 2003;88:F209–13.
94. Resch B, Gusenleitner W, Muller WD. Procalcitonin and interleukin-6 in the diagnosis of early-onset sepsis of the neonate. Acta Paediatr 2003;92:243–5.
95. Genel F, Atlihan F, Gulez N, et al. Evaluation of adhesion molecules CD64, CD11b and CD62L in neutrophils and monocytes of peripheral blood for early diagnosis of neonatal infection. World J Pediatr 2012;8:72–5.
96. Pammi M, Brocklehurst P. Granulocyte transfusions for neonates with confirmed or suspected sepsis and neutropenia. Cochrane Database Syst Rev 2011;(10):CD003956.
97. Ng PC, Ang IL, Chiu RW, et al. Host-response biomarkers for diagnosis of late-onset septicemia and necrotizing enterocolitis in preterm infants. J Clin Invest 2010;120:2989–3000.
98. Daniels JP, Gray J, Pattison HM, et al. Intrapartum tests for group B streptococcus: accuracy and acceptability of screening. BJOG 2011;118:257–65.
99. Polin RA, Denson S, Brady MT. Strategies for prevention of health care-associated infections in the NICU. Pediatrics 2012;129:e1085–93.
100. Kilbride HW, Wirtschafter DD, Powers RJ, et al. Implementation of evidence-based potentially better practices to decrease nosocomial infections. Pediatrics 2003;111:e519–33.
101. Bloom BT, Craddock A, Delmore PM, et al. Reducing acquired infections in the NICU: observing and implementing meaningful differences in process between high and low acquired infection rate centers. J Perinatol 2003;23:489–92.
102. Andersen C, Hart J, Vemgal P, et al. Prospective evaluation of a multi-factorial prevention strategy on the impact of nosocomial infection in very-low-birthweight infants. J Hosp Infect 2005;61:162–7.

103. Shah P, Shah V. Continuous heparin infusion to prevent thrombosis and catheter occlusion in neonates with peripherally placed percutaneous central venous catheters. Cochrane Database Syst Rev 2005;(3):CD002772.
104. Birch P, Ogden S, Hewson M. A randomised, controlled trial of heparin in total parenteral nutrition to prevent sepsis associated with neonatal long lines: the Heparin in Long Line Total Parenteral Nutrition (HILLTOP) trial. Arch Dis Child Fetal Neonatal Ed 2010;95:F252–7.
105. Fanaroff AA, Korones SB, Wright LL, et al. A controlled trial of intravenous immune globulin to reduce nosocomial infections in very-low-birth-weight infants. National Institute of Child Health and Human Development Neonatal Research Network. N Engl J Med 1994;330:1107–13.
106. Ohlsson A, Lacy J. Intravenous immunoglobulin for suspected or subsequently proven infection in neonates. Cochrane Database Syst Rev 2010;(3):CD001239.
107. Brocklehurst P, Farrell B, King A, et al. Treatment of neonatal sepsis with intravenous immune globulin. N Engl J Med 2011;365:1201–11.
108. Vernachio J, Bayer AS, Le T, et al. Anti-clumping factor A immunoglobulin reduces the duration of methicillin-resistant *Staphylococcus aureus* bacteremia in an experimental model of infective endocarditis. Antimicrob Agents Chemother 2003;47:3400–6.
109. Patti JM, Allen BL, McGavin MJ, et al. MSCRAMM-mediated adherence of microorganisms to host tissues. Annu Rev Microbiol 1994;48:585–617.
110. Weisman LE, Thackray HM, Steinhorn RH, et al. A randomized study of a monoclonal antibody (pagibaximab) to prevent staphylococcal sepsis. Pediatrics 2011;128:271–9.
111. Benjamin DK, Schelonka R, White R, et al. A blinded, randomized, multicenter study of an intravenous *Staphylococcus aureus* immune globulin. J Perinatol 2006;26:290–5.
112. Bloom B, Schelonka R, Kueser T, et al. Multicenter study to assess safety and efficacy of INH-A21, a donor-selected human staphylococcal immunoglobulin, for prevention of nosocomial infections in very low birth weight infants. Pediatr Infect Dis J 2005;24:858–66.
113. Shah PS, Kaufman DA. Antistaphylococcal immunoglobulins to prevent staphylococcal infection in very low birth weight infants. Cochrane Database Syst Rev 2009;(2):CD006449.
114. Carr R, Brocklehurst P, Dore CJ, et al. Granulocyte-macrophage colony stimulating factor administered as prophylaxis for reduction of sepsis in extremely preterm, small for gestational age neonates (the PROGRAMS trial): a single-blind, multicentre, randomised controlled trial. Lancet 2009;373:226–33.
115. Poindexter BB, Ehrenkranz RA, Stoll BJ, et al. Effect of parenteral glutamine supplementation on plasma amino acid concentrations in extremely low-birth-weight infants. Am J Clin Nutr 2003;77:737–43.
116. Tubman TR, Thompson SW, McGuire W. Glutamine supplementation to prevent morbidity and mortality in preterm infants. Cochrane Database Syst Rev 2008;(1):CD001457.
117. Alfaleh K, Anabrees J, Bassler D, et al. Probiotics for prevention of necrotizing enterocolitis in preterm infants. Cochrane Database Syst Rev 2011;(3):CD005496.
118. Bonsante F, Iacobelli S, Gouyon JB. Routine probiotic use in very preterm infants: retrospective comparison of two cohorts. Am J Perinatol 2012. [Epub ahead of print].
119. Deshpande G, Rao S, Patole S, et al. Updated meta-analysis of probiotics for preventing necrotizing enterocolitis in preterm neonates. Pediatrics 2010;125: 921–30.

120. Manzoni P, Rinaldi M, Cattani S, et al. Bovine lactoferrin supplementation for prevention of late-onset sepsis in very low-birth-weight neonates: a randomized trial. JAMA 2009;302:1421–8.
121. Kaufman D, Boyle R, Hazen KC, et al. Fluconazole prophylaxis against fungal colonization and infection in preterm infants. N Engl J Med 2001;345:1660–6.
122. Manzoni P, Stolfi I, Pugni L, et al. A multicenter, randomized trial of prophylactic fluconazole in preterm neonates. N Engl J Med 2007;356:2483–95.
123. Kaufman DA, Cuff AL, Wamstad JB, et al. Fluconazole prophylaxis in extremely low birth weight infants and neurodevelopmental outcomes and quality of life at 8 to 10 years of age. J Pediatr 2011;158:759–765.e1.
124. Kicklighter SD, Springer SC, Cox T, et al. Fluconazole for prophylaxis against candidal rectal colonization in the very low birth weight infant. Pediatrics 2001;107:293–8.
125. Healy CM, Campbell JR, Zaccaria E, et al. Fluconazole prophylaxis in extremely low birth weight neonates reduces invasive candidiasis mortality rates without emergence of fluconazole-resistant *Candida* species. Pediatrics 2008;121:703–10.
126. Pappas PG, Kauffman CA, Andes D, et al. Clinical practice guidelines for the management of candidiasis: 2009 update by the Infectious Diseases Society of America. Clin Infect Dis 2009;48:503–35.
127. Cotten CM, Taylor S, Stoll B, et al. Prolonged duration of initial empirical antibiotic treatment is associated with increased rates of necrotizing enterocolitis and death for extremely low birth weight infants. Pediatrics 2009;123:58–66.
128. Kuppala VS, Meinzen-Derr J, Morrow AL, et al. Prolonged initial empirical antibiotic treatment is associated with adverse outcomes in premature infants. J Pediatr 2011;159:720–5.
129. Arslan U, Erayman I, Kirdar S, et al. *Serratia marcescens* sepsis outbreak in a neonatal intensive care unit. Pediatr Int 2010;52:208–12.
130. Dashti AA, Jadaon MM, Gomaa HH, et al. Transmission of a *Klebsiella pneumoniae* clone harbouring genes for CTX-M-15-like and SHV-112 enzymes in a neonatal intensive care unit of a Kuwaiti hospital. J Med Microbiol 2010;59:687–92.
131. Golan Y, Doron S, Sullivan B, et al. Transmission of vancomycin-resistant enterococcus in a neonatal intensive care unit. Pediatr Infect Dis J 2005;24:566–7.
132. Linkin DR, Fishman NO, Patel JB, et al. Risk factors for extended-spectrum beta-lactamase-producing Enterobacteriaceae in a neonatal intensive care unit. Infect Control Hosp Epidemiol 2004;25:781–3.
133. Maraki S, Scoulica E, Manoura A, et al. *Chryseobacterium meningosepticum* colonization outbreak in a neonatal intensive care unit. Eur J Clin Microbiol Infect Dis 2009;28:1415–9.
134. Touati A, Achour W, Cherif A, et al. Outbreak of *Acinetobacter baumannii* in a neonatal intensive care unit: antimicrobial susceptibility and genotyping analysis. Ann Epidemiol 2009;19:372–8.
135. Patel SJ, Oshodi A, Prasad P, et al. Antibiotic use in neonatal intensive care units and adherence with Centers for Disease Control and Prevention 12 Step Campaign to Prevent Antimicrobial Resistance. Pediatr Infect Dis J 2009;28:1047–51.
136. Tamma PD, Cosgrove SE. Antimicrobial stewardship. Infect Dis Clin North Am 2011;25:245–60.
137. Patel SJ, Saiman L, Duchon JM, et al. Development of an antimicrobial stewardship intervention using a model of actionable feedback. Interdiscip Perspect Infect Dis 2012;2012:150367.

138. Chen SC, Slavin MA, Sorrell TC. Echinocandin antifungal drugs in fungal infections: a comparison. Drugs 2011;71:11–41.
139. Smith PB, Walsh TJ, Hope W, et al. Pharmacokinetics of an elevated dosage of micafungin in premature neonates. Pediatr Infect Dis J 2009;28:412–5.
140. Heresi GP, Gerstmann DR, Reed MD, et al. The pharmacokinetics and safety of micafungin, a novel echinocandin, in premature infants. Pediatr Infect Dis J 2006;25:1110–5.
141. Benjamin DK Jr, Smith PB, Arrieta A, et al. Safety and pharmacokinetics of repeat-dose micafungin in young infants. Clin Pharmacol Ther 2010;87:93–9.

Otitis Media

Michael E. Pichichero, MD

KEYWORDS

- Otitis media • Antibiotics • Aminopenicillins • Cephalosporins
- Pneumococcal conjugate vaccine • *Streptococcus pneumoniae*
- *Haemophilus influenzae* • Tympanocentesis

KEY POINTS

- The diagnosis of acute otitis media (AOM) requires visualization of a tympanic membrane that is full or bulging, with middle ear effusion present.
- Recent antibiotic pressure and vaccination with the pneumococcal conjugate vaccine have resulted in the emergence of β-lactamase–producing *Haemophilus influenzae* and *Moraxella catarrhalis* as the leading organisms causing AOM, followed by *Streptococcus pneumoniae*.
- Current American Academy of Pediatrics guidelines endorse amoxicillin as the preferred treatment of AOM, but the recent increase in amoxicillin-resistant *H influenzae* and *M catarrhalis* would suggest high-dose amoxicillin-clavulanate as a preferred treatment.
- Cefdinir, cefuroxime, and cefpodoxime proxetil are the preferred oral cephalosporins for the treatment of AOM. Among these, cefdinir is the most palatable.
- Recent evidence suggests cellular and humoral immunodeficiency against AOM-causing organisms in children with recurrent AOM.
- Antibiotic prophylaxis is no longer recommended as a preventative strategy for AOM recurrences.

DEFINITIONS

Otitis media is a broad term that includes acute otitis media (AOM), otitis media with effusion (OME), and chronic otitis media with effusion. This article focuses on AOM and OME.

EPIDEMIOLOGY

AOM is an infectious disease that primarily affects young children. Onset of AOM in the first 6 months is not common because infants in this age group are still protected from infection by maternal antibodies acquired transplacentally. If a child experiences AOM in the first 6 months of life, then frequent AOM likely will occur throughout the first few years of life.[1] Most AOM occurs between 6 and 24 months of age; the peak incidence

---

Center for Infectious Diseases and Immunology, Rochester General Hospital Research Institute, Rochester General Hospital, 1425 Portland Avenue, Rochester, NY 14621, USA
E-mail address: Michael.pichichero@rochestergeneral.org

Pediatr Clin N Am 60 (2013) 391–407
http://dx.doi.org/10.1016/j.pcl.2012.12.007 **pediatric.theclinics.com**

is between 9 and 15 months of age.[1] AOM occurs with modest frequency between 2 and 3 years of age but its appearance quickly diminishes between 3 and 5 years of age.[1] AOM can occur at any age, including adolescence and adulthood, but it is not a common infectious disease in those years of life. The frequency of AOM and OME events in children is shown in **Fig. 1**.[2]

ORIGIN

The bacteria that cause AOM vary from country to country because of vaccination and antibiotic prescribing habits. In North America virtually all vaccinations against pneumococcus in children are with the 13-valent pneumococcal conjugate vaccine (PCV13). Most children are treated with antibiotics, predominantly amoxicillin in a standard dose (40 mg/kg/d divided twice daily) or a high dose (80 mg/kg/d divided twice daily) for 10 days. As a consequence of PCV and amoxicillin use, the etiology of AOM continues to change over time.[3]

Health care providers must be cautious when they read reports of the etiology of AOM if the study was conducted outside of North America. The availability and extent of use of 7-valent pneumococcal conjugate vaccine (PCV7) varies and the introduction of PCV13 varies. The use of antibiotics at all (observation option), and the primary choice, dose, and routine duration of antibiotics all influence the bacterial etiology and the extent of antibiotic resistance.

The most recent data on the distribution of bacteria causing AOM in North America are shown in **Table 1** (J Casey and ME Pichichero, unpublished data). The mix of organisms and the resistance to amoxicillin among the otopathogens as shown in **Table 1**, and the in vitro activity of antibiotic choices available (**Fig. 2**)[4] suggest that a β-lactamase–stable aminopenicillin (amoxicillin/clavulanate) in high dosage would be the preferred treatment (discussed later).

Much confusion surrounds the role of upper respiratory infection (URI) viruses as a cause of AOM and OME. Although no doubt exists that viral URI plays a key role in the pathogenesis of AOM and OME, the role is more facilitation of bacterial AOM than a primary origin for these viruses (see section on Immunology). Respiratory syncytial virus, influenzae, parainfluenzae, rhinovirus, metapneumovirus, and others can be detected in the nasopharyngeal secretions of children with an URI, followed by AOM or OME. The nasopharyngeal secretions can reflux from the nasopharyngeal region via the eustachian tube into the middle ear space. Therefore, detection of the

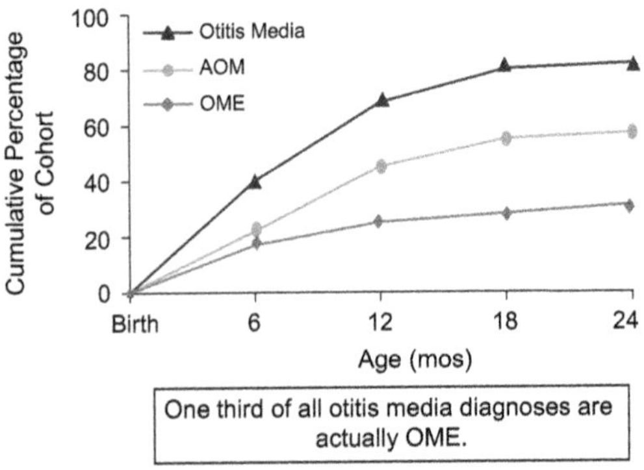

Fig. 1. Frequency of the anticipated diagnosis of AOM compared with the frequency of anticipated diagnosis of OME in children from birth to 2 years of age. (*From* Faden H, Duffy L, Boeve M. Otitis media: back to basics. Pediatr Infect Dis J 1998;17:1105–13; with permission.)

Table 1
Bacteria causing AOM in North America, 2012[a]

	% of Total Pathogen
Streptococcus pneumoniae	12
Amoxicillin-resistant	20
Haemophilus influenzae	56
Amoxicillin-resistant	50
Moraxella catarrhalis	22
Amoxicillin-resistant	100

[a] Based on results from Legacy Pediatrics, Rochester, NY, 2011–2012 respiratory season.

virus in middle ear fluid (MEF) using tympanocentesis does not inform on whether the virus causes AOM. With modern polymerase chain reaction (PCR) techniques, the DNA or RNA of viruses can be detected in the nasopharyngeal region and MEF of many children with AOM and OME. The presence of a respiratory virus without a bacterial otopathogen simultaneously detected is uncommon, probably occurring in around 2% to 10% of cases.[5] Even with that low detection rate, studies have not systematically used PCR molecular methods for both viral and bacterial detection in the same nasopharyngeal and MEF samples.

OME can persist after an AOM for some time. Approximately half of the children who experience AOM will have OME 1 month after initial diagnosis, one-third will have OME 2 months after AOM, and 10% will have OME 3 months after AOM (**Fig. 3**). Years ago,

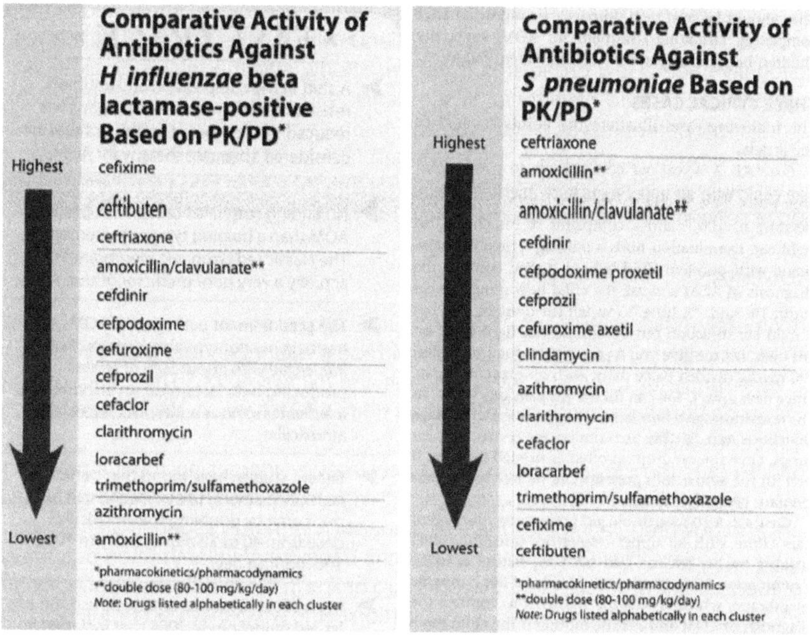

Fig. 2. Comparative activity of selected antibiotics with a US Food and Drug Administration approval for AOM regarding anticipated effectiveness against β-lactamase–producing *Haemophilus influenzae* and penicillin-resistant *Streptococcus pneumoniae*. (*From* Pichichero ME. Acute otitis media: part II. Treatment in an era of increasing antibiotic resistance. Am Fam Physician 2000;61(8):2410–6; with permission.)

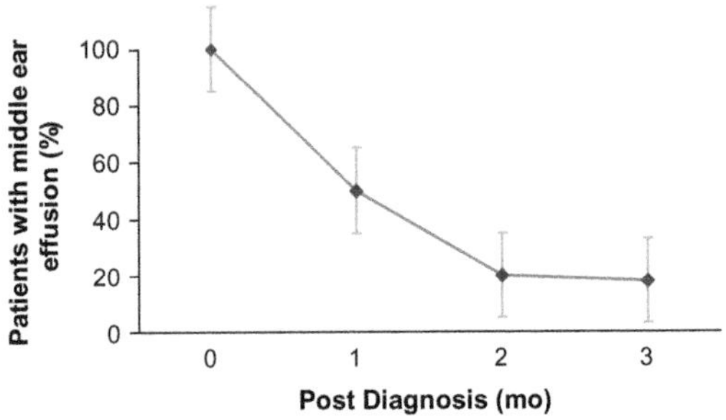

Fig. 3. Middle ear effusions gradually disappear over time after diagnosis of AOM.

health care providers would ask for a follow-up visit 2 weeks after diagnosis of AOM to determine that the infection had resolved. When they observed the tympanic membrane and found OME, they presumed a treatment failure had occurred and would prescribe more and stronger antibiotics. That practice is no longer followed, largely because of the discovery that OME persists so long after AOM and can easily be confused with persistent AOM.

OME can become chronic (>3 months in duration). When this occurs, ample evidence suggests that the common otopathogens form biofilms.[6] Biofilms comprise microbes in a colony, which reduces their process of dividing, slows their metabolism, and allows them to communicate with each other to share survival mechanisms through a process called *quorum sensing*. Biofilm colonies exist in a matrix of DNA, and cover themselves with a shield of biomaterial that prevents the penetration of antibiotics and antibodies. Most clinicians are familiar with biofilms as bacteria that grow on implanted catheters. Biofilms of the *Pseudomonas* sp form in patients with cystic fibrosis. Biofilm colonies occasionally shed a few organisms from the colony, and the microbes change their biology and are termed *planktonic*. When biofilms form in chronic OME they consist of the major otopathogens as single-species colonies or as polymicrobial colonies consisting of 2 or even 3 species of otopathogen. Because the biofilms do not elicit an immune response, little clinical evidence shows that they exist because minimal inflammation is seen in the middle ear when the biofilms is present.

PATHOGENESIS

Approximately 90% to 95% of AOM and OME cases are preceded by a viral URI. Upper airway allergy may cause eustachian tube dysfunction and lead to OME, and much less frequently to AOM. OME precedes and follows AOM.[7] This concept is fairly new. Most health care providers were taught that OME follows AOM, but not that OME also precedes AOM.

Viral URI sets the stage for AOM and OME through increasing mucus production, slowing the beat of cilia in the nasopharyngeal region, creating nasopharyngeal inflammation, and downregulating the innate and adaptive immune response (see section on Immunology). Next, the eustachian tube closes because of inflammation occurring as part of the viral URI process. Negative pressure builds in the middle ear space, resulting in a retracted tympanic membrane. The distortion of the tympanic membrane caused by retraction can easily be confused with bulging. The middle ear also produces mucus to keep the surface of the middle ear cells moist. With the eustachian tube closed, the mucus builds up and causes fluid to be visible behind the tympanic membrane; this is OME. However, when OME develops, the middle ear is still sterile and the absence of a virus or bacteria results in the tympanic membrane remaining generally translucent.

The secretions in the nasopharyngeal region are then literally sucked into the middle ear space when the eustachian tube temporarily relaxes for a part of a second. Once the secretions and accompanying virus and bacteria that were in the nasopharyngeal region gain entry to the middle ear space, the environment is free of immune control factors, and the bacteria begin to divide. In response to the local bacteria invasion the innate immune response is activated, resulting in the influx of neutrophils. The neutrophils release mediators of inflammation, and the health care provider observes that pathogenic process when glimpsing the tympanic membrane that has become thickened with edema, perhaps red, but most importantly observes bulging from the pressure of an inflammatory response (see sections on Clinical Manifestations and Diagnosis).

CLINICAL MANIFESTATIONS

Because nearly all AOM and OME events occur in the context of a viral URI, the clinical manifestations of AOM and OME often include those of a viral URI (**Table 2**).[8] That is, children with AOM and OME often have rhinorrhea, nasal congestion, and elevated body temperature. When children have a cold they are cranky, feed poorly, and sleep poorly. URI causes increased mucus production in the nasopharyngeal region that drips into the stomach, sometimes causing the child to vomit. Altogether it is apparent that the clinical manifestations of a viral URI are indistinct from those of AOM or OME.

Two-thirds of children with AOM have fever, but that means one-third do not. OME is not associated with fever, but if the child has a concurrent viral URI, that may cause fever. Therefore, ample evidence now confirms that the diagnosis of AOM or OME cannot rely on clinical manifestations.

Health care providers often presume that a child pulling at the ears has an AOM. This is not correct. Even pulling the ear is not a clear clinical manifestation of AOM or OME. When the tympanic membrane becomes retracted, the change in its position causes sensory nerve receptors to fire off, and this is associated with discomfort or even pain and ear tugging. For confirmation of this evidence, the reader is encouraged to recall an airplane ride and a child crying suddenly when the cabin was given positive pressure as the plane ascended. Several small children on board may have begun to cry as their eardrums began to retract from the pressure.

Table 2
Sensitivity and specificity of symptoms and signs to predict AOM

Source and Symptoms	Sensitivity (%)	Specificity (%)
Ear pain	54	82
Ear rubbing	42	87
Fever	40	48
Cough	47	45
Rhinitis	75	43
Excessive crying	55	69
Poor appetite	36	66
Vomiting	11	89
Sore throat	13	74
Headache	9	76

Abbreviation: NA, not applicable.

Data from Routhman R, Owens T, Simel DL. Does this child have acute otitis media? JAMA 2003;290(12):1633–40.

DIAGNOSIS

AOM is a visual diagnosis based on viewing the tympanic membrane.[7–9] Stated another way, it is not possible to diagnose AOM accurately without visualizing the tympanic membrane. The examination is difficult and training in diagnosis often is limited and much outdated.

A glimpse of a small portion of the tympanic membrane is not sufficient to diagnose AOM. The clinician is advised to make an effort to clear all or nearly all of the ear canal cerumen to view all or nearly all of the tympanic membrane.

The key diagnostic feature of AOM is a bulging or full appearance of the tympanic membrane (**Fig. 4**).[6] The bulging is from pressure behind the tympanic membrane caused by inflammation in the middle ear space. AOM is not associated with a retracted tympanic membrane, and therefore a determination of retraction of the tympanic membrane is a viral-mediated phenomenon or associated with OME (**Fig. 5**).[6] A bulging tympanic membrane can be difficult to distinguish from one that is retracted. Use of pneumatic otoscopy is helpful in this setting because positive pressure on insufflation will result in movement backward by a bulging tympanic membrane, and negative pressure will result in movement forward by a retracted tympanic membrane.

Because of the inflammation in the middle ear space during AOM, typically the tympanic membrane becomes thickened and nontranslucent or completely opaque. A translucent tympanic membrane is unlikely to be associated with AOM (**Fig. 6**). With a translucent or semitranslucent tympanic membrane and MEF visualized behind the tympanic membrane, the likely diagnosis is OME (see **Fig. 5**).[6]

Redness of the tympanic membrane is no longer considered a valuable diagnostic sign of AOM. Redness occurs from inflammation, but can also occur from fever or the child crying (and most children of the age at which they would experience AOM cry during the examination). Furthermore, when an otoscope speculum is inserted into the external auditory canal, sometimes the tympanic membrane will turn red. The presence of only one red tympanic membrane suggests inflammation and is consistent with the diagnosis of AOM if fluid is visualized behind it. Most likely this examination represents early AOM before inflammation has persisted long enough to cause the tympanic membrane to become more yellowish and opaque.

OME is not associated with inflammation, and therefore it was previously taught that OME occurred without symptoms other than hearing loss. It is now realized that a child with OME may experience discomfort, and may feel popping noises as air gains entry via the eustachian tube into the middle ear space, which may cause the child to pull

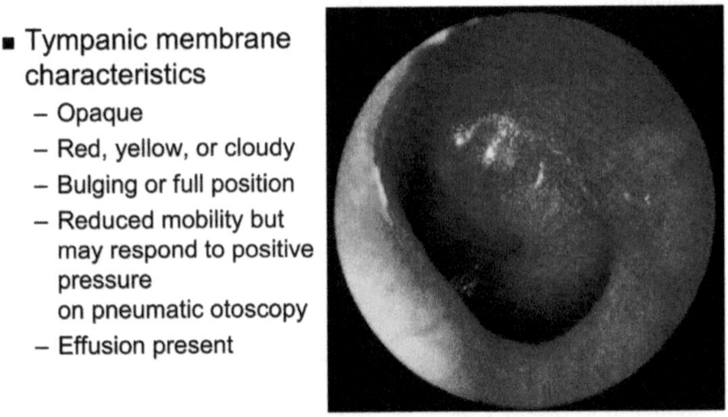

▪ Tympanic membrane characteristics
– Opaque
– Red, yellow, or cloudy
– Bulging or full position
– Reduced mobility but may respond to positive pressure on pneumatic otoscopy
– Effusion present

Fig. 4. AOM tympanic membrane appearance in children.

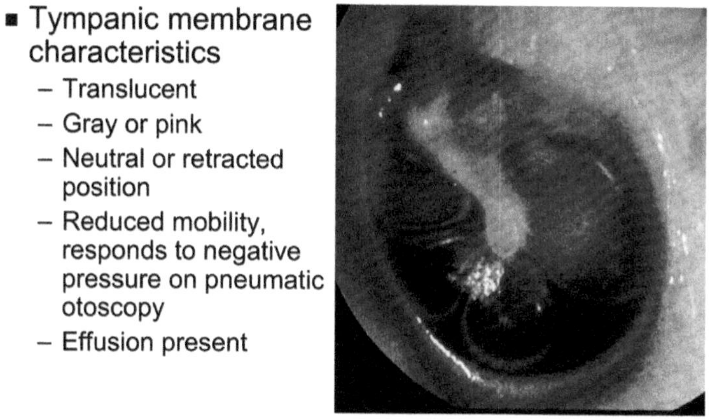
Tympanic membrane characteristics
– Translucent
– Gray or pink
– Neutral or retracted position
– Reduced mobility, responds to negative pressure on pneumatic otoscopy
– Effusion present

Fig. 5. OME tympanic membrane appearance in children.

and tug at the ear or even cry. However, the visual examination is distinct from AOM, as outlined earlier.

As an adjunct to the examination, 2 instruments are available to help diagnose AOM and OME, although neither is superior to pneumatic otoscopy.[10,11] Tympanometry requires a seal of the inserted speculum-like device in the external auditory canal. In children younger than 2 years, when AOM is most common, the child often moves and a seal cannot be obtained. Furthermore, if a child is crying, a tympanogram reading cannot be obtained. The tympanogram identifies the movement of the tympanic membrane in response to positive and negative pressure. If no movement occurs with applied pressure and the seal is adequate, then the tympanogram readout is flat; this is the typical case for AOM. In some cases the tympanic membrane will be full or bulging, also called a *positive pressure tympanogram readout*. This finding occurs early in the AOM pathogenesis. In some cases, the tympanic membrane will be retracted, also called a *negative pressure tympanogram readout*. This finding occurs during a viral URI, sometimes with concomitant MEF, and is consistent with OME.

Another instrument to help diagnose AOM and OME is the acoustic reflectometer, also called the *acoustic otoscope*. This device is not as readily available because it

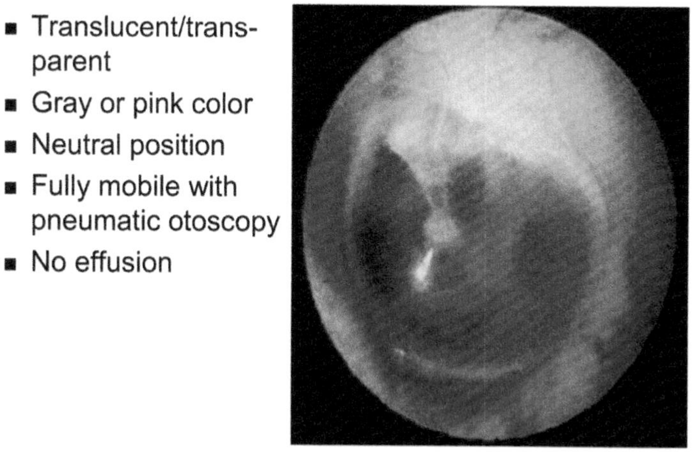
Translucent/transparent
Gray or pink color
Neutral position
Fully mobile with pneumatic otoscopy
No effusion

Fig. 6. Normal tympanic membrane appearance in children.

has come in and out of ownership by several companies with variable marketing efforts. This instrument does not require a seal in the external auditory canal, and readings can be obtained in the crying child. The main limitation is the presence of wax in the external auditory canal. Cerumen that blocks the sonar wave emitted by the acoustic reflectometer is misinterpreted by the device and false readings occur. Therefore, the wax must be removed to the extent possible. The sonar wave emitted from the device is programmed to go through the tympanic membrane, bounce off the posterior bony wall of the middle ear space, and then bounce back to the emitter device to produce a reading. If the sonar wave is impeded by cerumen, a false readout occurs. If the wave passes through a thickened tympanic membrane, the wave is slowed, giving a higher reading, such as level 5, consistent with a middle ear effusion risk of 92% (**Table 3**).[12] If the wave passes through fluid of any type it slows the wave, with thicker fluid (pus) impeding the wave more than thinner fluid (OME).

When fluid is present in the middle ear space it can cause diminished hearing. An audiogram can help establish the extent of hearing loss for both AOM and OME. Testing for hearing in young children is difficult in clinical settings other than audiology practices that can use brainstem-evoked responses. Thus, although a potential useful tool to quantify hearing loss, audiometry is not often used in the first few years of life when AOM and OME most frequently occur. This paradox is problematic in terms of compliance with national recommendations for management of OME, wherein the presence of unilateral hearing loss of 6 months' duration or bilateral hearing loss of 3 months' duration to greater than 30 dB thresholds in the speech range (500–2000 Hz) is a primary criterion for recommending insertion of tympanostomy tubes.

TREATMENT

The principal treatment of AOM in North America is antibiotics. Guidelines have been promulgated recommending as preferred treatment a high dose of amoxicillin (80 mg/kg/d in 2 divided doses) for 5 to 10 days.[13,14] The selection of high-dose amoxicillin has been made based on its long-term safety, a primary intention of treating penicillin-resistant *Streptococcus pneumoniae* because that organism can cause the most morbidity, and the recognition that overdiagnosis of AOM is common and that as a consequence, emergence of antibiotic resistant microbes occurs more rapidly. The recommendations of the American Academy of Pediatrics (AAP) are presented in **Table 4**.[13]

The best choice of antibiotic based on current otopathogen mix and antibiotic resistance would be high-dose amoxicillin/clavulanate (80 mg/kg/d divided twice daily) (see **Fig. 2**). Amoxicillin would not be considered the most effective antibiotic for empiric selection because it has no activity against β-lactamase–producing bacteria, which are currently much more common than penicillin-resistant *S pneumoniae* (see **Table 1**). The addition of clavulanate as a β-lactamase–neutralizing product would

Table 3
Acoustic reflectometry readouts

Gradient Angle	Predicted Risk of MEE	*n*	% of Ears with Documented MEE
<49°	Low	383	3.4
49°–59°	Low to moderate	279	15.8
60°–69°	Moderate	82	34.2
70°–95	Moderate to high	76	57.9
>95°	High	50	92.0

Abbreviation: MEE, middle ear effusion.

Table 4
American Academy of Pediatrics/American Academy of Family Physicians treatment recommendations for AOM

Criteria	Initial Management		Treatment Failure at 48–72 h	
Temperature ≥39°C or moderate to severe otalgia	Recommended antimicrobial agents[a]	Alternatives for penicillin allergy	Recommended antimicrobial agents[a]	Alternatives for penicillin allergy
No	Amoxicillin, 80–90 mg/kg/d	Non–type I: cefdinir cefuroxime cefpodoxime Type 1: azithromycin clarithromycin	Amoxicillin/ clavulanate (90 mg/kg/d of amoxicillin with 6.4 mg/kg/d of clavulanate)	Non–type I: ceftriaxone 3 d Type I: clindamycin
Yes	Amoxicillin/ clavulanate (90 mg/kg/d of amoxicillin with 6.4 mg/kg/d of clavulanate)	Ceftriaxone 1 or 3 d	Ceftriaxone 3 d	Tympanocentesis clindamycin

[a] If a child is initially observed and symptoms persist or worsen at 48 to 72 hours, antimicrobial agents are recommended.

Data from American Academy of Pediatrics Subcommittee on Management of Acute Otitis Media. Diagnosis and management of acute otitis media. Pediatrics 2004;113:1451–65.

provide anticipated efficacy against β-lactamase–producing *Haemophilus influenzae* and *Moraxella catarrhalis* while maintaining excellent antimicrobial activity against penicillin-resistant *S pneumoniae*. Amoxicillin/clavulanate has 2 disadvantages: in suspension formulation it has a marginal taste that can cause nonadherence to the prescribed regimen, and it causes more loose stools and diarrhea than many cephalosporin alternatives.

The preferred oral cephalosporins for treating AOM according to the AAP are cefdinir, cefuroxime axetil, and cefpodoxime proxetil (see **Table 4**).[13] Among these choices in North America, cefdinir has emerged as the most frequently used, largely because the other 2 drugs have a bitter taste and are associated with taste aversion by children. Cefdinir can be dosed once or divided twice daily (14 mg/kg/d). The duration of treatment with cefdinir can be 5 days with twice-daily dosing or 10 days with once-daily dosing. In a head-to-head comparison of amoxicillin/clavulanate, 80 mg/kg/d divided twice daily for 10 days versus cefdinir, 14 mg/kg/d divided twice daily for 5 days, amoxicillin/clavulanate showed superior efficacy.[15] However, outside the context of a clinical trial, the adherence characteristics favor cefdinir (better taste and less diarrhea). The taste of cefuroxime and cefpodoxime can be masked with chocolate syrup, but the addition of flavorings at the pharmacy should not be advised because these antibiotics have been shown to precipitate with changes in pH and chemical reactions between the active drug and the flavoring ingredients.

Ceftriaxone by injection (50 mg/kg per dose) is among the preferred antibiotics for AOM (see **Table 4**).[12] It is effective as a single injection against all penicillin-susceptible *S pneumoniae* and against β-lactamase–producing *H influenzae* and *Moraxella*. Penicillin-resistant *S pneumoniae* that cause AOM are more effectively and consistently eradicated by 3 sequential doses of ceftriaxone on 3 sequential days.

In light of the long half-life of ceftriaxone, the sequential doses may be spaced every other day, or even every third day if weekends or holidays dictate an alternative regimen.

Clindamycin is also included as a treatment alternative for AOM after failure of other preferred first-and second-line agents (see **Table 4**).[13] However, even after treatment with an antibiotic that should have eradicated a specific bacteria based on in vitro susceptibility testing, about half the time the susceptible organism is not eradicated. Most often this failure to correlate in vitro with in vivo effects is caused by altered pharmacokinetics (the drug is not fully absorbed) or pharmacodynamics (the drug does not reach the site of infection in adequate concentrations). Because clindamycin is ineffective against β-lactamase–producing *H influenzae* and *Moraxella* and only effective against penicillin-susceptible and penicillin-resistant *S pneumoniae*, its use might best be limited to cases in which a tympanocentesis has been performed and the persisting bacteria identified.

Tympanocentesis can be used to treat AOM if performed in association with evacuation of pus, microbes, and proinflammatory fluid. Not all tympanocenteses are performed with evacuation of MEF, and that fact complicates the interpretation of available clinical studies of the therapeutic benefit of the procedure and confuses the clinician.[16] Tympanocentesis can be performed in an office practice setting without anesthesia or conscious sedation. Instillation of 8% tetracaine into the external canal after an otowick has been inserted to assure the anesthetic reaches the tympanic membrane is effective for allowing the procedure to occur without the child experiencing pain. However, the child must be restrained to avoid head movement during the procedure, and children typically cry when they are restrained. Tympanocentesis is not a frequently performed procedure because most clinicians have not received training, and those who have been trained become concerned about its use as a standard of care despite the AAP[13] and Centers for Disease Control and Prevention[14] recommending its selected use in AOM management.

In 2004 the AAP endorsed a recommendation for watchful waiting as an option for managing AOM in selected cases (**Table 5**).[9] The main concept was to allow observation as an option when the diagnosis was uncertain (unlikely AOM) as long as the child was older than 2 years, because by that age the immune system is stronger and an infection would be unlikely to progress beyond a more certain examination to confirm AOM. In older children who are verbal and can describe their symptoms, especially pain, watchful waiting was allowed as long as the child did not complain of pain.

Table 5
Criteria for initial treatment or observation in children with AOM

Age	Certain Diagnosis	Uncertain Diagnosis
<6 mo	Antibacterial therapy	Antibacterial therapy
6 mo–2 y	Antibacterial therapy	Antibacterial therapy if severe illness Observe[a] if nonsevere illness
≥2 y	Antibacterial therapy if severe illness Observe[a] if nonsevere illness	Observe[a]

Certain diagnosis of AOM if all 3 criteria are met: (1) rapid onset, (2) sign of middle ear effusion, and (3) signs and symptoms of middle ear inflammation. Severe illness is considered moderate to severe otalgia or temperature of 39°C (102°F) or greater. Nonsevere illness is considered mild otalgia and temperature of less than 39°C (102°F) in the past 24 hours.

[a] Observation is an appropriate option only when follow-up can be assured and antibacterial agents are started if symptoms persist or worsen.

Data from American Academy of Pediatrics Subcommittee on Management of Acute Otitis Media. Diagnosis and management of acute otitis media. Pediatrics 2004;113:1451–65.

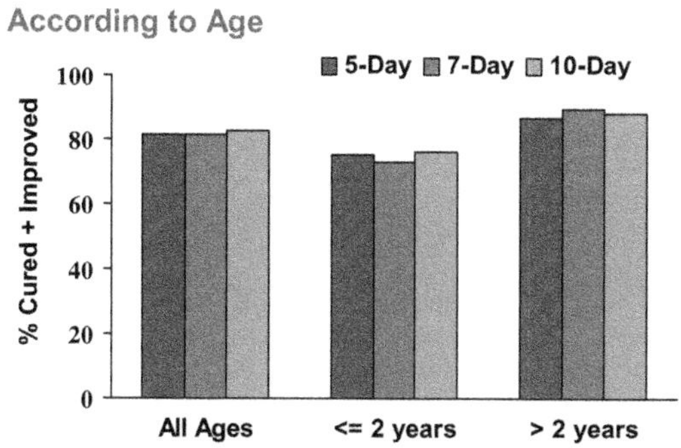

Fig. 7. Comparison of cured + improved outcome after AOM diagnosis treated with approved antibiotics for 5, 7, and 10 days, divided according to age of the child at diagnosis. (*Data from* Pichichero ME, Marsocci SM, Murphy ML, et al. A prospective observational study of 5-, 7-, and 10-day antibiotic treatment for acute otitis media. Otolaryngol Head Neck Surg 2001;124(4):381–7.)

However, the studies that the AAP used to make this recommendation were flawed.[17] Two recent studies proved that amoxicillin/clavulanate provides superior outcomes compared with observation.[18,19]

Pain management for AOM has received attention more recently. A child with suspected or confirmed AOM should be given pain treatment. Usually this would involve acetaminophen or ibuprofen in weight-appropriate doses. Ototopical ear drops also can be considered, although evidence of efficacy is limited.

The optimal duration of antibiotic treatment in North America is generally considered to be 10 days. This recommendation is not evidence-based,[20,21] but rather grew from the evidence-based recommendation for 10 days' treatment of group A streptococcal pharyngitis with penicillin. Outside of North America, the treatment duration of AOM with antibiotics varies widely. Treatment regimens of 1, 3, 5, 7, and 10 days are all standard in different countries. The recent AAP guidelines endorse 10 days' treatment as the standard for most AOM, but acknowledge that shorter treatment regimens may be as effective. The AAP recommendation for 7 days' treatment of children aged 5 years

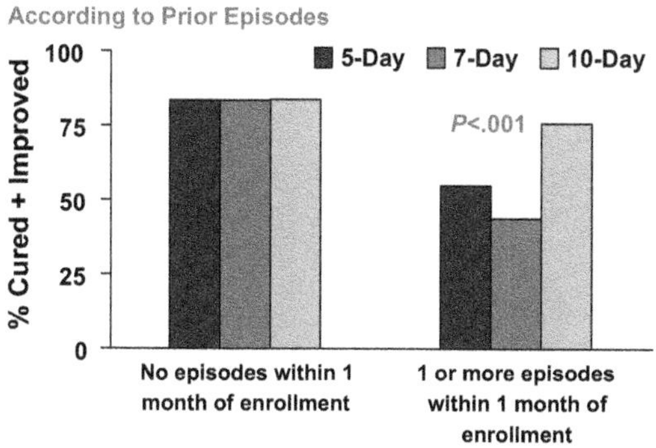

Fig. 8. Comparison of cured + improved outcome after AOM diagnosis treated with approved antibiotics for 5, 7, and 10 days, divided according to number of recent prior episodes of AOM diagnosis. (*Data from* Pichichero ME, Marsocci SM, Murphy ML, et al. A prospective observational study of 5-, 7-, and 10-day antibiotic treatment for acute otitis media. Otolaryngol Head Neck Surg 2001;124(4):381–7.)

Table 6
Cross-reactivity between penicillins and cephalosporins based on side chain structure similarity

Seven-position side chain

Similar side chain/ cross-reactivity possible within group[a,b]	Similar side chain/ cross-reactivity possible with group	Similar side chain/ cross-reactivity possible with group	Completely dissimilar side chains/unlikely cross-reactivity with each other[b,c]	
Cephaloridine (first-generation) Cephalothin (first-generation) Penicillin G	Cefaclor (second-generation) Cephradine (first-generation) Cephalexin (first-generation) Cefadroxil (first-generation) Amoxicillin Ampicillin	Cefepime (fourth-generation) Ceftizoxime (third-generation) Cefpirome (fourth-generation) Cefotaxime (third-generation) Cefpodoxime (third-generation) Ceftriaxone (third-generation)	Cefoperazone (third-generation) Cefotetan (second-generation) Cefazolin (first-generation) Cefuroxime (second-generation) Cefdinir (third-generation) Cefditoren (third-generation)	Cefixime (third-generation) Cefprozil (second-generation) Cefmetazole (second-generation) Ceftibuten (third-generation) Ceftazidime (third-generation) Cefoxitin (second-generation)

Three-position side chain

Similar side chain/ cross-reactivity possible within group[b,d]	Similar side chain/ cross-reactivity possible within group	Similar side chain/ cross-reactivity possible within group	Similar side chain/ cross-reactivity possible within group	Similar side chain/ cross-reactivity possible within group	Similar side chain/ cross-reactivity possible within group	Dissimilar side chain/ unlikely cross-reactivity with each other[b,e]

Cefadroxil (first-generation) Cephalexin (first-generation)	Cefmetazole (second-generation) Cefoperazone (third-generation) Cefotetan (second-generation)	Cefotaxime (third-generation) Cephalothin (first-generation)	Ceftibuten (third-generation) Ceftizoxime (third-generation)	Cefuroxime (second-generation) Cefoxitin (second-generation)	Cefdinir (third-generation) Cefixime (third-generation)	Cefpodoxime (third-generation) Cefprozil (second-generation) Ceftibuten (third-generation) Ceftriaxone (third-generation) Cefepime (fourth-generation) Cefpirome (fourth-generation) Cefazolin (first-generation) Cefaclor (second-generation) Ceftazidime (third-generation)

[a] Based on the 7-position side chain structure similarity, allergic cross-reactivity might occur among these 3 drugs: cephaloridine (second-generation cephalosporin), cephalothin (first-generation cephalosporin), and penicillin. The same interpretation applies to the subsequent 4 columns.

[b] To apply this table clinically, check the antibiotic for cross-reactivity possibilities based on both the 7-position and 3-position side chains. If either side chain position is shared between antibiotics to avoid a possible cross-allergy reaction, this use would not be recommended. If neither of the side chains shares structured similarity between antibiotics, then cross-reactivity is highly unlikely and these antibiotics can be recommended without anticipated increased risk of a cross-allergy reaction.

[c] Based on the 7-position side chain structure uniqueness of these cephalosporins, allergic cross-reactivity with each other and with all other cephalosporins and penicillins would be highly unlikely.

[d] Based on the 3-position side chain structure similarity, allergic cross-reactivity might occur between these 2 drugs: cefadroxil (first-generation cephalosporin) and cephalexin (first-generation cephalosporin). The same interpretation applies to the subsequent 6 columns.

[e] Based on the 3-position side chain structure uniqueness of these cephalosporins, allergic cross-reactivity with each other and with all other cephalosporins and penicillins would be highly unlikely.

Data from Pichichero ME. Use of selected cephalosporins in penicillin-allergic patients: a paradigm shift. Diagn Microbiol Infect Dis 2007;57(3 Suppl 1):S13–8.

and older has no evidence base. A systematic analysis and meta-analysis concluded that 5 days of antibiotics is as effective as 10 days in all children older than 2 years, and only marginally inferior to 10 days in children younger than 2 years. A comparison of 5-, 7-, and 10- days' treatment of AOM concluded that 5 days was equivalent to 7 and 10 days for all ages (**Fig. 7**),[22] unless the child had a perforated tympanic membrane or had been treated for AOM within the preceding month (**Fig. 8**),[23] because that information was associated with more frequent causation of AOM by resistant bacteria and with a continued inflamed middle ear mucosa.

Antibiotics not listed in the AAP guidelines are omitted because of poor efficacy, poor adherence, or safety concerns. Therefore, alternatives not included in the guideline should be used after consideration of the information provided earlier and the rationale documented in the patient chart.

The use of cephalosporins in penicillin-allergic children was recently reevaluated. The selection of cephalosporins by the AAP (see **Table 4**) took into consideration the likelihood of cross-reaction with penicillin.[23] Second- and third-generation cephalosporins have chemical side chain structures sufficiently distinct from penicillin and amoxicillin that they may be used in children allergic to penicillin and amoxicillin. The structure accountable for allergy is not the β-lactam ring, but rather the side chains. Some cross-reactivity occurs among cephalosporins based on their shared chemical side chain structure (**Table 6**).[24] The possibility of allergy to all penicillins and cephalosporins has never been confirmed, and statistically the likelihood is very small.

Antihistamines and decongestants taken orally or intranasally are not recommended for treatment of AOM or OME because they either have been shown to be nonefficacious or were not studied at all.

The 2 treatment options recommended for persistent OME are watchful waiting and insertion of tympanostomy tubes.[24] Use of oral systemic steroids is not recommended because the evidence supporting their use was deemed insufficient by the guideline review panel. When used, oral steroids in a burst similar to that used in the management of an acute asthma exacerbation might be considered (1–2 mg/kg/d in the morning for 5–7 days) before referral to an ear, nose, and throat (ENT) specialist for tympanostomy tube insertion. The indications to move from watchful waiting to ENT referral are persisting OME for 6 months in 1 ear or 3 months in both ears, associated with a 30-dB hearing loss in the speech range.[25]

RECURRENT AOM

Some children experience repeated AOM episodes and reach a threshold at which they are termed *otitis prone*. The definition of otitis prone has varied among investigators in the field; however, the most frequently used definition currently is 3 episodes of AOM within 6 months or 4 episodes within 4 months. Children with recurrent AOM are generally treated with broader-spectrum antibiotics as additional cases of infection occur, leading to a concerning cycle of escalation of the antimicrobial resistance of bacteria causing AOM in children with recurrent infections. The immune response of children who are otitis prone is not as mature as that of those who are not otitis prone.

IMMUNOLOGY

Why do some children experience recurrent AOM whereas others experience infrequent episodes of AOM or no AOM at all? Anatomic dysfunction has been identified as a key element of susceptibility to frequent AOM infections in some children based on observations of those with poor eustachian tube function, such as children with a cleft palate and Down syndrome. However, recently the immune response to

AOM has been increasingly studied and new evidence has emerged to explain susceptibility to an increased frequency of AOM in otitis-prone children.

Essentially, children who experience frequent episodes of AOM have immature immune systems. These children have poor antibody[26] and cellular[27] immune responses to AOM infections. After an episode of AOM, the immune system of the otitis-prone child fails to generate an immune memory response.[26,27] Therefore, the child remains susceptible to another episode of AOM after antibiotic treatment, even by the same otopathogen residing in the nasopharyngeal region that caused a preceding episode of AOM.

PREVENTION

In North America, virtually all children who receive a pneumococcal vaccine are vaccinated with PCV13. The predecessor vaccine PCV7 was shown to be effective in preventing AOM because of the 7 serotypes contained in the vaccine. Escape serotypes replaced the 7 serotypes in PCV7 over time.[28] Based on the emergence of escape serotypes, the newer product PCV13 was developed to include the original 7 serotypes and the 6 additional serotypes that had emerged as fairly common. The predominant serotype that emerged in the PCV7 era of vaccine use was a serotype 19A.[28] The new PCV13 vaccine contains serotype 19A. A trial is ongoing to determine if the 6 additional serotypes included in PCV13 are effective in preventing AOM, similar to the efficacy of PCV13 in invasive pneumococcal disease.

Antibiotic prophylaxis has fallen into disfavor over the past decade as a prevention strategy for AOM recurrences. The emergence of antimicrobial-resistant otopathogens and their escalation in prevalence caused a reconsideration of the ecologic cost of antibiotic prophylaxis as a prevention strategy.

Influenza vaccination can prevent at least one episode of AOM each winter that might occur in the context of an influenzae illness. Future vaccines against respiratory viruses will likely produce the same prevention benefit.

COMPLICATIONS

The principle complication of AOM and OME is hearing loss. The loss is temporary until the infection clears after AOM or the fluid clears from the middle ear after OME. The child may experience temporary speech delay and/or poor educational performance associated with hearing loss. The notion that AOM and/or OME causes permanent educational problems is no longer viewed as valid based on recent evidence-based research.[29]

Suppurative complications after AOM are uncommon. Acute mastoiditis is the most frequent complication to be considered. More serious complications include meningitis and other local infections that result from extension to adjacent tissues and locations.

REFERENCES

1. Klein JO. Otitis media. Clin Infect Dis 1994;19:823–33.
2. Faden H, Duffy L, Boeve M. Otitis media: back to basics. Pediatr Infect Dis J 1998;17:1105–13.
3. Casey JR, Adlowitz DG, Pichichero ME. New patterns in the otopathogens causing acute otitis media six to eight years after introduction of pneumococcal conjugate vaccine. Pediatr Infect Dis J 2010;29(4):304–9.
4. Pichichero ME. Acute otitis media: part II. Treatment in an era of increasing antibiotic resistance. Am Fam Physician 2000;61(8):2410–6.

5. Revai K, Dobbs LA, Nair S, et al. Incidence of acute otitis media and sinusitis complicating upper respiratory tract infections: the effect of age. Pediatrics 2007;119:e1408–12.
6. Post JC. Direct evidence of bacterial biofilms in otitis media. Laryngoscope 2001; 111:2083–93.
7. Pichichero ME. Acute otitis media: part I. Improving diagnostic accuracy. Am Fam Physician 2000;61:2051–6.
8. Routhman R, Owens T, Simel DL. Does this child have acute otitis media? JAMA 2003;290(12):1633–40.
9. Pelton SI. Otoscopy for the diagnosis of otitis media. Pediatr Infect Dis J 1998;17: 540–3.
10. Helenius KK, Laine MK, Tuhtinen PA, et al. Tympanometry in discrimination of otoscopic diagnoses in young ambulatory children. Pediatr Infect Dis J 2012; 31(10):1003–6.
11. Laine MK, Tahtinen PA, Helenius KK, et al. Acoustic reflectometry in discrimination of otoscopic diagnoses in young ambulatory children. Pediatr Infect Dis J 2012;31(10):1007–11.
12. Block SL, Mandel E, McLinn S, et al. Spectral gradient acoustic reflectometry for the detection of middle ear effusion by pediatricians and parents. Pediatr Infect Dis J 1998;17:560–4.
13. American Academy of Pediatrics Subcommittee on Management of Acute Otitis Media. Diagnosis and management of acute otitis media. Pediatrics 2004;113: 1451–65.
14. Dowell SF, Butler JC, Giebink GS, et al. Acute otitis media: management and surveillance in the era of pneumococcal resistance—a report from the Drug-Resistant Streptococcus Pneumoniae Therapeutic Working Group. Pediatr Infect Dis J 1999;18:1–9.
15. Casey JR, Block S, Hedrick J, et al. Comparison of amoxicillin/clavulanic acid high dose with cefdinir in the treatment of acute otitis media. Drugs 2012; 72(16):1–7.
16. Pichichero ME, Casey JR. Comparison of study designs for acute otitis media trials. Int J Pediatr Otorhinolaryngol 2008;72:737–50.
17. Pichichero ME, Casey JR. Diagnostic inaccuracy and subject exclusions render placebo and observational studies of acute otitis media inconclusive. Pediatr Infect Dis J 2008;27:958–62.
18. Hoberman A, Paradise JL, Rockette HE, et al. Treatment of acute otitis media in children under 2 years of age. N Engl J Med 2011;364(2):105–15.
19. Tahtinen PA, Laine MK, Huovinen P, et al. A placebo-controlled trial of antimicrobial treatment for acute otitis media. N Engl J Med 2011;364(2): 116–26.
20. Pichichero ME. Short-course antibiotic therapy for respiratory infections: a review of the evidence. Pediatr Infect Dis J 2000;19:929–37.
21. Kozyrskyj AL, Hildes-Ripstein E, Longstaffe SE, et al. Treatment of acute otitis media with a shortened course of antibiotics. A meta-analysis. JAMA 1998; 279(21):1736–42.
22. Pichichero ME, Marsocci SM, Murphy ML, et al. A prospective observational study of 5-, 7-, and 10-day antibiotic treatment for acute otitis media. Otolaryngol Head Neck Surg 2001;124(4):381–7.
23. Pichichero ME. A review of evidence supporting the American Academy of Pediatrics recommendation for prescribing cephalosporin antibiotics in penicillin-allergic patients. Pediatrics 2005;115:1048–57.

24. Pichichero ME. Use of selected cephalosporins in penicillin-allergic patients: a paradigm shift. Diagn Microbiol Infect Dis 2007;57(3 Suppl 1):S13–8.
25. The Otitis Media guideline panel. Managing otitis media with effusion in young children. Pediatrics 1994;94:766–73.
26. Sharma SK, Casey JR, Pichichero ME. Reduced memory CD4+T-cell generation in the circulation of young children may contribute to the otitis-prone condition. J Infect Dis 2011;204:645–53.
27. Sharma SK, Casey JR, Pichichero ME. Reduced serum IgG responses to pneumococcal antigens in otitis-prone children may be due to poor memory B-cell generation. J Infect Dis 2012;205(8):1225–9.
28. Pichichero ME, Casey JR. Emergence of a multiresistant serotype 19A pneumococcal strain not included in the 7-valent conjugate vaccine as an otopathogen in children. JAMA 2007;298(15):1772–8.
29. Paradise JL, Feldman HM, Campbell TF, et al. Tympanostomy tubes and developmental outcome at 9 to 11 years of age. N Engl J Med 2007;356:248–61.

Acute Sinusitis in Children

Itzhak Brook, MD, MSc

KEYWORDS

- Rhinosinusitis • Anaerobes • *Streptococcus pneumoniae* • *Haemophilus influenzae*
- Antimicrobials

KEY POINTS

- Viral infection of the upper respiratory tract is the most common presentation of rhinosinusitis and the vast majority of cases resolve spontaneously.
- Only a small proportion develops a secondary bacterial infection that will benefit from antimicrobial therapy.
- The most common bacterial isolates from acute rhinosinusitis are *Streptococcus pneumoniae, Haemophilus influenzae, Moraxella catarrhalis,* Group A beta-hemolytic streptococci, and *Staphylococcus aureus.*
- The proper choice of antibiotic therapy depends on the likely infecting pathogens, bacterial antibiotic resistance, and the pharmacologic profiles of the antibiotics.
- Continuous monitoring of the evolving bacterial etiology of acute bacterial rhinosinusitis is of great importance.

INTRODUCTION

Acute rhinosinusitis is one of the most common health problems in children and has increased in prevalence and incidence.[1] It causes significant physical symptoms, negatively affects quality of life, and can substantially impair daily functioning. Prospective longitudinal studies performed in young children (6–35 months of age) illustrated that viral upper respiratory tract infection (URTI) occurred with an incidence of 6 episodes per patient-year, and that 8% (0.5 episodes per patient-year) were complicated by acute rhinosinusitis.[2] The pathophysiological cause of rhinosinusitis may be obstruction of sinus drainage pathways (sinus ostia), ciliary impairment, and altered mucus quantity and quality.

Acute rhinosinusitis is defined as an inflammation of the mucosal lining of the nasal passage and paranasal sinuses lasting up to 4 weeks, and can be caused by various factors, including environmental irritants, allergy, and viral infection, bacteria, or fungi.

Department of Pediatrics and Medicine, Georgetown University School of Medicine, 4431 Albemarle Street Northwest, Washington, DC 20016, USA
E-mail address: ib6@georgetown.edu

Pediatr Clin N Am 60 (2013) 409–424
http://dx.doi.org/10.1016/j.pcl.2012.12.002 **pediatric.theclinics.com**
0031-3955/13/$ – see front matter

HISTORY

Suspicion of acute bacterial rhinosinusitis (ABRS) is based on clinical symptoms and signs when at least 2 major or 1 major and 2 minor criteria are present (**Table 1**).[3] The most common presentation is a persistent (and nonimproved) nasal discharge or cough (or both) lasting more than 10 days.[4] Typical clinical manifestations of ABRS in children are cough that worsens at night (80%), nasal symptoms (anterior or posterior discharge, obstruction, and/or congestion) (76%), and fever for more than 3 days (63%). Malodorous fetid breath is common, whereas facial pain and swelling, sore throat, and headache are rare in children. There is only one study of children that correlated the presence of respiratory signs and symptoms with the findings of sinus aspiration.[5]

Differentiating viral URTI from ABRS is critical and remains difficult. The main feature of viral URTI is the presence of nasal symptoms (discharge and congestion/obstruction) or cough or both, and sometimes also a scratchy throat. Fever is absent in most patients and when present it occurs early in the illness. Fever and constitutional symptoms generally disappear within 24 to 48 hours, after which the respiratory symptoms predominate. Most with acute viral rhinosinusitis improved spontaneously after 7 to 12 days. Generally, the nasal discharge is clear and watery initially, but often its quality changes over time. In most individuals, the discharge turns thicker and more mucoid and purulent.[6] After several days, these changes are reversed, with the purulent discharge turning mucoid and then clear, or dry. These changes occur in uncomplicated viral URTIs without the use of antimicrobials.

The characteristic presenting symptoms that are commonly associated with a bacterial rather than viral infection were evaluated by 5 consensus panels, created by 5 national societies.[7–10] The panels highlighted 3 clinical presentations that should prompt consideration of ABRS rather than a viral URTI:

1. Onset with persistent symptoms (respiratory symptoms that are present for more than 10 but fewer than 30 days with no improvement). The criterion of duration of symptoms for 10 or more days or signs and worsening of symptoms within 10 days after initial improvement (double-sickening) is used to differentiate between bacterial versus viral acute rhinosinusitis.[8] Patients manifest low-grade or nonresolving respiratory symptoms. Nasal discharge and daytime cough are common, whereas headache, facial pain, and fever are variable.

Table 1
Major and minor clinical criteria suggestive of bacterial sinusitis[a]

Major Criteria	Minor Criteria
Facial pain or pressure (requires a second major criterion to constitute a suggestive history)	Headache
Facial congestion or fullness	Fever (for subacute and chronic sinusitis)
Nasal congestion or obstruction	Halitosis
Nasal discharge, purulence, or discolored postnasal drainage	Fatigue
Hyposmia or anosmia	Dental pain
Fever (for acute sinusitis, requires a second major criterion to constitute a strong history)	Cough
Purulence on intranasal examination	Ear pain, pressure, or fullness

[a] A strongly suggestive history requires the presence of 2 major criteria or 1 major and 2 or more minor criteria. A suggestive history requires the presence of 1 major criterion or 2 or more minor criteria.[3]

Confirmation of bacterial infection by sinus aspiration was possible in only about two-thirds of adults with symptoms lasting longer than 7 to 10 days.[11,12] This suggests that additional qualifying clinical features are needed to differentiate viral from ABRS.

2. Onset with severe symptoms (an ill appearance with fever of at least 39°C [102°F] and purulent nasal discharge for at least 3–4 consecutive days at the beginning of illness) (**Table 2**). The onset of fever, headache, and facial pain differs from an uncomplicated viral URTI, as the elevated temperature and purulent nasal discharge in ABRS occur at the beginning of the illness.[13]
3. Worsening symptoms after initial improvement with a new onset of fever, an increase in nasal discharge or cough, or the onset of severe headache (also called "double-sickening").

The symptoms and signs of acute bacterial infection can be divided into nonsevere and severe (see **Table 2**).[14] The severe form carries a higher risk of complications and mandates earlier use of antimicrobial therapy. The combination of high fever and purulent nasal discharge that lasts for at least 3 to 4 days suggests ABRS.

Individuals with ABRS often have edema of nasal mucous membranes, mucopurulent nasal discharge, persistent postnasal drip, fever, and malaise. The quality of the nasal discharge varies, and can be thin or thick, clear mucoid, or purulent. Tenderness and pain of the involved sinus can be induced by percussion of the affected sinus. Cellulitis can also be present overlying the affected sinus. Other findings, especially in acute ethmoiditis, are periorbital cellulitis, edema, and proptosis. Failure to transilluminate the sinus and the presence of nasal voice can be present in many patients. Direct smear of nasal secretions usually shows the predominance of neutrophils, and the observation of numerous eosinophils suggests allergy.

The symptoms are generally protracted and vary considerably in subacute or chronic bacterial sinusitis. Fever can be of low grade or absent. The patient may complain of malaise, easy fatigability, irregular nasal or postnasal discharge, frequent headaches, difficulty in mental concentration, anorexia, and pain or tenderness to palpation over the affected sinus. Cough and nasal congestion can persist, and a sore throat (because of mouth-breathing) is frequent.

BACTERIAL ETIOLOGY

The most common bacteria recovered from pediatric and adult patients with community-acquired, ABRS are *Streptococcus pneumoniae,* nontypeable *Haemophilus influenzae, Moraxella catarrhalis,* Group A beta-hemolytic streptococci, and *Staphylococcus aureus.*[11,15–19] The vaccination of children with the 7-valent pneumococcal vaccine, introduced in 2000 in the United States, brought about the decline in the recovery rate of *S pneumoniae* and an increase in *H influenzae.*[20,21] *S aureus* is

Table 2
Severity of symptoms and signs in acute bacterial sinusitis

Nonsevere	Severe
Rhinorrhea (of any quality)	Purulent (thick, colored, opaque) rhinorrhea
Nasal congestion	Nasal congestion
Cough	Facial pain or headache
Headache, facial pain, and irritability (variable)	Periorbital edema (variable)
Low-grade or no fever	High fever (temperature ≥39°C)

a common pathogen in sphenoid sinusitis.[17] Recent data illustrate a significant increase in the rate of recovery of methicillin-resistant *S aureus* (MRSA) in patients with ABRS.[22,23]

The infection is polymicrobial in about a third of the patients. Enteric bacteria are rarely isolated, and anaerobes account for about 8% of isolates and are usually recovered from ABRS associated with an odontogenic origin, mainly as an extension of the infection from the roots of the premolar or molar teeth.[15,24] *Pseudomonas aeruginosa* and other aerobic and facultative gram-negative rods are mainly recovered from nosocomial rhinosinusitis (mostly in those with nasal tubes or catheters), the immunocompromised, and those with human immunodeficiency virus (HIV) infection[25] or cystic fibrosis.[26]

The dynamics of sinusitis, as well as otitis media, progress through several phases (**Fig. 1**). The early phase is generally viral (mostly rhinovirus, adenovirus, influenza, and parainfluenza viruses) and lasts up to 10 days when complete recovery occurs in 99% of individuals.[27] In a small number of patients, a secondary acute bacterial infection may emerge, generally caused by aerobic bacteria (ie, *S pneumoniae*, *H influenzae*, or *M catarrhalis*). If resolution does not take place, anaerobic bacteria from the oropharyngeal flora become predominant over time.[28] The mechanism by which viruses predispose to bacterial sinusitis may involve viral-bacterial synergy, induction of local inflammation that blocks the sinus ostia, increase of bacterial attachment to the epithelial cells, and disruption of the local immune defense.

DIAGNOSIS

History

Past medical history should evaluate for previous episodes of sinusitis and other respiratory tract infections, previous use of antibiotics, the potential of nasal foreign bodies, attendance at a day care center, immunizations, history of allergy, exposure to cigarette smoke, comorbidities, and previous hospitalization. The presence of any swelling and pain, especially in the facial, forehead, temporal, or orbital area or any other site in the head, should be noted. Information about what makes the symptoms worse or better should be obtained. The length of symptoms, such as cough, nasal secretions, headaches, pain, fever, hyposmia, or dental pain or problems, should be recorded.

Physical Examination

Physical examination should include the following:

- A thorough and complete general and head and neck examination (including the orbit, extraocular motility, the response of the pupils, vision, and cranial nerve function).

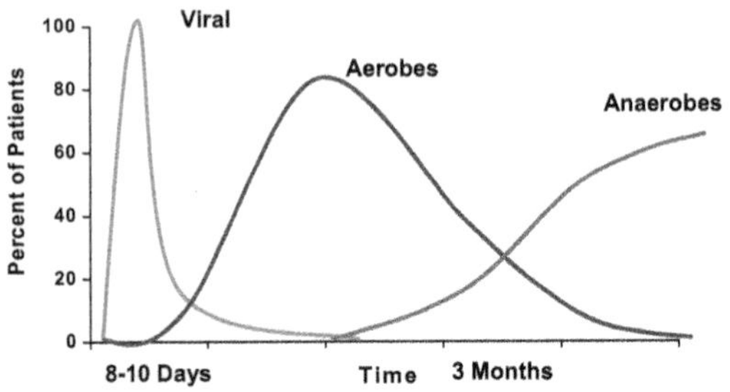

Fig. 1. The chronology of viral and bacterial causes of sinusitis.

- Palpation and/or percussion (over the frontal sinuses, cheeks [maxillary sinuses], and medial orbit [ethmoid sinuses]).
- The nasopharynx should be assessed for postnasal drip and obstruction caused by adenoid hypertrophy, choanal atresia, malignancy, polyps, and septal deviation.
- Nasal examination, including anterior rhinoscopy with a good light source looking for edema, erythema, crusting, purulent secretion, and presence of a foreign body.
- Bending the patient's head forward (when sitting) and holding it at knee level for 45 to 60 seconds can elicit a sensation of fullness and pain at the involved sites (compliance in young patients may be difficult).
- Endoscopic examination performed by an otolaryngologist may localize pus within the nasal cavity, directing the examiner to the involved sinus(es). Bacterial cultures can also be obtained; however, the specimens may contain nasal mucosal flora.
- Transillumination is infrequently used because the findings do not always correlate with the disorder, and reproducibility between observers is poor.
- Indications for referral to an otolaryngologist for maxillary sinus aspiration are the following: failure to improve on antimicrobial therapy, severe facial pain, orbital or intracranial complications, and in the immunocompromised host (because of their unique microbiology).
- The ears should be otoscopically examined, the oral cavity should be observed for any postnasal drip, all teeth (especially the upper molars and premolars) should be inspected for cavities and tenderness, and pressure should be applied on the maxillary sinuses by the examiner's thumbs.

Signs of sinus infection that can be observed by physical examination are the following:

- Mucopurulent nasal or posterior pharyngeal discharge.
- Erythematous nasal mucosa that can be pale and boggy.
- Signs of throat infection that can be associated with malodorous breath.
- Acute otitis media can be present in association with ABRS.
- Cervical lymphadenitis is rarely present.
- Facial tenderness is inconsistent and nonspecific.
- Periorbital edema with skin discoloration may be present, especially with ethmoid sinusitis.
- Upper molar teeth pathology may be the source of maxillary sinusitis.

Clinical Findings

The location of the facial pain can point to the involved sinus. Maxillary rhinosinusitis is commonly associated with cheeks, frontal with forehead pain, ethmoid with medial canthus, and sphenoid with occipital pain. In patients with chronic infection, changes in motion or position can worsen or alleviate the sinus symptoms.

The gold standard for the diagnosis of ABRS is the isolation of bacteria in high density ($\geq 10^4$ colony-forming units/mL) from the paranasal sinus cavity. Improper decontamination of the paranasal mucosa before aspiration may lead to misinterpretation of results.[5,29–31] Sinus aspiration is an invasive and painful procedure that is impractical in the office setting. Endoscopically guided middle meatus cultures can be used as a surrogate for sinus aspirates in patients with ABRS.[32] The validity of these cultures in children has not been well established, however.

Imaging

Imaging studies, such as plain radiographs or computed tomography (CT), are often used for the diagnosis of ABRS; however, they are nonspecific and cannot differentiate viral from bacterial rhinosinusitis.[33]

More than 50% of children with viral URTI had abnormal maxillary sinus radiographs.[34] Sinus CTs are often abnormal in healthy children,[34,35] and those having CT for nonrespiratory reasons.[36] CT performed on young adults recovering from a cold illustrated that 87% had significant maxillary sinus abnormalities.[36] Magnetic resonance imagining (MRI) illustrated that 68% of symptomatic children with URTI[37] and 42% of healthy children[38] had significant sinus abnormalities.

These findings illustrate that imaging studies in most children with uncomplicated viral URTI will show major abnormalities that are indistinguishable from those associated with ABRS. Therefore, these studies can be useful only when they are negative, as they confirm the absence of ABRS; however, abnormal radiographic studies cannot assist in ABRS diagnosis, and are therefore not required in uncomplicated ABRS. Imaging can be helpful in determining disease location and extent beyond the site of the original source. It may help in supporting the diagnosis or determining the degree of mucosal involvement.[39]

CT or MRI should be generally performed only in children with recurrent or complicated sinusitis or when suppurative complications are suspected. Suppurative complications of ABRS are infrequent, occurring in 3.7% to 11.0% of hospitalized children with sinusitis. They are mainly associated with potential orbital and intracranial complications of sinusitis.[40] CT is best for the assessment of bony and anatomic changes associated with sinusitis and is also helpful in surgical planning and for intraoperative image-guided navigation. MRI is most effective in evaluating the extent of soft tissue inflammation and abnormalities.[41–47]

The American College of Radiology criteria for the adequacy of imaging examinations for ABRS in children[48] stated that both CT and MRI are complementary for the evaluation of suspected orbital and/or intracranial complication of sinusitis. However, the Infectious Diseases Society of America (IDSA) panel favored contrast-enhanced CT over MRI because of its greater value, relative availability, speed, and lack of need for sedation.[49] CT is especially advantageous in children because their sinuses are often asymmetrical and smaller than those in adults.[50]

Differential Diagnosis

Differentiation must be made between allergic rhinitis, other causes of head or facial pain, asthma, and dental disorders. An allergic etiology can be confirmed by history of nasal symptoms and a history of allergy.[14]

ABRS has to be differentiated chronologically from other types of rhinosinusitis. These include recurrent acute, subacute, chronic, and acute exacerbation of chronic rhinosinusitis.

The symptoms and signs of ABRS can be divided into nonsevere and severe forms (see **Table 2**).[14] The severe form has a greater risk of complications and mandates earlier use of antimicrobial treatment. In children with subacute or chronic bacterial sinusitis, the symptoms are protracted, fever is uncommon, cough and nasal congestion persist, and a sore throat is common.

TREATMENT

The medical management of ABRS includes the use of antibiotics and adjuvants. The goals of therapy are to eliminate infection, decrease the severity and duration of symptoms, and prevent complications.

The management of sinusitis has become a challenging endeavor because the choice of appropriate antimicrobial agents has become more complex in recent years.

This is because many of the predominant bacterial pathogens have developed resistance to commonly used antibiotics.[51]

Culture obtained through direct aspiration or endoscopy can direct the selection of antimicrobials in the treatment of patients who fail to respond.[28]

The emerging antimicrobial resistance among respiratory pathogens leads to the empiric overuse of broad-spectrum antibiotics, which generates selective pressure that promotes the emergence of greater antimicrobial resistance.[52,53]

Several practice guidelines for the treatment of ABRS have been published in the United States within the past decade.[13,54–60] These guidelines present varying opinions about the clinical criteria for initiation and choice of empiric antimicrobial regimens. The most recent guideline, developed by the IDSA,[49] addresses some of the more controversial areas concerning initial choice of empiric management of ABRS in children and adults.

Empiric antimicrobial therapy should be started as soon as the clinical diagnosis of ABRS is made. Pharmacokinetic/pharmacodynamic principles should guide adequate dosing for respiratory tract infections.[61] The utility of these diagnostic criteria for initiating antibiotic treatment has been validated by 3 randomized clinical trials in children.[62–64] These studies demonstrated significantly higher cure rates in those treated with antibiotics compared with placebo. Some children with mild but persistent symptoms can be observed without giving antimicrobial therapy.[64] These children need close observation and antimicrobials should be administered if improvement has not occurred within 3 days.

Amoxicillin is no longer considered to be adequate for the initial empiric treatment of ABRS in children.[49] The addition of clavulanate improves the amoxicillin coverage against beta-lactamase–producing pathogens in ABRS, estimated to be present in about a quarter of patients. These include 25% to 35% of *H influenzae* and more than 90% of *M catarrhalis*.[65]

The "standard-dose" of amoxicillin-clavulanate is 45 mg/kg/d orally 3 times a day or twice a day or 500 mg orally 3 times a day, and the "high-dose" amoxicillin-clavulanate is 90 mg/kg/d orally twice a day, or 2 g orally twice a day. The primary disadvantages of using the "high-dose" amoxicillin-clavulanate is the added cost and potentially higher incidence of adverse effects. "High-dose" amoxicillin-clavulanate is recommended for children with ABRS from locations with high rates of penicillin-nonsusceptible *S pneumoniae*, recent hospitalization, or antibiotic use within the past month; those with severe infection; those with evidence of systemic toxicity (eg, fever of 39°C [102°F] or higher); those with comorbidities; or those who are immunocompromised.[66,67]

Studies determining *S pneumoniae* penicillin resistance using the revised Clinical Laboratory Standards Institute breakpoints defining penicillin-intermediate (minimal inhibitory concentration [MIC] 4 μg/mL; treatable with "high-dose" amoxicillin) and penicillin-resistant *S pneumoniae* (MIC ≥8 μg/mL; untreatable with amoxicillin), illustrated a higher rate of penicillin susceptibility (89%–93%) than those using earlier breakpoints.[51,65,68,69] These studies suggest that unless the rate of penicillin-nonsusceptible *S pneumoniae* in the community is high (>10%), "standard-dose" amoxicillin-clavulanate should be adequate for the treatment of nonmeningitic *S pneumoniae* infections, including ABRS.

Oral cephalosporins are inactive against penicillin-resistant *S pneumoniae*.[70,71] The activity of second-generation and third-generation oral cephalosporins (ie, cefaclor, cefuroxime axetil, cefpodoxime, cefprozil, cefdinir, and cefixime) is variable against penicillin-intermediate and resistant *S pneumoniae*. Cefpodoxime, cefuroxime axetil, and cefidnir are moderately active against this organism (<50% susceptible), and cefixime is less effective.[65,70–72] The parenteral third-generation cephalosporins, cefotaxime and ceftriaxone, are active against all *S pneumoniae,* including penicillin-resistant ones and are the recommended second-line empiric therapy (in place of high-dose amoxicillin-clavulanate) for hospitalized children. The most active oral cephalosporin against both *H influenzae* and *M catarrhalis* (beta-lactamase positive and negative) is cefpodoxime, followed by cefixime, cefuroxime, and cefdinir.[70,73] Cefaclor and cefprozil are least effective.

Because of the variable activity of second-generation and third-generation oral cephalosporins against *S pneumoniae* and *H influenzae,* they are no longer adequate as monotherapy for the initial empiric treatment of ABRS. If an oral cephalosporin is used, a third-generation cephalosporin (eg, cefpodoxime or cefixime) combined with clindamycin is recommended in regions with high isolation rates of penicillin-nonsusceptible *S pneumoniae* ($\geq$10%).

The increased recovery of MRSA in ABRS requires consideration of the need for coverage against these organisms.[74] A comparison of the rate of recovery of MRSA between 2001–2003 and 2004–2006 in 244 patients with ABRS illustrated a significant increase in the rate of recovery of this organism in patients (from 3% of patients to 10%, $P<.01$).[23] This finding suggests the use of greater index of suspicion for the presence of MRSA in sinusitis and greater use of sinus cultures, especially in patients who do not improve or fail antimicrobial treatment after 48 hours of therapy. Because the nose can be a reservoir for *S aureus*, there is a concern that the recovery of *S aureus* could be attributable to contamination by the nasal flora during sinus aspiration or acquisition of middle meatus cultures. Accurate diagnosis of MRSA rhinosinusitis by microbiological cultures is essential for appropriate antimicrobial treatment.

Currently there is insufficient evidence to support the empiric coverage for MRSA in ABRS; however, in seriously ill individuals with suspected orbital or intracranial complication, and hospitalized patients with nosocomial sinusitis, empiric coverage for MRSA is helpful. Although vancomycin is considered the gold standard for therapy of MRSA, the increasing in vitro resistance to vancomycin[74] and reports of clinical failures underscore the need for alternative therapies. Other agents with good in vitro activity include trimethoprim-sulfamethoxazole, clindamycin, linezolid, quinupristin-dalfopristin, daptomycin, and tigecycline.

For children with a history of immediate-type hypersensitivity response to penicillin, levofloxacin is recommended as an alternative to amoxicillin-clavulanate. In those with a history of non–type I hypersensitivity reaction to penicillin, a third-generation oral cephalosporin (eg, cefixime or cefpodoxime) in combination with clindamycin is recommended. Cefixime or cefpodoxime are active against most strains of *H influenzae* and *M catarrhalis,* whereas clindamycin is active against *S pneumoniae,* including penicillin-intermediate and penicillin-resistant strains.[65]

The current treatment guidelines for ABRS that generally recommend a course of antimicrobial therapy for 10 to 14 days are derived from the length of therapy in many of the randomized controlled studies in adults.[10] Some recommend treatment for 7 days beyond the time symptoms had resolved.[75] Data in children, about the optimal duration of therapy, are nonconclusive because the efficacy of shorter courses has not been studied in a rigorous randomized manner.[76] In children with ABRS, the longer treatment duration of 10 to 14 days is still recommended.[49]

Clinically, improvement is expected within 3 to 5 days following initiation of effective antimicrobials.[64] Complete resolution of symptoms occurred in 45% of children with ABRS on antibiotics compared with 11% of those on placebo.[63] A study that compared "high-dose" amoxicillin-clavulanate to placebo illustrated that 19 (83%) of the 23 of children failed in the placebo group and 4 (17.4%) in the antibiotic group failed to improve or worsened within 3 days.[64]

Most pathogens are eliminated from the maxillary sinuses by the third day of adequate antimicrobial therapy.[57,77–80] A correlation was noted between time to bacterial eradication and time to clinical resolution.[78] If symptoms and signs worsen despite 3 days of initial empiric antimicrobial therapy, the potential reasons for treatment failure must be evaluated. These include the presence of resistant pathogens, structural abnormalities, or a noninfectious etiology. Similarly, if there is no clinical improvement within 3 to 5 days despite initial empiric antimicrobial therapy, an alternate management strategy should be considered.

Consecutive endoscopic cultures from the maxillary sinus were performed of aspirates obtained from 20 patients with ABRS who failed initial empiric antimicrobial therapy.[81] Increased level of resistance with MIC at least twofold higher than for the pretreatment isolate was identified in half of patients. These findings show that bacterial resistance should be considered in all patients who fail to respond to initial empiric antimicrobial therapy.

In choosing a second-line treatment in those who failed initial antimicrobial choice, an agent with a broader spectrum of activity and in a different antimicrobial class should be considered.[75,82] Antimicrobials selected should be active against penicillin-nonsusceptible *S pneumoniae* and ampicillin-resistant *H influenzae,* as well as other beta-lactamase–producing respiratory pathogens.

The recommended second-line antimicrobial agents suitable for children with treatment failure to first-line agents are amoxicillin-clavulanate (90 mg/kg/d orally twice a day); clindamycin (30–40 mg/kg/d by mouth 3 times a day) *plus* cefixime (8 mg/kg/d orally twice a day) *or* cefpodoxime (10 mg/kg/d orally twice a day); or ceftriaxone (50 mg/kg/d intramuscularly).

It is advisable that cultures be obtained from the involved sinuses in those who have failed to respond to empiric antimicrobial therapy. Identification and susceptibility testing of the isolates can guide the choice of the second-line agent(s). Endoscopically guided middle meatus cultures can be considered as an alternative in older children[83]; however, their reliability in young children has not been established. Sinus puncture can be performed in children whose endoscopic cultures show no growth. Nasopharyngeal cultures are unreliable and are not recommended for the microbiologic diagnosis of ABRS.[32]

ADJUVANT THERAPIES

In addition to antibiotics, other therapies have been used in the management of bacterial sinusitis. These therapies included topical and systemic decongestants, corticosteroids, anti-inflammatory agents, mucolytic agents, humidification, antihistamines, nasal irrigation, saline nasal spray, spicy food, and hot dry air.[84] These agents induce rapid vasoconstriction, improve ostial potency, reduce swelling and congestion of the turbinates, and decrease inflammation at the osteomeatal, thus facilitating sinus drainage. Use of any intranasal medications in children may not be well tolerated.

Neither topical nor oral decongestants and/or antihistamines are recommended as adjunctive treatment in patients with ABRS. Topical decongestants may induce rebound congestion and inflammation, whereas oral antihistamines may induce drowsiness, xerostomia, and other adverse effects.

Even though decongestants and antihistamines are frequently used by those with ABRS, there is minimal evidence supporting that they enhance recovery.[49] Although patients may subjectively feel improvement after using these agents, objective rhinometric measurements do not support this impression.[85–89]

The recommendation against the use of decongestants or antihistamines as adjunctive therapy in ABRS places a relatively high value on avoiding their adverse effects, and a relatively low value on the incremental clinical improvement. These agents may still provide symptom relief in some individuals with viral rhinosinusitis, however.

Reduction in the viscosity and improvement in the quality of mucus can assist in resolution of the infection. Several methods achieve this goal, including nasal saline spray or irrigation, air humidification, adequate hydration, and mucolytic agents.[90,91]

Antihistamines are generally not used to treat bacterial sinusitis, because they can thicken and dry the secretions, which leads to crusting and further blocks the osteomeatal complex. They can be useful, however, if the underlying cause is allergic.

Intranasal corticosteroids offer modest symptomatic improvement and minimal adverse effects with short-term use.[92] They are recommended as an adjunct to antibiotics in the empiric treatment of ABRS, mainly in those with a history of allergic rhinitis. Steroids have a delayed onset of action, and clinical improvement may take 7 to 10 days. They are always used in conjunction with antimicrobial therapy.

Systemic corticosteroids are rarely necessary in the treatment of allergic rhinitis, because of the generally good efficacy of topical corticosteroids.[93]

SURGICAL TREATMENT

Surgical drainage may be needed in those who fail medical therapy, especially when complications occur. The goals of surgery are to allow drainage of purulent material and prevent persistence, recurrence, progression, and complications. This is accomplished by removing diseased tissue, and promoting drainage (or obliteration if this is not possible) while considering the cosmetic outcome. Functional endoscopic sinus surgery has become the main surgical technique used. Endoscopic surgery achieves success in more than three-fourths of patients in both adults and children.[94,95] Radical procedures are used when rhinosinusitis is complicated by orbital or intracranial involvement.

COMPLICATIONS

When not treated promptly and properly, sinus infection can spread via anastomosing veins or by direct extension to nearby structures.[96] Orbital complications are categorized[97] into 5 stages according to their severity. Contiguous spread to the orbital area can result in periorbital cellulitis, subperiosteal abscess, orbital cellulitis, and abscess. Sinusitis can extend to the central nervous system, where it can cause cavernous sinus thrombosis; retrograde meningitis; and epidural, subdural, and brain abscesses.[96,97] Orbital symptoms often precede intracranial extension.[96] Osteomyelitis of the frontal bone often originates from a spreading thrombophlebitis.[96] A periostitis of the frontal sinus causes an osteitis and a periostitis of the outer membrane, which produces a tender, puffy swelling of the forehead.

Complications of sinusitis are rare, but can be life threatening. Diagnosis is assisted by observing local tenderness and dull pain, and is confirmed by CT and nuclear isotope scanning. The most common bacterial causes are anaerobic bacteria and *S aureus*. Management includes surgical drainage and antimicrobial therapy that covers all ABRS organisms, *S aureus* including MRSA, and anaerobes.[96] For central nervous system infections, drugs that penetrate the central nervous system and cover the likely organisms should be used (eg, a combination of vancomycin, ceftriaxone, and metronidazole). Antibiotics should be administered for at least 6 weeks.

SUMMARY

Viral infection of the upper respiratory tract is the most common presentation of rhinosinusitis and the vast majority of cases resolve spontaneously. Only a small proportion develops a secondary bacterial infection that will benefit from antimicrobial therapy. ABRS is generally diagnosed in the presence of more than 7 to 10 days and fewer than 30 days of nasal discharge. The most common bacterial isolates from acute rhinosinusitis are *S pneumoniae, H influenzae, M catarrhalis,* Group A beta-hemolytic streptococci, and *S aureus.* Aerobic gram-negative rods, including *P aeruginosa,* are common in nosocomial sinusitis, the immunocompromised, and those with HIV infection or cystic fibrosis. Fungus and *P aeruginosa* are common causes of sinusitis in neutropenic patients. The proper choice of antibiotic therapy depends on the likely infecting pathogens, bacterial antibiotic resistance, and the pharmacologic profiles of the antibiotics. In addition to antibiotics, adjuvant therapies and surgery are used in the management of bacterial sinusitis.

Because there are currently no good markers that define viral rhinosinusitis from ABRS, many clinicians elect when in doubt to administer antimicrobials to their patients; however, this approach is one of the main contributors to the increase of resistance to antimicrobials of respiratory pathogens that has made the management of true bacterial rhinosinusitis more challenging. The introduction of new vaccinations against *S pneumoniae* and the expected new vaccines against other potential sinus pathogens (ie, non–type b *H influenzae*) may change the bacterial etiology of ABRS. The increased recovery of MRSA is an example of such a change. Continuous monitoring of the evolving bacterial etiology of ABRS is therefore of great importance.

REFERENCES

1. Benninger MS, Sedory Holzer SE, Lau J. Diagnosis and treatment of uncomplicated acute bacterial rhinosinusitis: summary of the Agency for Health Care Policy and Research evidence-based report. Otolaryngol Head Neck Surg 2000;122:1–7.
2. Revai K, Dobbs LA, Nair S, et al. Incidence of acute otitis media and sinusitis complicating upper respiratory tract infection: the effect of age. Pediatrics 2007;119:e1408–12.
3. Lanza DC, Kennedy DW. Adult rhinosinusitis defined. Otolaryngol Head Neck Surg 1997;117:51–7.
4. Wald ER, Guerra N, Byers C. Upper respiratory tract infections in young children: duration of and frequency of complications. Pediatrics 1991;87:129–33.
5. Wald ER, Milmoe GJ, Bowen AD, et al. Acute maxillary sinusitis in children. N Engl J Med 1981;304:749–54.
6. Brook I. Aerobic and anaerobic bacteriology of purulent nasopharyngitis in children. J Clin Microbiol 1988;26:592–4.
7. Meltzer EO, Bachert C, Staudinger H. Treating acute rhinosinusitis: comparing efficacy and safety of mometasone furoate nasal spray, amoxicillin, and placebo. J Allergy Clin Immunol 2005;116:1289–95.
8. Meltzer EO, Hamilos DL, Hadley JA, et al. Rhinosinusitis: developing guidance for clinical trials. Otolaryngol Head Neck Surg 2006;135:S31–80.
9. Meltzer EO, Hamilos DL, Hadley JA, et al. Rhinosinusitis: establishing definitions for clinical research and patient care. J Allergy Clin Immunol 2004;114:155–212.
10. Rosenfeld RM, Singer M, Jones S. Systematic review of antimicrobial therapy in patients with acute rhinosinusitis. Otolaryngol Head Neck Surg 2007;137:S32–45.

11. Gwaltney JM Jr, Scheld WM, Sande MA, et al. The microbial etiology and antimicrobial therapy of adults with acute community-acquired sinusitis: a fifteen-year experience at the University of Virginia and review of other selected studies. J Allergy Clin Immunol 1992;90:457–62.
12. Hadley JA, Mosges R, Desrosiers M, et al. Moxifloxacin five-day therapy versus placebo in acute bacterial rhinosinusitis. Laryngoscope 2010;120:1057–62.
13. Rosenfeld RM, Andes D, Bhattacharyya N, et al. Clinical practice guideline: adult sinusitis. Otolaryngol Head Neck Surg 2007;137:S1–31.
14. Clement PA, Bluestone CD, Gordts F, et al. Management of rhinosinusitis in children. Consensus Meeting, Brussels, Belgium, September 13, 1996. Arch Otolaryngol Head Neck Surg 1998;124:31–4.
15. Brook I. Microbiology of acute and chronic maxillary sinusitis associated with an odontogenic origin. Laryngoscope 2005;115:823–5.
16. Brook I. Bacteriology of acute and chronic frontal sinusitis. Arch Otolaryngol Head Neck Surg 2002;128:583–5.
17. Brook I. Bacteriology of acute and chronic sphenoid sinusitis. Ann Otol Rhinol Laryngol 2002;111:1002–4.
18. Brook I. Acute and chronic frontal sinusitis. Curr Opin Pulm Med 2003;9:171–4.
19. Wald ER, Reilly JS, Casselbrant M, et al. Treatment of acute maxillary sinusitis in childhood—a comparative study of amoxicillin and cefaclor. J Pediatr 1984;104: 297–302.
20. Brook I, Foote PA, Hausfeld JN. Frequency of recovery of pathogens causing acute maxillary sinusitis in adults before and after introduction of vaccination of children with the 7-valent pneumococcal vaccine. J Med Microbiol 2006;55: 943–6.
21. Brook I, Gober AE. Frequency of recovery of pathogens from the nasopharynx of children with acute maxillary sinusitis before and after the introduction of vaccination with the 7-valent pneumococcal vaccine. Int J Pediatr Otorhinolaryngol 2007; 71:575–9.
22. Brook I. Role of methicillin-resistant *Staphylococcus aureus* in head and neck infections. J Laryngol Otol 2009;11:1–7.
23. Brook I, Foote PA, Hausfeld JN. Increase in the frequency of recovery of meticillin-resistant *Staphylococcus aureus* in acute and chronic maxillary sinusitis. J Med Microbiol 2008;57:1015–7.
24. Brook I, Frazier EH, Gher ME Jr. Microbiology of periapical abscesses and associated maxillary sinusitis. J Periodontol 1996;67:608–10.
25. Decker CF. Sinusitis in the immunocompromised host. Curr Infect Dis Rep 1999; 1:27–32.
26. Shapiro ED, Milmoe GJ, Wald ER, et al. Bacteriology of the maxillary sinuses in patients with cystic fibrosis. J Infect Dis 1982;146:589–93.
27. Sande MA, Gwaltney JM. Acute community-acquired bacterial sinusitis—continuing challenges and current management. Clin Infect Dis 2004;39(Suppl 3):S151–8.
28. Brook I, Frazier EH, Foote PA. Microbiology of the transition from acute to chronic maxillary sinusitis. J Med Microbiol 1996;45:372–5.
29. Evans FO Jr, Sydnor JB, Moore WE, et al. Sinusitis of the maxillary antrum. N Engl J Med 1975;293:735–9.
30. Hamory BH, Sande MA, Sydnor A Jr, et al. Etiology and antimicrobial therapy of acute maxillary sinusitis. J Infect Dis 1979;139:197–202.
31. Gwaltney JM Jr, Wiesinger BA, Patrie JT. Acute community-acquired bacterial sinusitis: the value of antimicrobial treatment and the natural history. Clin Infect Dis 2004;38:227–33.

32. Benninger MS, Appelbaum PC, Denneny JC, et al. Maxillary sinus puncture and culture in the diagnosis of acute rhinosinusitis: the case for pursuing alternative culture methods. Otolaryngol Head Neck Surg 2002;127:7–12.
33. Kovatch AL, Wald ER, Ledesma-Medina J, et al. Maxillary sinus radiographs in children with nonrespiratory complaints. Pediatrics 1984;73:306–8.
34. Shopfner CE, Rossi JO. Roentgen evaluation of the paranasal sinuses in children. Am J Roentgenol Radium Ther Nucl Med 1973;118:176–86.
35. Diament MJ, Senac MO Jr, Gilsanz V, et al. Prevalence of incidental paranasal sinuses opacification in pediatric patients: a CT study. J Comput Assist Tomogr 1987;11:426–31.
36. Gwaltney J Jr, Phillips CD, Miller RD, et al. Computed tomographic study of the common cold. N Engl J Med 1994;330:25–30.
37. Kristo A, Uhari M, Luotonen J, et al. Paranasal sinus findings in children during respiratory infection evaluated with magnetic resonance imaging. Pediatrics 2003;111:e586–9.
38. Kristo A, Alho OP, Luotonen J, et al. Cross-sectional survey of paranasal sinus magnetic resonance imaging findings in schoolchildren. Acta Paediatr 2003;92: 34–6.
39. Slavin RG, Spector SL, Bernstein IL, et al. The diagnosis and management of sinusitis: a practice parameter update. J Allergy Clin Immunol 2005;116:S13–47.
40. Younis RT, Lazar RH, Anand VK. Intracranial complications of sinusitis: a 15-year review of 39 cases. Ear Nose Throat J 2002;81:636–8, 640–2, 644.
41. Hurley MC, Heran MK. Imaging studies for head and neck infections. Infect Dis Clin North Am 2007;21:305–53, vi.
42. Mafee MF, Tran BH, Chapa AR. Imaging of rhinosinusitis and its complications: plain film, CT, and MRI. Clin Rev Allergy Immunol 2006;30:165–86.
43. Sievers KW, Dietrich U, Zoller E, et al. Diagnostic aspects of isolated sphenoid sinusitis. HNO 1992;40:464–7.
44. Younis RT, Anand VK, Davidson B. The role of computed tomography and magnetic resonance imaging in patients with sinusitis with complications. Laryngoscope 2002;112:224–9.
45. McIntosh D, Mahadevan M. Failure of contrast enhanced computed tomography scans to identify an orbital abscess. The benefit of magnetic resonance imaging. J Laryngol Otol 2008;122:639–40.
46. Herrmann BW, Forsen JW Jr. Simultaneous intracranial and orbital complications of acute rhinosinusitis in children. Int J Pediatr Otorhinolaryngol 2004; 68:619–25.
47. Adame N, Hedlund G, Byington CL. Sinogenic intracranial empyema in children. Pediatrics 2005;116:e461–7.
48. Karmazyn BK. ACR appropriateness criteria—sinusitis. Expert Panel on Pediatric Imaging. American College of Radiology 2009;1–5.
49. Chow AW, Benninger MS, Brook I, et al. IDSA practical guidelines for acute bacterial rhinosinusitis in children and adults—a GRADE approach to recommendations. Clin Infect Dis 2012;54:e72–112.
50. Aalokken TM, Hagtvedt T, Dalen I, et al. Conventional sinus radiography compared with CT in the diagnosis of acute sinusitis. Dentomaxillofac Radiol 2003;32:60–2.
51. Critchley IA, Brown SD, Traczewski MM, et al. National and regional assessment of antimicrobial resistance among community-acquired respiratory tract pathogens identified in a 2005-2006 U.S. Faropenem surveillance study. Antimicrob Agents Chemother 2007;51:4382–9.

52. Austin DJ, Kristinsson KG, Anderson RM. The relationship between the volume of antimicrobial consumption in human communities and the frequency of resistance. Proc Natl Acad Sci U S A 1999;96:1152–6.
53. Magee JT, Pritchard EL, Fitzgerald KA, et al. Antibiotic prescribing and antibiotic resistance in community practice: retrospective study, 1996-8. BMJ 1999;319: 1239–40.
54. Brook I, Gooch WM 3rd, Jenkins SG, et al. Medical management of bacterial sinusitis. Recommendation of Clinical Advisory Committee on Pediatric and Adult Sinusitis. Ann Otol Rhinol Laryngol Suppl 2000;182:1–20.
55. Agency for Health Care Research and Quality. Update on acute bacterial rhinosinusitis. Evidence Report/Technology Assessment: Number 124, Contract No. 290-02-0022. 2005. 1–7. Available at: http://www.ahrq.gov/.
56. American Academy of Pediatrics, Subcommittee on Management of Sinusitis and Committee on Quality Improvement. Clinical practice guideline: management of sinusitis. Pediatrics 2001;108:798–808.
57. Anon JB, Jacobs MR, Poole MD, et al. Antimicrobial treatment guidelines for acute bacterial rhinosinusitis. Otolaryngol Head Neck Surg 2004;130:1–45.
58. Hickner JM, Bartlett JG, Besser RE, et al. Principles of appropriate antibiotic use for acute rhinosinusitis in adults: background. Ann Intern Med 2001;134:498–505.
59. Snow V, Mottur-Pilson C, Hickner JM. Principles of appropriate antibiotic use for acute sinusitis in adults. Ann Intern Med 2001;134:495–7.
60. Institute for Clinical Systems Improvement (ICSI). Healthcare guidelines: diagnosis and treatment of respiratory illness in children and adults. 2nd edition. Rochester (MN): ICSI; 2008.
61. Craig WA. The hidden impact of antibacterial resistance in respiratory tract infection. Re-evaluating current antibiotic therapy. Respir Med 2001;95(Suppl A):S12–9.
62. Garbutt JM, Goldstein M, Gellman E, et al. A randomized, placebo-controlled trial of antimicrobial treatment for children with clinically diagnosed acute sinusitis. Pediatrics 2001;107:619–25.
63. Wald ER, Chiponis D, Ledesma-Medina J. Comparative effectiveness of amoxicillin and amoxicillin-clavulanate potassium in acute paranasal sinus infections in children: a double-blind, placebo-controlled trial. Pediatrics 1986;77:795–800.
64. Wald ER, Nash D, Eickhoff J. Effectiveness of amoxicillin/clavulanate potassium in the treatment of acute bacterial sinusitis in children. Pediatrics 2009;124:9–15.
65. Harrison CJ, Woods C, Stout G, et al. Susceptibilities of *Haemophilus influenzae, Streptococcus pneumoniae*, including serotype 19A, and *Moraxella catarrhalis* paediatric isolates from 2005 to 2007 to commonly used antibiotics. J Antimicrob Chemother 2009;63:511–9.
66. Jacobs MR. Antimicrobial-resistant *Streptococcus pneumoniae*: trends and management. Expert Rev Anti Infect Ther 2008;6:619–35.
67. Lynch JP III, Zhanel GG. *Streptococcus pneumoniae*: epidemiology, risk factors, and strategies for prevention. Semin Respir Crit Care Med 2009;30:189–209.
68. Centers for Disease Control and Prevention. Effects of new penicillin susceptibility breakpoints for *Streptococcus pneumoniae*—United States, 2006–2007. MMWR Morb Mortal Wkly Rep 2008;57:1353–5.
69. Sahm DF, Brown NP, Draghi DC, et al. Tracking resistance among bacterial respiratory tract pathogens: summary of findings of the TRUST Surveillance Initiative, 2001–2005. Postgrad Med 2008;120:8–15.
70. Sader HS, Jacobs MR, Fritsche TR. Review of the spectrum and potency of orally administered cephalosporins and amoxicillin/clavulanate. Diagn Microbiol Infect Dis 2007;57:5S–12S.

71. Fenoll A, Gimenez MJ, Robledo O, et al. In vitro activity of oral cephalosporins against pediatric isolates of *Streptococcus pneumoniae* non-susceptible to penicillin, amoxicillin or erythromycin. J Chemother 2008;20:175–9.
72. Fenoll A, Gimenez MJ, Robledo O, et al. Influence of penicillin/amoxicillin non-susceptibility on the activity of third-generation cephalosporins against *Streptococcus pneumoniae*. Eur J Clin Microbiol Infect Dis 2008;27:75–80.
73. Jansen WT, Verel A, Beitsma M, et al. Surveillance study of the susceptibility of *Haemophilus influenzae* to various antibacterial agents in Europe and Canada. Curr Med Res Opin 2008;24:2853–61.
74. Howden BP, Johnson PD, Ward PB, et al. Isolates with low-level vancomycin resistance associated with persistent methicillin-resistant *Staphylococcus aureus* bacteremia. Antimicrob Agents Chemother 2006;50:3039–47.
75. Wald ER. Sinusitis. Pediatr Ann 1998;27:811–8.
76. Pichichero ME. Short course antibiotic therapy for respiratory infections: a review of the evidence. Pediatr Infect Dis J 2000;19:929–37.
77. Ambrose PG, Anon JB, Bhavnani SM, et al. Use of pharmacodynamic endpoints for the evaluation of levofloxacin for the treatment of acute maxillary sinusitis. Diagn Microbiol Infect Dis 2008;61:13–20.
78. Ambrose PG, Anon JB, Owen JS, et al. Use of pharmacodynamic end points in the evaluation of gatifloxacin for the treatment of acute maxillary sinusitis. Clin Infect Dis 2004;38:1513–20.
79. Anon JB, Paglia M, Xiang J, et al. Serial sinus aspirate samples during high-dose, short-course levofloxacin treatment of acute maxillary sinusitis. Diagn Microbiol Infect Dis 2007;57:105–7.
80. Ariza H, Rojas R, Johnson P, et al. Eradication of common pathogens at days 2, 3 and 4 of moxifloxacin therapy in patients with acute bacterial sinusitis. BMC Ear Nose Throat Disord 2006;6:8.
81. Brook I, Gober AE. Resistance to antimicrobials used for therapy of otitis media and sinusitis: effect of previous antimicrobial therapy and smoking. Ann Otol Rhinol Laryngol 1999;108:645–7.
82. Scheid DC, Hamm RM. Acute bacterial rhinosinusitis in adults: part II. Treatment. Am Fam Physician 2004;70:1697–704.
83. Benninger MS, Payne SC, Ferguson BJ, et al. Endoscopically directed middle meatal cultures versus maxillary sinus taps in acute bacterial maxillary rhinosinusitis: a meta-analysis. Otolaryngol Head Neck Surg 2006;134:3–9.
84. Scarupa MD, Kaliner MA. Adjuvant therapies in the treatment of acute and chronic rhinosinusitis. Clin Allergy Immunol 2007;20:251–62.
85. Sipila J, Suonpaa J, Silvoniemi P, et al. Correlations between subjective sensation of nasal patency and rhinomanometry in both unilateral and total nasal assessment. ORL J Otorhinolaryngol Relat Spec 1995;57:260–3.
86. Inanli S, Ozturk O, Korkmaz M, et al. The effects of topical agents of fluticasone propionate, oxymetazoline, and 3% and 0.9% sodium chloride solutions on mucociliary clearance in the therapy of acute bacterial rhinosinusitis in vivo. Laryngoscope 2002;112:320–5.
87. McCormick DP, John SD, Swischuk LE, et al. A double-blind, placebo-controlled trial of decongestant-antihistamine for the treatment of sinusitis in children. Clin Pediatr (Phila) 1996;35:457–60.
88. Wiklund L, Stierna P, Berglund R, et al. The efficacy of oxymetazoline administered with a nasal bellows container and combined with oral phenoxymethylpenicillin in the treatment of acute maxillary sinusitis. Acta Otolaryngol Suppl 1994;515:57–64.

89. Bende M, Fukami M, Arfors KE, et al. Effect of oxymetazoline nose drops on acute sinusitis in the rabbit. Ann Otol Rhinol Laryngol 1996;105:222–5.
90. Tomooka LT, Murphy C, Davidson TM. Clinical study and literature review of nasal irrigation. Laryngoscope 2000;110:1189–93.
91. Wang YH, Yang CP, Ku MS, et al. Efficacy of nasal irrigation in the treatment of acute sinusitis in children. Int J Pediatr Otorhinolaryngol 2009;73:1696–701.
92. Barlan IB, Erkan E, Bakir M, et al. Intranasal budesonide spray as an adjunct to oral antibiotic therapy for acute sinusitis in children. Ann Allergy Asthma Immunol 1997;78:598–601.
93. Meltzer EO, Teper A, Danzig M. Intranasal corticosteroids in the treatment of acute rhinosinusitis. Curr Allergy Asthma Rep 2008;8:133–8.
94. Criddle MW, Stinson A, Savliwala M, et al. Pediatric chronic rhinosinusitis: a retrospective review. Am J Otol 2008;29:372–8.
95. Siedek V, Stelter K, Betz CS, et al. Functional endoscopic sinus surgery—a retrospective analysis of 115 children and adolescents with chronic rhinosinusitis. Int J Pediatr Otorhinolaryngol 2009;73:741–5.
96. Brook I. Microbiology and antimicrobial treatment of orbital and intracranial complications of sinusitis in children and their management. Int J Pediatr Otorhinolaryngol 2009;73:1183–6.
97. Chandler JR, Langenbrunner DJ, Stevens EF. The pathogenesis of orbital complications in acute sinusitis. Laryngoscope 1970;80:1414–28.

Bone and Joint Infections

Markus Pääkkönen, MD, PhD[a,*], Heikki Peltola, MD, PhD[b]

KEYWORDS

• Septic arthritis • Osteomyelitis • Arthrocentesis • Trepanation • Clindamycin

KEY POINTS

- The treatment of childhood acute osteoarticular infections can be simplified.
- For the treatment of uncomplicated childhood osteoarticular infections, in which fever and symptoms resolve rapidly, 2 to 4 days of intravenous antibiotics can be followed by high-dose oral antibiotics, for a total antibiotic course of 3 weeks for osteomyelitis and 2 weeks for septic arthritis.
- Oral antibiotics should be well absorbed, provide good bone penetration, and be given in sufficiently high doses. Clindamycin or first-generation cephalosporins should be given 4 times a day.
- Serum C-reactive protein measurements are reliable and inexpensive in the diagnosis and follow-up of osteomyelitis and septic arthritis.

INTRODUCTION

In contrast to developing countries, acute ostearticular infections (AOI) of children, osteomyelitis (OM), septic arthritis (SA), and OM with adjacent SA (OM+SA), are rare diseases in high-income settings.[1–3] The annual incidence of AOI varies regionally between 10 and 25 per 100,000 population, of which OM constitutes two-thirds.[1,4,5] The incidence is increased in immunocompromised patients and those with sickle-cell disease. The infection is considered acute if the time from the onset of symptoms to the presentation to a hospital is less than 2 weeks. Most cases are hematogenous in origin, although direct inoculation from trauma or spread from an adjacent tissue occurs as well. Boys predominate girls with an approximate ratio of 2:1.[1,4,5]

Funding Sources: Dr Pääkkönen: Foundation for Pediatric Research, Finland. Turku University Hospital Foundation for Education and Research; Dr Peltola: Foundation for Pediatric Research, Finland.

Conflict of Interest: Dr Pääkkönen: Nil; Dr Peltola: Works as a consultant for Serum Institute of India Ltd.

[a] Department of Orthopaedics and Traumatology, Turku University Hospital, University of Turku, PO Box 52, Kiinamyllynkatu 4–8, Turku 20521, Finland; [b] Department of Pediatrics, Children's Hospital, Helsinki University Central Hospital, University of Helsinki, PO Box 281, 11 Stenbäck Street, Helsinki 00029, Finland
* Corresponding author.
E-mail address: Markus.Paakkonen@helsinki.fi

Pediatr Clin N Am 60 (2013) 425–436
http://dx.doi.org/10.1016/j.pcl.2012.12.006
pediatric.theclinics.com
0031-3955/13/$ – see front matter

Cultures frequently fail to disclose the causative agent, but when tested positive, almost all cases show only a single organism.[1,4,6] Overwhelmingly, the most common agent is *Staphylococcus aureus*, followed by respiratory pathogens *Streptococcus pyogenes, Streptococcus pneumoniae* (pneumococcus), and *Haemophilus influenzae* type b (Hib).[7–13] *Kingella kingae* is a common cause of OM and SA in some areas and requires special culture techniques or real-time polymerase chain reaction for diagnosis.[14] Current vaccinations have caused decreased incidence of Hib and pneumococcus in some countries.[12,13] *Salmonella* spp are a common agent in the tropics and in children with sickle-cell disease,[15] and neonates may be affected by bacteria such as *Streptococcus agalactiae*.[1]

PATIENT HISTORY

The classical presentation of AOI is a locally swollen, warm limb or joint combined with high fever with no prior history of trauma. In a high-income setting the time from onset of symptoms is 2 to 5 days, and rarely more than a week.[6,16–19] Focal symptoms are not always remarkable, especially in OM, and fever of unknown origin may be the only remarkable sign present in an OM patient visiting the emergency department.[20] Prior trauma is documented in one-third of the cases.[5]

PHYSICAL EXAMINATION

The limb or joint may be too painful to allow thorough palpation or testing of joint motion, but plenty of useful information may be obtained from the disease history and mere observation of the patient. The child may be limping or refuse to use an extremity. Newborns may be irritable and may present as pseudoparalytic, whereas older children show more clear signs such as focal tenderness.[1] Fever may be absent or high, up to 40°C.[5,21] Generally, children with SA are clinically more ill than those with OM, which has a more insidious onset. Mild reddish color with no swelling may be the only visible focal sign in OM. Gonococcal arthritis, previously more common than today in the western settings, may present in the newborn only with unspecific irritability and poor feeding.[1]

Focal symptoms and signs vary according to localization, causative organism, and the age of the child (**Table 1**). *S aureus* causes clear focal symptoms compared with the insidious onset of *K kingae*, and culture-negative cases tend to present milder symptoms.[6,14] Spinal osteomyelitis may manifest as unspecific back pain. The diagnosis of pelvic osteomyelitis is difficult; the mean diagnostic delay in 1 study was 12 days.[22] OM in a long bone of a child beyond the neonatal age might show local pinpoint tenderness, which can be provoked by percussing the bone away from the affected area. Calcaneal osteomyelitis is characterized by slowly developing symptoms, and thus, late presentation.[23] Sacroilitis may present as pain in the sacrum or lower back, provoked by digital dorsal compression in rectal examination.[1] The swelling in hip arthritis of a neonate may pass detection unless the child has sought a characteristic position, with the affected hip flexed and externally rotated. Pain is elicited by compression of the head of the femur into the acetabulum.

DIAGNOSTIC EVALUATION

Further evaluation is warranted whenever an acute AOI is suspected. **Box 1** summarizes the commonly performed tests, and **Box 2** lists some of the examinations to be considered in the differential diagnosis. Blood tests are used to assess the extent of inflammation. Blood leukocyte count (white blood cell count) is unspecific

Table 1
Characteristics of osteomyelitis (OM) versus septic arthritis (SA), diseases caused by *Staphylococcus aureus* versus *Kingella kingae*, and symptoms and signs of newborns versus older children

	OM	**SA**
Fever >38.5°C	Suggestive if present	Suggestive
Malaise	Usually	Usually
Swollen joint/limited motion	Not unless concurrent arthritis	Nearly always
Edema overlying bone	Often	Absent
Back pain	Suggestive of spinal OM	Rare
Difficulty weight-bearing	Lower limb affected	Lower limb affected
	S aureus	***K kingae***
Age	Any age group	Often <4 y
Fever	>38°C	Afebrile on admission
CRP	Elevated	May be normal
WBC	Elevated	May be normal
	Neonates	**Children and Adolescents**
Systemic effects	Poor feeding/ irritability	Malaise and fever
Pain	Nonspecific limp/pseudoparalysis	Often focal
Joint involvement	Common	Possible

Abbreviations: CRP, C-reactive protein; WBC, white blood cell count.

and elevated only in 20% of cases.[24,25] Erythrocyte sedimentation rate with a cutoff of 20 mm/h is sensitive in the diagnostics, but is inferior to C-reactive protein (CRP) measurements in monitoring the course of the illness because of slow normalization.[25] Procalcitonin is more useful in OM than SA,[26] but is considerably more costly than CRP and does not offer more information. CRP with a cutoff of 20 mg/L is sensitive in the diagnosis of OM and SA.[25] The levels of CRP not only

Box 1
Diagnostic armamentarium for childhood acute osteoarticular infections

- Parameters of inflammation/infection: C-reactive protein, procalcitonin, erythrocyte sedimentation rate, white blood cell count
- Plain X ray
- Ultrasound
- Scintigram
- Magnetic resonance imaging
- Blood cultures
- Synovial fluid cytology
- Synovial fluid/bone sample; Gram-staining, culture

Box 2
Differential diagnoses of osteomyelitis and septic arthritis

Osteomyelitis

- Traumatic fracture
- Septicemia
- Rheumatic fever
- Cellulitis
- Thrombophlebitis
- Pyomyositis
- Leukemia
- Benign/malignant tumors
- Child abuse
- Scurvy
- Stress fracture

Septic arthritis

- Transient synovitis
- Viral arthritis
- Tuberculosis
- Henoch-Schönlein purpura
- Perthes disease
- Septic bursitis
- Slipped capital femoral epiphysis
- Reactive arthritis
- Juvenile rheumatoid arthritis
- Sickle cell anemia

increase rapidly (doubling time is 6 hours) but also descend quickly enough (the level is halved in 24 hours if the recovery is uneventful) to be useful later in the monitoring of the patient.[25] CRP is especially high in OM complicated by SA, but because of considerable overlapping, OM, SA, and OM+SA cannot be distinguished from each other with CRP alone.[25,27]

In OM, plain radiographs are notoriously normal on admission in most cases because the characteristic "rat bites" appear only in 2 to 3 weeks in long bones and even after 6 weeks in flat bones. Traditional radiographs are still of value in ruling out other pathologic abnormalities, such as a fracture, Perthes disease, or slipped capital femoral epiphysis.[5]

In SA, radiographs are of lesser importance and may at most show an enlarged joint space. Instead, ultrasound (US) may find joint effusion, but, conditions permitting, magnetic resonance imaging (MRI) is the most accurate diagnostic tool especially useful in OM.[28–30] Contrast enhancement does not improve sensitivity or specificity of MRI in OM, but increases reader confidence if bone or soft tissue edema is found on unenhanced images.[31] Computed tomography is another valuable option, along with technetium 99 bone scintigraphy (bone scan), which is still useful, especially in major long bones, or if the symptoms are poorly localized.[32–34]

The symptoms, signs, routine blood tests, and vaccination history against Hib or pneumococcus may give a hint toward the possible causative organism.[12,13] *S aureus* OM or SA often develops in a short time and causes high fever, which is not typical of *K kingae* infection (see **Table 1**).[14,21] These generalizations may be valuable in the primary evaluation, but bacterial culture or other identification (polymerase chain reaction) remains pivotal in terms of the choice of treatment and for an antibiogram. In SA, the aspirated synovial fluid sample before treatment is essential for bacteriology.[17] Spontaneous clotting, high white blood cell count, and low glucose concentration suggest SA, but values overlap with other types of arthritides causing problems with interpretation.[35]

Joint puncture is always recommended in SA, although even 70% of synovial cultures may remain culture-negative.[6] In OM the need for a bone sample is more contentious because the diagnosis by MRI is reliable.[30–32] The authors strive to identify the agent also in OM and emphasize the importance of blood cultures, which yield bacteria in one-third of the cases.[19] A sample for bacteriology is obtainable by needle aspiration of soft tissue in neonates, subperiosteal aspiration in infants, or drilling in older children.[1,6]

TREATMENT

Choosing the Antibiotic

The major role of *S aureus* among the agents causing AOIs[1,8,9] influences the choice of the initial antibiotic, provided the local resistance pattern is known.[1,19,36] **Table 2** summarizes some current recommendations for methicillin-sensitive *S aureus* and methicillin-resistant *S aureus* (MRSA).[16,19,36–39] *S pyogenes* and pneumococcus do not pose a similar challenge, because both are sensitive to first-generation cephalosporins and clindamycin. The authors prefer to use clindamycin for staphylococcal infection, but anti-staphylococcal penicillins are also widely used.[16,19] Of note, *K kingae* is resistant to clindamycin and vancomycin, but sensitive to cephalosporins and penicillins.[14,40] In countries where Hib is still common in SA (Hib rarely causes OM), an unvaccinated child should receive concomitant ampicillin or amoxicillin (200 mg/kg/d divided in 4 equal doses) until the agent is identified.[13] Gonococcal arthritis can be treated with ceftriaxone or cefotaxime.[39,41] These agents are also appropriate for salmonella AOIs. In developing countries one may have to resort to cheaper agents such as chloramphenicol or possibly trimethoprim-sulfamethoxazole.[42] An antibiogram would be of paramount importance in these situations.

Duration of Intravenous and Oral Treatment

For decades recommendations stated that the medication for AOIs should start with a long intravenous phase and treatment lasting a minimum of 4 to 6 weeks.[43,44] A lack of prospective trials led to stagnation until in the last decade more than 1 study showed that a short intravenous period suffices.[16,45,46] In the authors' largest to date, prospective, and randomized trial, the intravenous administration was only 2 to 4 days, after which the treatment was switched to oral medication, provided the first signs of recovery were observed and level of CRP began to descend.[17–19]

Fig. 1 demonstrates the short antibiotic courses tested in recent trials on OM and SA. The entire course of antibiotic was approximately 3 weeks for uncomplicated OM,[18] and 10 to 14 days for SA.[17] The key points of this treatment have been exceptionally high doses (see **Table 2**) of well-absorbed first-generation cephalosporins or clindamycin, antibiotics that penetrate bone and soft tissue well, in intravenous and oral administration, and equal doses 4 times a day, because time-dependent

Table 2
Empiric antibiotic treatment of acute osteoarticular infections targeting primarily methicillin-sensitive (MSSA) and methicillin-resistant (MRSA) *Staphylococcus aureus*

Local Resistance	Antibiotic	Dose	Reference
>90% of strains in community MSSA[a]	1st gen. CEPH	≥150 mg/kg/d q.i.d.[b]	Peltola et al,[19] 2011
	Or		
	Flucloxacillin	≥200 mg/kg/d q.i.d.	Jadogzinski et al,[16] 2009
	Or		
	Clindamycin	≥40 mg/kg/d q.i.d.[b]	Peltola et al,[19] 2012
>10% of strains MRSA[c] + Clindamycin resistance <10%	Clindamycin	≥40 mg/kg/d q.i.d.	Liu et al,[38] 2011
>10% of strains MRSA + Clindamycin resistance 10%–25%	Vancomycin	≥40 mg/kg/d q.i.d.	Liu et al,[38] 2011
	Or		
	Clindamycin	≥40 mg/kg/d q.i.d.[b]	Harik and Smeltzer,[36] 2010
	Or		
	TMP-SMX[d]	≥16 mg/kg/d b.i.d.[e]	Messina et al,[39] 2011
>10% of strains MRSA + Clindamycin resistance >25%	Vancomycin	≥40 mg/kg/d q.i.d.	Harik and Smeltzer,[36] 2010
	Or		
	TMP-SMX	≥16 mg/kg/d b.i.d.	Messina et al,[39] 2011
Resistant to vancomycin/ TMP-SMX	Linezolid	≥30 mg/kg/d t.i.d.	Chen et al,[37] 2007

Abbreviations: b.i.d., divided into 2 equal doses each per 24 hours; 1st gen. CEPH, first-generation cephalosporin; q.i.d., divided into 4 equal doses each per 24 hours; t.i.d., divided into 3 equal doses each per 24 hours.

[a] Methicillin-sensitive strains.
[b] Author's choice.
[c] Methicillin-resistant strains.
[d] Trimethoprim-sulfamethoxazole.
[e] Dosage of trimethoprim component.

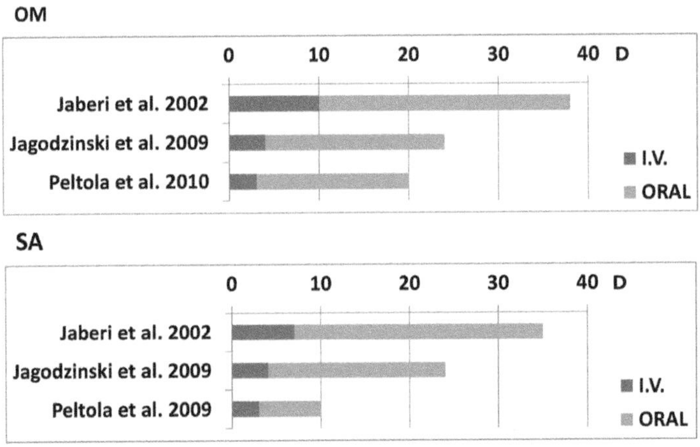

Fig. 1. Short courses of antibiotic for osteoarticular infections that have been tried successfully in the last 10 years. D, days; I.V., intravenous; OM, osteomyelitis; SA, septic arthritis. (*Data from* Refs.[16–18,45])

antibiotics do better with shorter intervals between doses.[47] For convenience and to ensure good compliance of the parents, the treatment was modify slightly so that the day's last dose is given before bedtime and the first at wake up. The efficiency of the approach in the past decades has been widely documented in both OM and SA.[17–19]

Adjuvant Medication

Nonsteroidal anti-inflammatory agents are given at the clinician's discretion and in large enough doses to relieve pain and fever.[17,18] A 4-day course of low-dose dexamethasone provides some relief in the symptoms of SA without a shown effect in the rate of sequelae.[48,49] A potential effect of large-dose adjuvant paracetamol has not been studied in AOIs, but in bacterial meningitis it seems to be beneficial.[50]

Surgical Treatment

No consensus prevails in the timing, procedures, extent, or even the overall need for surgical intervention in OM.[51] In 1 patient series with aggressive surgical approach, 17% of the patients went on to develop chronic OM.[52] On the other hand, conservative treatment with antibiotics has cured as many as 90% the patients with an early OM.[51,53] Surgery may benefit the patient if an abscess or a sequestra has already developed, but the issue is unclear even in cases in which pus has elevated the periosteum, as subperiosteal collections greater than 3 mm wide have resolved spontaneously with adequate antibiotic treatment.[44,54,55] In pelvic osteomyelitis an abscess greater than 20 mm may benefit from surgery.[29] The decision to drain a collection cannot be based solely on size but on the clinical grounds, which take into account the response to antibiotic therapy.[5] Persistent fevers and persistent elevation of the CRP in a patient with a periosteal abscess are indications for surgical drainage. Patients whose treatment has been instituted after more than a week from the onset of symptoms seem more likely to require open trepanation.[44,53,54,56] Thus, the need for surgery in a resource-poor environment is more likely than in the standard western setting.

A septic joint can be drained by aspiration (under US or fluoroscopic control, conditions permitting), arthroscopy, or open arthrotomy.[28,57–59] Traditionally, routine open arthrotomy has been considered essential in shoulder and hip arthritis.[57,58] Arthroscopy and repeated US-guided aspirations have been introduced more recently.[28,58] Eighty-one percent of children in the authors' series of 62 children with SA of the hip were treated without arthrotomy with uneventful recovery in all cases.[59]

Some caveats should be noted in applying minimally invasive surgery or a conservative approach in SA. Patients presenting in the early stages of disease usually recover uneventfully with no surgery at all, but the outcome starts to worsen if the history is 5 days or more.[57–59] There are no good data on success without surgical intervention in neonates, who are deemed to be at greater risk of sequelae than older children.[57]

PREVENTION

Hib was the second most common pathogen in SA of young children through the 1980s, but practically vanished from regions where large-scale Hib vaccination has been adopted. Hib vaccination had implications for treatment because adjuvant ampicillin or amoxicillin for children less than 5 years was no longer used.[13] Similar success might be expected with the *S pneumoniae* conjugate vaccines,[12] but the path has not been as smooth as with Hib vaccination. For example, the incidence of AOI caused by nonvaccine serotype 19A increased significantly in France after the use of the heptavalent pneumococcal vaccine was started.[12] This snag may be averted with newer vaccines that cover the serotype in question.

TREATMENT RESISTANCE AND COMPLICATIONS

Increased pneumococcal resistance to penicillin has not led to an increase in the rate of complications, but the rise of MRSA in many, although not all, countries has had an impact in the treatment of bone and joint infections.[7–11] Staphylococcal infections are no more problematic in terms of treatment and outcomes than other AOIs when caused by methicillin-sensitive *S aureus*.[60] In contrast, MRSA seems to associate somewhat more frequently with complications.[7–10,61] In the United States, the strain USA300 is predominant and is associated with a longer duration of fever.[9,62] The patient seems to be at an elevated risk of a pathologic fracture when OM is caused by the USA300–0114 pulsotype.[62] Fortunately, most MRSA strains are still susceptible to clindamycin, but this resistance pattern needs to be monitored constantly[63] as some areas are reporting increased clindamycin resistance in MRSA. The Panton-Valentine leukocidin–coding gene is associated with MRSA and causes more severe local symptoms and somewhat greater systemic inflammatory response.[64]

Surprisingly the old-fashioned, and very cheap, antibiotic trimethoprim-sulfamethoxazole is experiencing a renaissance in the treatment of clindamycin-resistant cases, because this agent has excellent bioavailability, and, in many areas, 99% of the MRSA strains are susceptible.[39] In contrast to the pre-antibiotic era, death from AOI is rare in an immunocompetent host in high-income countries.[6–10,16–19] However, deep vein thrombosis (DVT) may be life-threatening. A recent review on AOI identified 93 children with DVT from 28 studies, and risk factors for DVT were OM, male sex, and MRSA.[65]

Relapse or chronic infection occurs if the eradication of the infection has failed.[3] Also reinfections caused by dissimilar agents, in contrast to recurrences, are possible, although very rare events.[17,66] Chronic OM is a major health problem among children in the resource-poor settings, where it is the commonest cause of pathologic fracture.[2] In SA, avascular necrosis of the femoral head and joint cartilage destruction are feared sequelae.[57–59] Unsurprisingly, patients who present after many days of symptoms are more prone to these complications than those arriving early in the disease process.[57,58]

EVALUATION OF OUTCOME

Rates of recrudescence and sequelae are used as the yardsticks of the quality of treatment.[17–19] In this regard, reinfections should not be interpreted as treatment failures.[17,66] Much more common are sequelae, which, however, may pass unnoticed if the follow-up is not long enough.[1,18,57] Therefore, the authors recommend a late checkup for all cases of AOIs approximately 12 months after hospitalization, with intermediate checkups at 2 weeks and 3 months from discharge.[17–19] A thorough clinical investigation is the key, combined with CRP measurements and, when needed, radiography.[17–19,25,59,60]

SUMMARY

Early diagnosis and prompt treatment remain pivotal in avoiding complications in acute bacterial bone and joint infections.[67] Causative agents and the resistance pattern vary in different regions and should dictate the choice of antibiotics. In uncomplicated OM or SA, in which fever and symptoms quickly resolve, initial intravenous treatment for 2 to 4 days, followed by high-dose oral antibiotics, leads to outcomes as good as or better than those with longer intravenous treatment. Exceptionally large doses of a well-absorbing and penetrating agent, and administration of equal doses 4 times a day are likely pivotal in the parenteral and oral treatment. The authors' prospective and randomized trials showed 3 weeks and 2 weeks to be safe in uncomplicated OM and SA, respectively.[17–19] CRP is useful in the diagnosis and monitoring the cause of illness and in quick detection of pending complications.[25,27] Overall, the treatment of most cases of childhood OM, SA, and OM+SA can still be much simplified from the regimen practiced in many hospitals.[68,69]

REFERENCES

1. Krogstad P. Osteomyelitis and septic arthritis. In: Feigin RD, Cherry JD, editors. Textbook of pediatric infectious diseases. 6th edition. Philadelphia: Saunders; 2009. p. 725–48.
2. Akinyoola AL, Orimolade EA, Yusuf BM. Pathologic fractures of long bones in Nigerian children. J Child Orthop 2008;2:475–9.
3. Mantero E, Carbone M, Calevo MG, et al. Diagnosis and treatment of pediatric chronic osteomyelitis in developing countries: prospective study of 96 patients treated in Kenya. Musculoskelet Surg 2011;95:13–8.
4. Riise ØR, Handeland KS, Cvancarova M, et al. Incidence and characteristics of arthritis in Norwegian children: a population based study. Pediatrics 2008;121: e299–306.
5. Dartnell J, Ramachandran M, Katchburian M. Haematogenous acute and subacute paediatric osteomyelitis: a systematic review of the literature. J Bone Joint Surg Br 2012;94:584–95.
6. Lyon RM, Evanich JD. Culture-negative septic arthritis in children. J Pediatr Orthop 1999;19:655–9.
7. Qwynne-Jones DP, Stott NS. Community-acquired methicillin-resistant Staphylococcus aureus: a cause of musculoskeletal sepsis in children. J Pediatr Orthop 1999;19:413–6.
8. Arnold SR, Elias D, Buckingham SC, et al. Changing patterns of acute hematogenous osteomyelitis and septic arthritis: emergence of community-associated methicillin-resistant Staphylococcus aureus. J Pediatr Orthop 2006;26:703–8.
9. Carrillo-Marquez MA, Hulten KG, Hammerman W, et al. USA300 is the predominant genotype causing Staphylococcus aureus septic arthritis in children. Pediatr Infect Dis J 2009;28:1076–80.
10. Vander Have KL, Karmazyn B, Verma M, et al. Community-associated methicillin-resistant Staphylococcus aureus in acute musculoskeletal infection in children: a game changer. J Pediatr Orthop 2009;29:927–31.
11. Bradley JS, Kaplan SL, Tan TQ, et al. Pediatric pneumococcal bone and joint infections. The Pediatric Multicenter Pneumococcal Surveillance Study Group (PMPSSG). Pediatrics 1998;102:1376–82.
12. Lemaître C, Ferroni A, Doit C, et al. Pediatric osteoarticular infections caused by Streptococcus pneumoniae before and after the introduction of the heptavalent pneumococcal conjugate vaccine. Eur J Clin Microbiol Infect Dis 2012;31: 2773–81.
13. Peltola H, Kallio MJ, Unkila-Kallio L. Reduced incidence of septic arthritis in children by Haemophilus influenzae type-b vaccination. Implications for treatment. J Bone Joint Surg Br 1998;80:471–3.

14. Ceroni D, Cherkaoui A, Ferey S, et al. Kingella kingae osteoarticular infections in young children: clinical features and contribution of a new specific real-time PCR assay to the diagnosis. J Pediatr Orthop 2010;30:301–4.
15. Lavy CB, Thyoka M, Pitani AD. Clinical features and microbiology in 204 cases of septic arthritis in Malawian children. J Bone Joint Surg Br 2005;87:1545–8.
16. Jagodzinski NA, Kanwar R, Graham K, et al. Prospective evaluation of a shortened regimen of treatment for acute osteomyelitis and septic arthritis in children. J Pediatr Orthop 2009;29:518–25.
17. Peltola H, Pääkkönen M, Kallio P, et al. Prospective, randomized trial of 10 days versus 30 days of antimicrobial treatment, including a short-term course of parenteral therapy, for childhood septic arthritis. Clin Infect Dis 2009;48:1201–10.
18. Peltola H, Pääkkönen M, Kallio P, et al. Short- versus long-term antimicrobial treatment for acute hematogenous osteomyelitis of childhood: prospective, randomized trial on 131 culture-positive cases. Pediatr Infect Dis J 2010;29:1123–8.
19. Peltola H, Pääkkönen M, Kallio P, et al. Clindamycin vs. first-generation cephalosporins for acute osteoarticular infections of childhood–a prospective quasi-randomized controlled trial. Clin Microbiol Infect 2012;18:582–9.
20. Chow A, Robinson JL. Fever of unknown origin in children: a systematic review. World J Pediatr 2011;7:5–10.
21. Ju KL, Zurakowski D, Kocher MS. Differentiating between methicillin-resistant and methicillin-sensitive Staphylococcus aureus osteomyelitis in children: an evidence-based clinical prediction algorithm. J Bone Joint Surg Am 2011;93: 1693–701.
22. Zvulunov A, Gal A, Segev Z. Acute hematogenous osteomyelitis of the pelvis in childhood: diagnostic clues and pitfalls. Pediatr Emerg Care 2003;19:29–31.
23. Leigh W, Crawford H, Street M, et al. Pediatric calcaneal osteomyelitis. J Pediatr Orthop 2010;30:888–92.
24. Lorrot M, Fitoussi F, Faye A, et al. Laboratory studies in pediatric bone and joint infections. Arch Pediatr 2007;14(Suppl 2):S86–90 [in French].
25. Pääkkönen M, Kallio MJ, Kallio PE. Sensitivity of erythrocyte sedimentation rate and C-reactive protein in childhood bone and joint infections. Clin Orthop Relat Res 2010;468:861–6.
26. Butbul-Aviel Y, Koren A, Halevy R, et al. Procacitonin as a diagnostic aid in osteomyelitis and septic arthritis. Pediatr Emerg Care 2005;21:828–32.
27. Unkila-Kallio L, Kallio MJ, Peltola H. The usefulness of C-reactive protein levels in the identification of concurrent septic arthritis in children who have acute hematogenous osteomyelitis. A comparison with the usefulness of the erythrocyte sedimentation rate and the white blood cell count. J Bone Joint Surg Am 1994;76: 848–53.
28. Givon U, Liberman B, Schindler A, et al. Treatment of septic arthritis of the hip joint by repeated ultrasound-guided aspirations. J Pediatr Orthop 2004;24: 266–70.
29. Connolly SA, Connolly LP, Drubach LA, et al. MRI for detection of abscess in acute osteomyelitis of the pelvis in children. AJR Am J Roentgenol 2007;189: 867–72.
30. Courtney PM, Flynn JM, Jaramillo D, et al. Clinical indications for repeat MRI in children with acute hematogenous osteomyelitis. J Pediatr Orthop 2010;30: 883–7.
31. Averill LW, Hernandex A, Gonzalez L, et al. Diagnosis of osteomyelitis in children: utility of fat-suppressed contrast-enhanced MRI. AJR Am J Roentgenol 2009;192: 1232–8.

32. Connolly LP, Connolly SA, Drubach LA, et al. Acute hematogenous osteomyelitis of children: assessment of skeletal scintigraphy-based diagnosis in the era of MRI. J Nucl Med 2002;43:1310–6.
33. Fayad LM, Carrino JA, Fishman EK. Musculoskeletal infection: role of CT in the emergency department. Radiographics 2007;27:1723–36.
34. Browne LP, Mason EO, Kaplan SL, et al. Optimal imaging strategy for community-acquired Staphylococcus aureus musculoskeletal infections in children. Pediatr Radiol 2008;38:841–7.
35. Kunnamo I, Kallio P, Pelkonen P, et al. Clinical signs and laboratory tests in the differential diagnosis of arthritis in children. Am J Dis Child 1987;141:34–40.
36. Harik NS, Smeltzer MS. Management of acute hematogenous osteomyelitis in children. Expert Rev Anti Infect Ther 2010;8:175–81.
37. Chen CJ, Chiu CH, Lin TY, et al. Experience with linezolid therapy in children with osteoarticular infections. Pediatr Infect Dis J 2007;26:985–8.
38. Liu C, Bayer A, Cosgrove SE, et al. Clinical practice guidelines by the infectious diseases society of America for the treatment of methicillin-resistant Staphylococcus aureus infections in adults and children. Clin Infect Dis 2011;52:e18–55.
39. Messina AF, Namtu K, Guild M, et al. Trimethoprim-sulfamethoxazole therapy for children with acute osteomyelitis. Pediatr Infect Dis J 2011;30:1019–21.
40. Yagupsky P, Katz O, Peled N. Antibiotic susceptibility of Kingella kingae isolates form respiratory carriers and patients with invasive infections. J Antimicrob Chemother 2001;47:191–3.
41. Rice PA. Gonococcal arthritis (disseminated gonococcal infection). Infect Dis Clin North Am 2005;19:853–61.
42. Peek AC, Lavy CB, Thyoka M. Does long-term chloramphenicol cause anemia in Malawi? Trop Doct 2006;36:114–5.
43. Green JH. Cloxacillin in treatment of acute osteomyelitis. Br Med J 1967;2(5549):414–6.
44. Cole WG, Dalziel RE, Leitl S. Treatment of acute osteomyelitis in childhood. J Bone Joint Surg Br 1982;64:218–23.
45. Jaberi FM, Shahcheraghi GH, Ahadzadeh M. Short-term intravenous antibiotic treatment of acute hematogenous bone and joint infection in children: a prospective randomized trial. J Pediatr Orthop 2002;22:317–20.
46. Prado SM, Lixama CM, Peña DA, et al. Short duration of initial intravenous treatment in 70 pediatric patients with osteoarticular infections. Rev Chilena Infectol 2008;25:30–6 [in Spanish].
47. Roberts JA, Paratz J, Paratz E, et al. Continous infusion of beta-lactam antibiotics in severe infections: a review of its role. Int J Antimicrob Agents 2007;30:11–8.
48. Odio CM, Ramirez T, Arias G, et al. Double blind, randomized, placepo-controlled study of dexamethasone therapy for hematogenous septic arthritis in children. Pediatr Infect Dis J 2003;22:883–8.
49. Harel L, Prais D, Bar-On E, et al. Dexamethasone therapy for septic arthritis in children: results of a randomized double-blind placebo-controlled study. J Pediatr Orthop 2011;31:211–5.
50. Pelkonen T, Roine I, Cruzeiro ML, et al. Slow initial β-lactam infusion and oral paracetamol to treat childhood meningitis: a randomized, controlled trial. Lancet Infect Dis 2011;11:613–21.
51. Copley L. Infections of the musculoskeletal system. In: Herring JA, editor. Tachdjian's pediatric orthopedics. 4th edition. Philadelphia: Saunders Elsevier; 2008. p. 2089–119.

52. Meller I, Manor Y, Bar-Ziv J, et al. Pediatric update #8. Acute hematogenous osteomyelitis in children. Long-term results of surgical treatment. Orthop Rev 1989; 18:824–31.
53. Vaughan PA, Newman NM, Rosman MA. Acute hematogenous osteomyelitis in children. J Pediatr Orthop 1987;7:652–5.
54. Mah ET, LeQuesne QW, Gent RJ, et al. Ultrasonic features of acute osteomyelitis in children. J Bone Joint Surg Br 1994;76:969–74.
55. Howard CB, Einhorn M, Dagan R, et al. Ultrasound in diagnosis and management of acute hematogenous osteomyelitis in children. J Bone Joint Surg Br 1993;75: 79–82.
56. Scott RJ, Christofersen MR, Roberson WW Jr, et al. Acute osteomyelitis in children: a review of 116 cases. J Pediatr Orthop 1990;10:649–52.
57. Fabry G, Meire E. Septic arthritis of the hip in children: poor results after late and indaquate treatment. J Pediatr Orthop 1983;3:461–6.
58. El-Sayed AM. Treatment of early septic arthritis of the hip in children: comparison of arthrotomy versus artroscopic drainage. J Child Orthop 2008;2:229–37.
59. Pääkkönen M, Kallio MJ, Peltola H, et al. Pediatric septic hip with or without arthrotomy: retrospective analysis of 62 consecutive nonneonatal culture-positive cases. J Pediatr Orthop B 2010;19:264–9.
60. Pääkkönen M, Kallio PE, Kallio MJ, et al. Management of osteoarticular infections caused by Staphylococcus aureus is similar to that of other etiologies: analysis of 199 staphylococcal bone and joint infections. Pediatr Infect Dis J 2012;31:436–8.
61. Hawkshead JJ 3rd, Patel NB, Steele RW, et al. Comparative severity of pediatric osteomyelitis attributable to methicillin-resistant versus methicillin sensitive Staphylococcus aureus. J Pediatr Orthop 2009;29:85–90.
62. Belthur MV, Birchansky SB, Verdugo AA, et al. Pathologic fractures in children with acute Staphylococcus aureus osteomyelitis. J Bone Joint Surg Am 2012; 94:34–42.
63. Martínez-Aguilar G, Hammerman WA, Mason EO Jr, et al. Clindamycin treatment of invasive infections caused by community-aqcuired, methicillin-resistant and methicillin-susceptible Staphylococcus aureus in children. Pediatr Infect Dis J 2003;22:593–8.
64. Bocchini CE, Hulten KG, Mason EO Jr, et al. Panton-Valentine leukocidin genes are associated with enhanced inflammatory response and local disease in acute hematogenous Staphylococcus aureus osteomyelitis in children. Pediatrics 2006; 117:433–40.
65. Mantadakis E, Plessa E, Vouloumanou EK, et al. Deep venous thrombosis in children with musculoskeletal infections: the clinical evidence. Int J Infect Dis 2012; 16:e236–43.
66. Uçkay I, Assal M, Legout L, et al. Recurrent osteomyelitis caused by infection with different bacterial strains without obvious source of reinfection. J Clin Microbiol 2006;44:1194–6.
67. Sukswai P, Kovitvanitcha D, Thumkunanon V, et al. Acute hematogenous osteomyelitis and septic arthritis in children: clinical characteristics and outcomes study. J Med Assoc Thai 2011;94(Suppl 3):S209–16.
68. Pääkkönen M, Peltola H. Simplifying the treatment of acute bacterial bone and joint infections in children. Expert Rev Anti Infect Ther 2011;9:1125–31.
69. Pääkkönen M, Kallio MJ, Kallio PE, et al. Shortened hospital stay for childhood bone and joint infections: Analysis of 265 prospectively collected culture positive cases in 1983-2005. Scand J Infect Dis 2012;44:683–8.

Approach to Common Bacterial Infections: Community-Acquired Pneumonia

Pui-Ying Iroh Tam, MD

KEYWORDS

- Community-acquired pneumonia • Pediatric pneumonia • Children • CAP • Cause
- Management

KEY POINTS

- The diagnosis of community-acquired pneumonia (CAP) in children is not very sensitive or specific.
- Causative pathogens are challenging to isolate, and age is the best predictor of cause.
- A substantial proportion of CAP is mixed bacterial and viral infections; overdiagnosis of mild to moderate CAP can lead to overtreatment.
- The difficulty in differentiating between bacterial and viral pneumonia often leads to unnecessary antibiotic use.
- Current guidelines by the Pediatrics Infectious Diseases Society (PIDS) and the Infectious Diseases Society of America (IDSA) recommend amoxicillin (90 mg/kg/d orally in 2 doses) as the primary therapy for presumed bacterial pneumonia and azithromycin (10 mg/kg on day 1, followed by 5 mg/kg once daily on days 2–5) as the primary therapy for presumed atypical pneumonia in children younger than 5 years or aged 5 years or older.
- For children aged 5 years or older with presumed bacterial CAP who do not have clinical, laboratory, or radiographic evidence that distinguish bacterial CAP from atypical CAP, PIDS/IDSA guidelines note that a macrolide can be added to the β-lactam antibiotic.
- Much of the pediatric CAP guidelines is based on evidence of poor to moderate quality, and there many gaps in the evidence remain.

INTRODUCTION

Community-acquired pneumonia (CAP) is fundamentally different in children and in adults. The evaluation, diagnosis, and treatment that distinguish the approach to management in children from that of adult disease is based on the differing causes of childhood pneumonia, and this microbial spectrum has changed over the past 3 decades with the introduction of conjugate vaccines and improved molecular diagnostic assays.

Disclosures: No potential conflicts of interest.
Division of Pediatric Infectious Diseases, Department of Pediatrics, University of Minnesota, 3-210 McGuire Translational Research Facility, 2001 6th Street Southeast, Minneapolis, MN 55455, USA
E-mail address: irohtam@umn.edu

Pediatr Clin N Am 60 (2013) 437–453
http://dx.doi.org/10.1016/j.pcl.2012.12.009
pediatric.theclinics.com

There are 2 main challenges in the diagnosis of CAP: the first is the definition of CAP, particularly in young children, in whom bacterial and viral infections can occur with similar frequencies, and in whom overdiagnosis of mild symptoms and signs may lead to unnecessary antibiotic use; the second is the identification of a causative pathogen, which is frequently impractical and inadequate in children, and in whom the failure to isolate an organism can result in unnecessary antibiotic use. These problems affect the management of CAP, and lead to emergence of resistance as a result of overtreatment. Management decisions are complicated because there are few randomized controlled trials in children that evaluate different antibiotic therapies and treatment duration. Although guidelines exist, they are often based on poor-quality evidence.

The challenge for the general pediatrician is to recognize lower respiratory tract illness, to refer for hospitalization when it is severe, and to appropriately treat with antibiotics if a bacterial pneumonia is suspected. This review focuses on practical issues of clinical relevance for the general pediatrician, including what to elicit from the patient history and examination, keeping in mind not only the infections that are commonly seen but also emerging infectious diseases and those that are less frequently seen but that are severe when they occur.

CAUSE AND EPIDEMIOLOGY

The first key clinical issue is to diagnose CAP in children, and then determine which pathogen is responsible. There are discrepant definitions of CAP depending on whether the consideration is epidemiologic, which has more sensitive criteria, or regulatory, which is more specific (**Table 1**). Causative agents in children have been difficult to identify; however, clues in the history may help point toward certain infectious pathogens (**Table 2**). The cause of pediatric pneumonia is usually based on age, because that is the best predictor available (**Table 3**).

Streptococcus pneumoniae and *Haemophilus influenzae* type b (Hib) have been characterized as 2 bacteria predominately responsible for cases of fatal pneumonia in children.[1] However, widespread introduction of Hib and pneumococcal conjugate vaccines has led to significant declines, especially of Hib, although *Streptococcus pneumoniae* is still the predominant bacteria isolated from bacterial CAP in children. There is increasing recognition of the prevalence of mixed bacterial and viral infections, which have been documented in 23% to 33% of cases of pneumonia.[2–4]

Atypical organisms (eg, *Mycoplasma pneumoniae, Chlamydia pneumoniae*) account for up to a third of cases.[5,6] A new *Chlamydia*-like organism, *Simkania negevensis*, has been associated with bronchiolitis and pneumonia in children,[7] and has also been

Table 1
Definitions of CAP in children

World Health Organization[79,80]	Cough or difficulty breathing Fast breathing: 2–12 mo: ≥50 breaths/min 12–60 mo: ≥40 breaths/min
British Thoracic Society[43]	Persistent or repetitive fever >38.5°C together with chest recession and an increased respiratory rate
Infectious Diseases Society of America[33]	Presence of signs and symptoms of pneumonia in a previously healthy child caused by an infection that has been acquired outside the hospital

Table 2
Clues to the cause of pneumonia from history and physical examination

Factor	Possible Agent(s)
Host factor	
Sickle cell disease	*Streptococcus pneumoniae*
Human immunodeficiency virus infection and CD4+ lymphocyte count of <200/μL	*Streptococcus pneumoniae, Haemophilus influenzae, Cryptococcus neoformans, Mycobacterium tuberculosis*
Structural lung disease (bronchiectasis)	*Pseudomonas aeruginosa*
Travel	
Travel to southeast Asia	*Burkholderia pseudomallei, Mycobacterium tuberculosis*
Travel to China, Taiwan, Toronto, Canada, Middle East	Coronavirus causing SARS
Travel to tuberculosis-endemic countries	*Mycobacterium tuberculosis*
Travel to desert regions of southwestern United States, and Central and South America	*Coccidioides immitis*
Travel to Ohio and St Lawrence River valleys	*Histoplasma capsulatum*
Travel to Peru	*Sporothrix schenckii*
Travel to Vancouver Island, Canada, and Pacific Northwest (camping, residence)	*Cryptococcus gattii*
Other environmental factors	
Pneumonia outbreak in a homeless shelter	*Streptococcus pneumoniae, Mycobacterium tuberculosis*
Lawn mowing in an endemic area, including southcentral and western states and Martha's Vineyard	*Francisella tularensis*
Exposure to parturient cats, sheep, goats, and cattle in an endemic area, including western and plains states where ranching and rearing of cattle are common	*Coxiella burnetii*
Sleeping in a rose garden, playing on bales of hay	*Sporothrix schenckii*
Exposure to windstorm in an endemic area	*Coccidioides immitis, Coxiella burnetii*
Exposure to bats, excavation or residence in an endemic area	*Histoplasma capsulatum*
Camping, cutting down trees in an endemic area, including the Mississippi River and Ohio River valley basins and around the Great Lakes	*Blastomyces dermatitidis*
Exposure to mouse droppings in an endemic area, including the Four Corners and Yosemite National Park	Hantavirus
Immunosuppressed and exposure to hot tub; grocery store mist machine; recent stay in a hotel; visit to or recent stay in a hospital with Legionellaceae-contaminated drinking water	*Legionella pneumophila*, other Legionellaceae

found in healthy, asymptomatic individuals and may be an opportunistic organism rather than a true pathogen.[8]

Viral pathogens are responsible for most clinical disease in younger children, accounting for 77% of clinical pneumonia in children younger than 1 year compared

Table 3
Microbial causes of CAP in childhood, according to age in descending order of frequency, and associated testing

Age Grouping, Cause	Associated Testing[33,81,82]
Birth–20 d	
Group B streptococci Gram-negative enteric bacteria *Listeria monocytogenes*	Blood cultures should not be routinely performed in fully immunized, nontoxic children in outpatient setting, but should be obtained if children fail to improve or have progressive symptoms or clinically deteriorate after starting antibiotic therapy; blood and pleural fluid culture are insensitive, but there are no established alternatives in children
3 wk–3 mo	
Chlamydia trachomatis	Quadrupling of acute and convalescent serology, NP culture or NP PCR; although IDSA does not recommend diagnostic testing, because reliable and readily available diagnostic tests do not exist
RSV PIV 3	NP swab for PCR or immunofluorescence, viral culture and DFA staining, acute and convalescent serology. Whereas influenza and RSV have winter-spring seasonality, PIV3 is present year-round
Streptococcus pneumoniae	Blood culture (yield <10%), urinary antigen (low specificity, many false-positives because of NP carriage), pneumolysin-based PCR of blood, pleural fluid and secretions
Bordetella pertussis	Culture, immunofluorescence assay, PCR assay of NP secretions
Staphylococcus aureus	Blood culture, pleural fluid culture
4 mo–4 y	
RSV, parainfluenza viruses, influenza virus, adenovirus, rhinovirus	NP swab for PCR or immunofluorescence, viral culture and DFA staining, acute and convalescent serology
Streptococcus pneumoniae	Blood culture (yield <10%), urinary antigen (low specificity, many false-positive results because of NP carriage), pneumolysin-based PCR of blood, pleural fluid and secretions
Haemophilus influenzae	Blood culture, pleural fluid culture
Mycoplasma pneumoniae	Quadrupling of acute and convalescent serology is diagnostic, IgM antibody in acute or early convalescent serum is helpful, throat or NP swab PCR (high specificity and positive predictive value)
Mycobacterium tuberculosis	Identify bacteria in culture of sputum or gastric aspirates, with positive tuberculin skin test or interferon γ release assay

(*continued on next page*)

Table 3
(*continued*)

Age Grouping, Cause	Associated Testing[33,81,82]
5–15 y	
Mycoplasma pneumoniae	Quadrupling of acute and convalescent serology is diagnostic, IgM antibody in acute or early convalescent serum is helpful, throat or NP swab PCR (high specificity and positive predictive value)
Chlamydia pneumoniae	Quadrupling of acute and convalescent serology, NP culture or NP PCR; although IDSA does not recommend diagnostic testing, because reliable and readily available diagnostic tests do not exist
Streptococcus pneumoniae	Blood culture (yield <10%), urinary antigen (low specificity, many false-positive results because of NP carriage), pneumolysin-based PCR of blood, pleural fluid, and secretions
Influenza A or B, adenovirus	NP swab for PCR or immunofluorescence, viral culture and DFA staining, acute and convalescent serology
Nontypeable *Haemophilus influenzae*	Blood culture, pleural fluid culture
Mycobacterium tuberculosis	Identify bacteria in culture of sputum or gastric aspirates, with positive tuberculin skin test or interferon γ release assay
All ages, severe pneumonia requiring admission to intensive care unit:	
Streptococcus pneumoniae, Staphylococcus aureus, group A streptococci, *Haemophilus influenzae* type b, *Mycoplasma pneumoniae,* adenovirus	
Uncommon causes of pediatric CAP:	
Viruses: varicella zoster virus, coronaviruses, enteroviruses (coxsackievirus and echovirus), cytomegalovirus, Epstein-Barr virus, mumps virus, herpes simplex virus (in newborns), bocaviruses, polyomaviruses, measles virus, hantavirus	Varicella zoster virus: quadrupling of acute and convalescent serology, immunofluorescent assay of skin secretions; cytomegalovirus, Epstein-Barr virus: quadrupling of acute and convalescent serology, IgM antibody in acute serum; measles virus: quadrupling of acute and convalescent serology, immunofluorescent assay of NP secretions; hantavirus: quadrupling of acute and convalescent serology, IgM antibody in acute serum NP secretions or antibody in serum; sufficiently uncommon that IgM or IgG antibody in serum is essentially diagnostic
Chlamydia: *Chlamydia psittaci*	Quadrupling of acute and convalescent serology is diagnostic
Coxiella: *Coxiella burnetii*	Quadrupling of acute and convalescent serology is diagnostic

(*continued on next page*)

Table 3
(continued)

Age Grouping, Cause	Associated Testing[33,81,82]
Bacteria: *Streptococcus pyogenes*, anaerobic mouth flora (*Streptococcus milleri, Peptostreptococcus*), nontype B (but typeable) *Haemophilus influenzae, Bordetella pertussis, Klebsiella pneumoniae, Escherichia coli, Listeria monocytogenes, Neisseria meningitides* (often group Y), *Legionella, Burkholderia pseudomallei, Francisella tularensis, Brucella abortus, Leptospira*	*Francisella tularensis:* quadrupling of acute and convalescent serology is diagnostic (blood or sputum culture requires special medium and may pose danger of infection to laboratory workers and they should be notified before handling specimen); *Legionella pneumophila* and other *Legionella* species: sputum or tracheal aspirate culture, urinary antigen (urinary antigen tests detect only *Legionella pneumophila* antigen); *Brucella abortus:* blood culture, quadrupling of acute and convalescent serology
Fungi: *Coccidioides immitis, Histoplasma capsulatum, Blastomyces dermatitidis*	Urinary *Histoplasma* or *Blastomyces* antigen, stain or culture of respiratory tract secretions, serum IgM antibody; quadrupling of acute and convalescent serology

Abbreviations: DFA, direct fluorescent antibody; IDSA, Infectious Diseases Society of America; NP, nasopharyngeal; PCR, polymerase chain reaction.

with 59% in those older than 2 years.[4,9] Viruses account for 30% to 67% of pediatric CAP, with influenza A, respiratory syncytial virus (RSV), and parainfluenza virus (PIV) 1, 2, and 3 most commonly identified.[4] A study by Singleton and colleagues[10] recovered respiratory viruses from 90% of Alaskan children younger than 3 years hospitalized with respiratory infections. In that case-control study of 865 children, RSV, PIV, human metapneumovirus (hMPV), and influenza were significantly more common in hospitalized cases than control children, but rhinovirus, adenovirus, and coronavirus were not.

The high occurrence of asymptomatic carriage, such as in up to a third of asymptomatic children harboring rhinovirus, complicates the frequent detection of these respiratory viruses[10–12]; the causative nature of many respiratory viruses in pneumonia, particularly ones identified by sensitive new molecular diagnostics, remain unclear. However, rhinovirus identification has been associated with bronchiolitis, asthma, and wheezing.[13,14] hMPV, isolated in 2001,[15] has been recovered in 3.8% to 8.3% of isolates of nasopharyngeal and throat specimens of hospitalized children or children with CAP.[16,17] Human bocavirus, first described in 2005, has been detected in up to 19% of clinical samples, mainly in infants and young children[18]; its detection in serum and stool suggests that the virus may cause systemic disease.[18] In 2007, WU and KI polyomaviruses were detected in the respiratory tract samples of adults and children,[19,20] and subsequently shown to be present in respiratory secretions in patients with acute respiratory illness.[21,22]

Severe acquired respiratory syndrome (SARS)-associated coronavirus was the first novel coronavirus to be characterized among a succession of other novel coronaviruses that decade.[23–25] Using sensitive reverse transcription polymerase chain reaction (PCR) assays, Dominguez and colleagues[26] detected coronavirus RNAs in 5% of pediatric respiratory specimens, and 41% of coronavirus-positive patients had evidence of a lower respiratory tract infection. Twenty-six percent of that group presented with vomiting or diarrhea, and 8% with meningoencephalitis or seizures, which suggests that coronavirus may have more systemic involvement than previously believed.

Fungal pathogens such as *Histoplasma, Coccidioides, Blastomyces,* and *Cryptococcus* can cause pneumonia the immunocompromised patient population and may cause clinical illness in immunocompetent hosts, but usually not with the presentation of CAP. *Blastomyces* can cause prolonged fever and respiratory symptoms that mimic a prolonged CAP; however. *Cryptococcus gattii,* which can infect immunocompetent hosts,[27] has caused an increasing number of infections in the US Pacific Northwest since 2004 and has been detected in the southeastern United States.[28] The pathogen can cause cryptococcomas in the lungs, and in 1 report, 54% of infected patients had documented pneumonia.[27] *Mycobacterium tuberculosis* and nontuberculous mycobacteria can likewise cause CAP, but tend to be limited to people with high-risk exposures. Similarly, other high-risk exposures suggest specific causes, as outlined in **Table 2**.

PATIENT HISTORY

Symptoms (fever, chills, cough) of pneumonia can overlap significantly with a spectrum of conditions, such as bacterial sepsis or severe anemia, making differentiation between these diagnoses challenging. Signs such as crackles and egophony are more specific, but are often absent in clinical pneumonia in children. Chest radiography is considered the gold standard for confirmation of pneumonia,[29] but is also of questionable benefit in children, as discussed later. The limitation in diagnosis is reflected in the various definitions of pediatric CAP that exist (see **Table 1**), none of which is considered sufficiently sensitive or specific, and few of which have been validated in children.[30] For example, the World Health Organization (WHO) criteria for mild to moderate CAP are based on cough or breathing difficulties and age-adjusted tachypnea; such a definition places CAP with all other types of lower respiratory tract disease.

PATIENT EXAMINATION

Clinical features in children with CAP vary with the age of the child, although none of them is very specific. Cevey-Macherel and colleagues[2] showed that more than a fifth of patients diagnosed with CAP as defined by WHO guidelines had completely normal breath sounds on admission, and auscultation was ruled to be poorly sensitive and specific in diagnosing WHO guideline-defined CAP in young children. However, WHO guidelines rely solely on respiratory rate and, using other criteria for a diagnosis of pneumonia or lower respiratory tract infection, respiratory rate has been shown to be less sensitive and specific in the first 3 days of illness.[31] In a study that defined pneumonia/lower respiratory tract infection as the presence of crepitations (crackles), wheeze, bronchial breathing, or chest radiograph (CXR) abnormalities, respiratory rates of less than 40 breaths/min were seen in 55% of children older than 35 months with a diagnosis of pneumonia.[32] Canadian guidelines regard oxygenation as a good indication of the severity of disease,[29] and oxygen saturation is recommended by the Infectious Diseases Society of America (IDSA) as a guide for referral of care and further diagnostic testing.[33]

Clinical features do not reliably distinguish between viral, bacterial, and atypical pneumonias.[34,35] Pneumococcal pneumonia has been associated with a history of fever and breathlessness and signs of tachypnea, indrawing, and toxic appearance, but these features can be indistinguishable from staphylococcal pneumonia at the beginning of illness. Similarly, mycoplasma pneumonia has been associated with cough, chest pain, and wheezing, symptoms being worse than the signs, as well as nonrespiratory symptoms such as arthralgia and headache, but studies have not successfully distinguished viral and bacterial CAP or between types of CAP by clinical signs alone.[36,37] In addition, many children with CAP have mixed bacterial and viral infections. *Mycoplasma* pneumonia is more common in children aged 5 years or younger, and is typically characterized by slow progression, sore throat, low-grade fever and cough developing over 3 to 5 days. Although some children have more abrupt onset of symptoms or higher fevers, this pattern may help to distinguish it from pneumococcal or staphylococcal pneumonia, and influence treatment decisions, because there are no rapid laboratory tests that allow clear distinction between classic bacterial and atypical pneumonia.

DIAGNOSTIC EVALUATION

Neither IDSA nor the British Thoracic Society (BTS) recommends CXRs for confirmation of suspected CAP in patients well enough to be treated in an outpatient setting. CXRs in children, unlike in adults with pneumonia, may not show any abnormalities, especially if taken at the onset of illness.[38] Beyond providing radiographic evidence of opacification, the use of a CXR is limited and has not been shown to correlate with clinical signs[39] or to help differentiate bacterial from viral pneumonia.[40] A prospective study in Switzerland enrolling 99 patients found that only 79% of patients had radiographic consolidation, with poor correlation between radiographic findings and diminished breath sounds, and no association with severity or cause of pneumonia.[2] A prospective study in the United Kingdom by Clark and colleagues[41] showed that lobar CXR changes were not associated with severity. In a study from Brazil, upper lobe involvement was shown to have 84% specificity and 65% positive predictive value for severity in children aged 1 year or younger hospitalized with CAP.[42]

Whereas IDSA guidelines support a posteroanterior (PA) and lateral CXR in patients with suspected or documented hypoxemia or significant respiratory distress, and in those who have failed an initial course of antibiotic therapy, BTS guidelines do not recommend that a lateral CXR should be performed routinely.[43] This recommendation was based on a retrospective study from the United States that indicated that a frontal CXR was 100% sensitive and specific for lobar consolidation but would underdiagnose nonlobar infiltrates in 15% of cases. The investigators considered the clinical implications to be unclear. However, patients hospitalized for management of CAP (**Box 1**) should have both PA and lateral CXRs, to ensure that all infiltrates are detected and to assess for pleural effusion. Follow-up CXRs are unnecessary in children who recover uneventfully from an episode of CAP, but should be obtained in children who do not improve clinically and in those with progressive symptoms or clinical deterioration after 48 to 72 hours of antibiotic therapy.[33,43]

Most patients with bacterial pneumonia present with a lobar infiltrate (**Fig. 1**). Interstitial infiltrates can be found in bacterial as well as viral and atypical pneumonia.[35] *Mycoplasma pneumoniae* pneumonia can have diffuse infiltrate radiologically out of proportion with clinical findings; lobar consolidation, atelectasis, nodular infiltration, and hilar adenopathy have also been described. *Streptococcus pneumoniae* pneumonia can present with round infiltrates (see **Fig. 1**B), as can also be seen with other bacteria.

Microbiologic recovery sampled directly from the infected region of lung is the gold standard, although less invasive sampling methods are usually used to achieve a diagnosis (see **Table 3**). For a child with suspected CAP in the community, there are no indications for any general investigations. However, if a child with CAP is hospitalized (see **Box 1**), testing for potential pathogens as well as obtaining acute phase reactants (white blood count [WBC], C-reactive protein [CRP], erythrocyte sedimentation rate [ESR], procalcitonin [PCT]) may be helpful for clinical management. No studies have

Box 1
Severe pediatric CAP and criteria for hospital admission

Indications of severe pediatric CAP[43]*:*

1. Temperature greater than 38.5°C
2. Respiratory rate: in infants, more than 70 breaths/min; in older children, more than 50 breaths/min
3. Moderate to severe recession
4. Nasal flaring
5. Cyanosis
6. Grunting respiration
7. In infants, intermittent apnea and not feeding
8. Tachycardia
9. Signs of dehydration
10. Capillary refill time 2 seconds or more

Criteria for hospital admission of a child with CAP[33,43]*:*

1. Hypoxemia with O_2 less than 90% at sea level
2. Infants younger than 3 to 6 months
3. Suspected or documented CAP caused by a pathogen with increased virulence, such as community-associated (CA) methicillin-resistant *Staphylococcus aureus* (MRSA)
4. Concern about careful observation at home; those who are unable to comply with therapy; those unable to be followed up

Transfer to intensive care should be considered if[33,43]*:*

1. Oxygen saturation is less than 92% on inspired oxygen of 50% or greater
2. Severe respiratory distress
3. Sustained tachycardia, inadequate blood pressure, or need for pharmacologic support of blood pressure or perfusion
4. Exhaustion
5. Apnea
6. Slow breathing
7. Altered mental status

found this to be definitively useful in differentiating the cause or severity of CAP.[44,45] Don and colleagues[46] studied 101 children and showed that an increase of 4 serum nonspecific inflammatory markers (WBC, CRP, ESR, PCT) was significantly associated with radiographic evidence of CAP; however, the role of these studies in the screening for bacterial and viral CAP was limited.

A study by Lahti and colleagues[47] involving children 6 months and older showed that inducing sputum production by inhalation of 5% hypertonic saline for 5 to 10 minutes and then aspirating or expectorating a sputum sample provided good-quality sputum specimens with 90% microbiological yield. However, the practicality of this relatively labor-intensive approach in a busy outpatient clinic is debatable. New molecular diagnostic tests have become available, particularly rapid antigen detection for respiratory viruses. Despite this development, one-quarter to one-third of patients still fail to yield an obvious cause.[48]

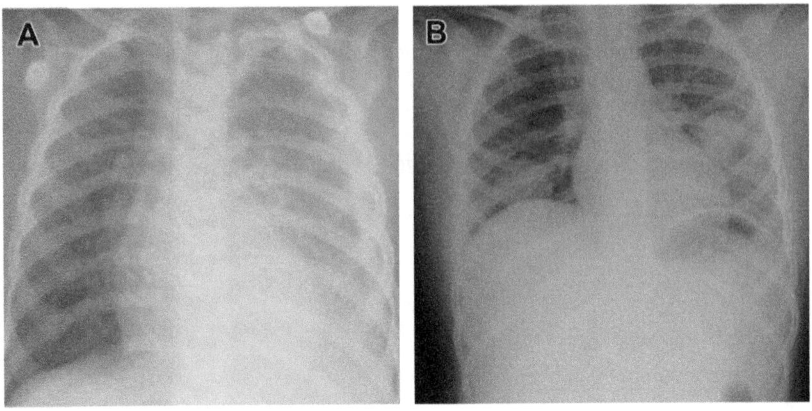

Fig. 1. CXRs of CAP in: (*A*) a 15-month-old patient with group A *Streptococcus* and (*B*) a 10-year-old patient with ulcerative colitis on immunosuppression, with *Legionella pneumophila*. Other causes of round pneumonia include *Streptococcus pneumoniae, Klebsiella pneumoniae, Haemophilus influenzae, Coxiella burnetii,* and *Mycobacterium tuberculosis*. Fungal infections, hydatid cysts, and lung abscesses may have a similar appearance.

Streptococcus pneumoniae is the most common bacterial pathogen in most studies but remains challenging to identify, because less than 10% of children with pneumonia are bacteremic and there are no definitive, noninvasive, and accurate tests.[3,49] Urinary antigen tests for *Streptococcus pneumoniae* are not recommended by IDSA for the diagnosis of pneumococcal pneumonia in children, because false-positive tests are common and likely attributable to nasopharyngeal carriage.[50] Diagnosis of *Mycoplasma pneumoniae* infection can be made by testing for IgM to *Mycoplasma pneumoniae* in serum or plasma by enzyme-linked immunosorbent assay (ELISA), or by PCR testing of nasal, throat, or sputum specimens. PCR seems to detect more *Mycoplasma* infections than IgM ELISA testing, but a single standardized test has not been used across studies, so definitive data are difficult to obtain. Rapid IgM testing kits are being assessed, and may be a promising way to more rapidly detect *Mycoplasma* infection, but none has been validated as highly sensitive and specific in multiple studies.[33]

TREATMENT

The main issue for a general pediatrician in management of suspected pediatric CAP is whether or not to treat with antibiotics. This decision is complicated because it is difficult to distinguish bacterial from viral pneumonia, and hence to decide whether antibiotics may be warranted. There are also few randomized controlled trials to guide antibiotic choice and duration. Because age is the best predictor of cause of pediatric pneumonia, guidelines for treatment are typically categorized by age and suspected pathogens.[33] BTS guidelines recommend that children with a clear clinical diagnosis of pneumonia should receive antibiotics, given that bacterial and viral pneumonia cannot be reliably differentiated. However, because viral pathogens are responsible for most of clinical disease in preschool-aged children with CAP, IDSA does not routinely recommend antimicrobial therapy for that group.

Streptococcus pneumoniae is the most prominent bacterial pathogen across all age groups, hence amoxicillin is recommended as first-line therapy for previously healthy, appropriately immunized patients.[33] Because the Hib vaccine offers no protection against nontypeable *Haemophilus influenzae,* there have not been alterations to choice of empiric antibiotic therapy for vaccinated children with suspected bacterial pneumonia. Atypical bacterial pathogens such as *Mycoplasma pneumoniae* are more prominent in school-aged children and older patients, and macrolide therapy is recommended for those with compatible findings, generally based on clinical findings. However, there are few high-quality data on the effectiveness of macrolide antibiotics in the treatment of children with *Mycoplasma* pneumonia, so the recommendation of treatment with a macrolide for this condition is listed as a weak recommendation in the PIDS/IDSA guidelines.[33] Bacterial-viral coinfections have been well documented to occur with influenza and *Streptococcus pneumoniae, Staphylococcus aureus,* and group A *Streptococcus*.[51] Hence, children with serious viral lower respiratory tract infections may still benefit from empiric therapy for bacterial agents. Adjunctive treatment with corticosteroids has been studied but has not shown proven benefit on outcomes.[52,53]

The summary PIDS/IDSA guidelines for CAP in children continue to recommend amoxicillin (90 mg/kg/d orally in 2 doses) as the primary therapy for presumed bacterial pneumonia and azithromycin (10 mg/kg on day 1, followed by 5 mg/kg once daily on days 2–5) as the primary therapy for presumed atypical pneumonia in children younger than 5 years or aged 5 years or older. For children aged 5 years or older with presumed bacterial CAP who do not have clinical, laboratory, or radiographic evidence to distinguish bacterial CAP from atypical CAP, PIDS/IDSA guidelines note that a macrolide can be added to the β-lactam antibiotic.[33] As noted earlier, there are no definitive clinical, laboratory, or radiographic findings that distinguish bacterial from atypical CAP, so the decision to use or add a macrolide remains based on an overall indication from the combined findings, rather than from a clearly defined set of criteria based on these findings.

Aside from influenza, there are no data from prospective, controlled studies for antiviral therapy against viruses associated with pediatric CAP. Adamantanes and neuraminidase inhibitors are effective against susceptible strains of influenza A, and neuraminidase inhibitors are effective for susceptible strains of influenza B. Because substantial genetic variation can occur in influenza from year to year, influenza virus strains can become resistant to either class of antiviral agents; most strains of influenza A isolated since the 2005 to 2006 season have been adamantine-resistant.[54] The recommended doses of antiviral agents for seasonal influenza were developed for fully susceptible strains[33] and evaluated in trials in which treatment was provided early, usually within 48 hours of onset of symptoms.[55] The degree of benefit provided by treatment after 48 hours of symptoms has not been defined.

Few studies have looked at the appropriate duration of antimicrobial therapy for CAP in children. Treatment courses of 10 days for β-lactams and 5 days for azithromycin have been best studied, although shorter courses have been studied showing no difference in acute cure or relapse rates between the groups.[56–58] Shorter courses are acknowledged to be just as effective, particularly for milder cases, although prolonged courses may be required for some pathogens, such as CA-MRSA.[59]

Similarly, there are no randomized controlled studies evaluating the optimum time to switch from parenteral to oral therapy; hence IDSA and BTS guidelines do not provide a statement recommendation, although Canadian guidelines recommend switching from parenteral to oral therapy after 2 to 4 days if the patients are afebrile without complications.[29]

TREATMENT RESISTANCE

Antimicrobial-resistant *Streptococcus pneumoniae* has been a recognized problem since the 1990s.[60] The hope that the heptavalent pneumococcal conjugate vaccine

(PCV7), which contains the 5 serotypes accounting for 89% of penicillin-resistant pneumococcal isolates in the United States,[61] would decrease antimicrobial-resistant pneumococci in the community has seen marginal success. One longitudinal surveillance program showed penicillin-resistant isolates decreasing from 21.5% to 14.6%, but intermediate penicillin resistance increasing from 2.7% to 17.9%, after introduction of PCV7.[62]

The effect of antibiotic resistance on clinical outcomes in children is less evident. Pneumococcal pneumonias that were penicillin-resistant or penicillin-sensitive were not associated with differences in outcome, hospital course, or complications.[63] No association between antimicrobial resistance and treatment failure has yet been shown in children. To minimize antimicrobial resistance, IDSA recommends limiting antibiotic exposure, using antibiotics with narrow spectrum activity and for shortest effective duration.[33] However none of these recommendations is based on strong-quality evidence.

Fluoroquinolones are generally avoided in children younger than 18 years because of concerns for arthropathy, but experience with its use to treat children for a variety of serious infectious diseases has led to consensus statements that fluoroquinolones can treat specific infections in children safely and effectively, and may be considered as an alternative therapy in serious infectious diseases.[64] Bradley and colleagues[65] enrolled 738 children from 6 months to 16 years with CAP in a noninferiority trial, which showed similar cure rates with levofloxacin as with a comparator drug. Fifty-two percent of children treated with levofloxacin experienced 1 or more adverse events, compared with 53% in the comparator-treated children; musculoskeletal adverse events (arthralgia, myalgia) were experienced in 4% versus 3% in the comparator group who received current standard of care antibiotics.[65] None of these differences was statistically significant. In an era of emerging drug resistance, fluoroquinolones may be an effective alternative therapy in treating children with CAP.

EVALUATION OF OUTCOME AND PREVENTION

Children with CAP who are on adequate therapy should clinically improve within 48 to 72 hours. If there is no improvement, possible complications to be considered include pleural effusions and empyema, necrotizing pneumonia, septicemia and metastatic infection (such as *Staphylococcus aureus* causing osteomyelitis or septic arthritis), and hemolytic-uremic syndrome. All of these complications require further investigation and possible hospitalization. Children with severe pneumonia, empyema, and lung abscess should be followed up after discharge until complete resolution clinically and on CXR.[43]

Vaccines play a crucial part in prevention of pneumonia. Pertussis causes pneumonia in about 5% of all reported cases, which doubles to 11.8% of reported cases for those younger than 6 months.[66] Pneumonia complicating measles occurs in up to 27% to 77%, depending if the study was based in the community or hospital setting.[67] Half of measles-related pneumonias are caused by bacterial superinfection, and it contributes to 56% to 86% of all deaths in measles.[67]

Influenza vaccines can prevent 87% of influenza-associated pneumonia hospitalizations,[68] including pneumococcal and CA-MRSA superinfection.[69,70] Pneumococcal conjugate vaccines have decreased radiologically confirmed pneumonia by 20% to 37% and 67% to 87% of vaccine-serotype bacteremic pneumonia.[71,72] The distribution of the 13-valent pneumococcal conjugate vaccine (PCV13) in 2010 may address the most common replacement serotypes that have been increasing since introduction of the 7-valent pneumococcal conjugate vaccine in the United States in 2000.[73]

Particularly, PCV13 contains the additional serotypes associated with empyema and necrotizing pneumonia,[74,75] and thus it is hoped that the number of these complications will decrease. For high-risk infants, RSV-specific monoclonal antibody can decrease the risk of severe pneumonia and hospitalization.

SUMMARY

Pneumonia occurs more often in early childhood than at any other age, with the exception of adults older than 75 years, and kills more children than any other disease worldwide.[76] The central clinical issue of CAP in children is that the diagnosis is typically not through microbiologic isolation, but rather through inference and deductions from clinical symptoms and signs, and supported by radiography and serum laboratory tests. This approach requires that the general pediatrician has a high level of suspicion and attempts to discern the cause as bacterial or viral, because this has implications for antimicrobial management.

CAP is changing, both in cause and in management approaches as more molecular diagnostics become available and well-performed trials are conducted. Despite this finding, although guidelines are available for patients with severe pediatric CAP, recommendations for mild to moderate cases, which constitute most cases seen by the general pediatrician, are based on evidence of poor to moderate quality.[77] This situation can lead to overtreatment[41] and, given the imprecise diagnostic methods available, unnecessary antibiotic treatment. There remain substantial gaps in the evidence for optimum management of pediatric CAP, from appropriate criteria for hospitalization to reference standards for identifying cases that need antibiotics, to what constitutes optimal antibiotic therapy.[78]

REFERENCES

1. Levine OS, O'Brien KL, Deloria-Knoll M, et al. The pneumonia etiology research for child health project: a 21st century childhood pneumonia etiology study. Clin Infect Dis 2012;54(Suppl 2):S93–101.
2. Cevey-Macherel M, Galetto-Lacour A, Gervaix A, et al. Etiology of community-acquired pneumonia in hospitalized children based on WHO clinical guidelines. Eur J Pediatr 2009;168(12):1429–36.
3. Juven T, Mertsola J, Waris M, et al. Etiology of community-acquired pneumonia in 254 hospitalized children. Pediatr Infect Dis J 2000;19(4):293–8.
4. Michelow IC, Olsen K, Lozano J, et al. Epidemiology and clinical characteristics of community-acquired pneumonia in hospitalized children. Pediatrics 2004; 113(4):701–7.
5. Baer G, Engelcke G, Abele-Horn M, et al. Role of *Chlamydia pneumoniae* and *Mycoplasma pneumoniae* as causative agents of community-acquired pneumonia in hospitalised children and adolescents. Eur J Clin Microbiol Infect Dis 2003;22(12):742–5.
6. Kurz H, Gopfrich H, Wabnegger L, et al. Role of *Chlamydophila pneumoniae* in children hospitalized for community-acquired pneumonia in Vienna, Austria. Pediatr Pulmonol 2009;44(9):873–6.
7. Heiskanen-Kosma T, Paldanius M, Korppi M. *Simkania negevensis* may be a true cause of community acquired pneumonia in children. Scand J Infect Dis 2008; 40(2):127–30.
8. Greenberg D, Banerji A, Friedman MG, et al. High rate of *Simkania negevensis* among Canadian Inuit infants hospitalized with lower respiratory tract infections. Scand J Infect Dis 2003;35(8):506–8.

9. Cilla G, Onate E, Perez-Yarza EG, et al. Viruses in community-acquired pneumonia in children aged less than 3 years old: high rate of viral coinfection. J Med Virol 2008;80(10):1843–9.
10. Singleton RJ, Bulkow LR, Miernyk K, et al. Viral respiratory infections in hospitalized and community control children in Alaska. J Med Virol 2010;82(7):1282–90.
11. Jansen RR, Wieringa J, Koekkoek SM, et al. Frequent detection of respiratory viruses without symptoms: toward defining clinically relevant cutoff values. J Clin Microbiol 2011;49(7):2631–6.
12. Peltola V, Waris M, Osterback R, et al. Rhinovirus transmission within families with children: incidence of symptomatic and asymptomatic infections. J Infect Dis 2008;197(3):382–9.
13. Iwane MK, Prill MM, Lu X, et al. Human rhinovirus species associated with hospitalizations for acute respiratory illness in young US children. J Infect Dis 2011; 204(11):1702–10.
14. Miller EK, Bugna J, Libster R, et al. Human rhinoviruses in severe respiratory disease in very low birth weight infants. Pediatrics 2012;129(1):e60–7.
15. van den Hoogen BG, de Jong JC, Groen J, et al. A newly discovered human pneumovirus isolated from young children with respiratory tract disease. Nat Med 2001;7(6):719–24.
16. Williams JV, Edwards KM, Weinberg GA, et al. Population-based incidence of human metapneumovirus infection among hospitalized children. J Infect Dis 2010;201(12):1890–8.
17. Wolf DG, Greenberg D, Shemer-Avni Y, et al. Association of human metapneumovirus with radiologically diagnosed community-acquired alveolar pneumonia in young children. J Pediatr 2010;156(1):115–20.
18. Schildgen O, Muller A, Allander T, et al. Human bocavirus: passenger or pathogen in acute respiratory tract infections? Clin Microbiol Rev 2008;21(2): 291–304 table of contents.
19. Allander T, Andreasson K, Gupta S, et al. Identification of a third human polyomavirus. J Virol 2007;81(8):4130–6.
20. Gaynor AM, Nissen MD, Whiley DM, et al. Identification of a novel polyomavirus from patients with acute respiratory tract infections. PLoS Pathog 2007;3(5):e64.
21. Lin F, Zheng M, Li H, et al. WU polyomavirus in children with acute lower respiratory tract infections, China. J Clin Virol 2008;42(1):94–102.
22. Yuan XH, Jin Y, Xie ZP, et al. Prevalence of human KI and WU polyomaviruses in children with acute respiratory tract infection in China. J Clin Microbiol 2008; 46(10):3522–5.
23. Ksiazek TG, Erdman D, Goldsmith CS, et al. A novel coronavirus associated with severe acute respiratory syndrome. N Engl J Med 2003;348(20):1953–66.
24. Kuiken T, Fouchier RA, Schutten M, et al. Newly discovered coronavirus as the primary cause of severe acute respiratory syndrome. Lancet 2003;362(9380): 263–70.
25. Rota PA, Oberste MS, Monroe SS, et al. Characterization of a novel coronavirus associated with severe acute respiratory syndrome. Science 2003;300(5624): 1394–9.
26. Dominguez SR, Robinson CC, Holmes KV. Detection of four human coronaviruses in respiratory infections in children: a one-year study in Colorado. J Med Virol 2009;81(9):1597–604.
27. Harris JR, Lockhart SR, Debess E, et al. *Cryptococcus gattii* in the United States: clinical aspects of infection with an emerging pathogen. Clin Infect Dis 2011; 53(12):1188–95.

28. Sellers B, Hall P, Cine-Gowdie S, et al. *Cryptococcus gattii*: an emerging fungal pathogen in the southeastern United States. Am J Med Sci 2012;343(6):510–1.
29. Jadavji T, Law B, Lebel MH, et al. A practical guide for the diagnosis and treatment of pediatric pneumonia. CMAJ 1997;156(5):S703–11.
30. Langley JM, Bradley JS. Defining pneumonia in critically ill infants and children. Pediatr Crit Care Med 2005;6(Suppl 3):S9–13.
31. Palafox M, Guiscafre H, Reyes H, et al. Diagnostic value of tachypnoea in pneumonia defined radiologically. Arch Dis Child 2000;82(1):41–5.
32. Cherian T, John TJ, Simoes E, et al. Evaluation of simple clinical signs for the diagnosis of acute lower respiratory tract infection. Lancet 1988;2(8603):125–8.
33. Bradley JS, Byington CL, Shah SS, et al. The management of community-acquired pneumonia in infants and children older than 3 months of age: clinical practice guidelines by the Pediatric Infectious Diseases Society and the Infectious Diseases Society of America. Clin Infect Dis 2011;53(7):e25–76.
34. Klig JE. Office pediatrics: current perspectives on the outpatient evaluation and management of lower respiratory infections in children. Curr Opin Pediatr 2006;18(1):71–6.
35. Korppi M, Don M, Valent F, et al. The value of clinical features in differentiating between viral, pneumococcal and atypical bacterial pneumonia in children. Acta Paediatr 2008;97(7):943–7.
36. Bettenay FA, de Campo JF, McCrossin DB. Differentiating bacterial from viral pneumonias in children. Pediatr Radiol 1988;18(6):453–4.
37. Isaacs D. Problems in determining the etiology of community-acquired childhood pneumonia. Pediatr Infect Dis J 1989;8(3):143–8.
38. Coote N, McKenzie S. Diagnosis and investigation of bacterial pneumonias. Paediatr Respir Rev 2000;1(1):8–13.
39. Hazir T, Fox LM, Nisar YB, et al. Ambulatory short-course high-dose oral amoxicillin for treatment of severe pneumonia in children: a randomised equivalency trial. Lancet 2008;371(9606):49–56.
40. Virkki R, Juven T, Rikalainen H, et al. Differentiation of bacterial and viral pneumonia in children. Thorax 2002;57(5):438–41.
41. Clark JE, Hammal D, Spencer D, et al. Children with pneumonia: how do they present and how are they managed? Arch Dis Child 2007;92(5):394–8.
42. Kin Key N, Araujo-Neto CA, Nascimento-Carvalho CM. Severity of childhood community-acquired pneumonia and chest radiographic findings. Pediatr Pulmonol 2009;44(3):249–52.
43. Harris M, Clark J, Coote N, et al. British Thoracic Society guidelines for the management of community acquired pneumonia in children: update 2011. Thorax 2011;66(Suppl 2):ii1–23.
44. Korppi M. Non-specific host response markers in the differentiation between pneumococcal and viral pneumonia: what is the most accurate combination? Pediatr Int 2004;46(5):545–50.
45. Korppi M, Remes S, Heiskanen-Kosma T. Serum procalcitonin concentrations in bacterial pneumonia in children: a negative result in primary healthcare settings. Pediatr Pulmonol 2003;35(1):56–61.
46. Don M, Valent F, Korppi M, et al. Differentiation of bacterial and viral community-acquired pneumonia in children. Pediatr Int 2009;51(1):91–6.
47. Lahti E, Peltola V, Waris M, et al. Induced sputum in the diagnosis of childhood community-acquired pneumonia. Thorax 2009;64(3):252–7.
48. Scott JA, Brooks WA, Peiris JS, et al. Pneumonia research to reduce childhood mortality in the developing world. J Clin Invest 2008;118(4):1291–300.

49. Vuori E, Peltola H, Kallio MJ, et al. Etiology of pneumonia and other common childhood infections requiring hospitalization and parenteral antimicrobial therapy. SE-TU Study Group. Clin Infect Dis 1998;27(3):566–72.
50. Dowell SF, Garman RL, Liu G, et al. Evaluation of Binax NOW, an assay for the detection of pneumococcal antigen in urine samples, performed among pediatric patients. Clin Infect Dis 2001;32(5):824–5.
51. Madhi SA, Klugman KP. A role for *Streptococcus pneumoniae* in virus-associated pneumonia. Nat Med 2004;10(8):811–3.
52. Gorman SK, Slavik RS, Marin J. Corticosteroid treatment of severe community-acquired pneumonia. Ann Pharmacother 2007;41(7):1233–7.
53. Weiss AK, Hall M, Lee GE, et al. Adjunct corticosteroids in children hospitalized with community-acquired pneumonia. Pediatrics 2011;127(2):e255–63.
54. Bright RA, Shay DK, Shu B, et al. Adamantane resistance among influenza A viruses isolated early during the 2005-2006 influenza season in the United States. JAMA 2006;295(8):891–4.
55. Heinonen S, Silvennoinen H, Lehtinen P, et al. Early oseltamivir treatment of influenza in children 1-3 years of age: a randomized controlled trial. Clin Infect Dis 2010;51(8):887–94.
56. Pakistan Multicentre Amoxycillin Short Course Therapy (MASCOT) pneumonia study group. Clinical efficacy of 3 days versus 5 days of oral amoxicillin for treatment of childhood pneumonia: a multicentre double-blind trial. Lancet 2002; 360(9336):835–41.
57. Agarwal G, Awasthi S, Kabra SK, et al. Three day versus five day treatment with amoxicillin for non-severe pneumonia in young children: a multicentre randomised controlled trial. BMJ 2004;328(7443):791.
58. Haider BA, Saeed MA, Bhutta ZA. Short-course versus long-course antibiotic therapy for non-severe community-acquired pneumonia in children aged 2 months to 59 months. Cochrane Database Syst Rev 2008;(2):CD005976.
59. Blaschke AJ, Heyrend C, Byington CL, et al. Molecular analysis improves pathogen identification and epidemiologic study of pediatric parapneumonic empyema. Pediatr Infect Dis J 2011;30(4):289–94.
60. Breiman RF, Butler JC, Tenover FC, et al. Emergence of drug-resistant pneumococcal infections in the United States. JAMA 1994;271(23):1831–5.
61. Richter SS, Heilmann KP, Coffman SL, et al. The molecular epidemiology of penicillin-resistant *Streptococcus pneumoniae* in the United States, 1994-2000. Clin Infect Dis 2002;34(3):330–9.
62. Richter SS, Heilmann KP, Dohrn CL, et al. Changing epidemiology of antimicrobial-resistant *Streptococcus pneumoniae* in the United States, 2004-2005. Clin Infect Dis 2009;48(3):e23–33.
63. Tan TQ, Mason EO Jr, Barson WJ, et al. Clinical characteristics and outcome of children with pneumonia attributable to penicillin-susceptible and penicillin-nonsusceptible *Streptococcus pneumoniae*. Pediatrics 1998;102(6):1369–75.
64. Committee on Infectious Diseases. The use of systemic fluoroquinolones. Pediatrics 2006;118(3):1287–92.
65. Bradley JS, Arguedas A, Blumer JL, et al. Comparative study of levofloxacin in the treatment of children with community-acquired pneumonia. Pediatr Infect Dis J 2007;26(10):868–78.
66. Centers for Disease Control and Prevention (CDC). Pertussis–United States, 1997-2000. MMWR Morb Mortal Wkly Rep 2002;51(4):73–6.
67. Duke T, Mgone CS. Measles: not just another viral exanthem. Lancet 2003; 361(9359):763–73.

68. Allison MA, Daley MF, Crane LA, et al. Influenza vaccine effectiveness in healthy 6- to 21-month-old children during the 2003-2004 season. J Pediatr 2006;149(6): 755–62.
69. Ampofo K, Bender J, Sheng X, et al. Seasonal invasive pneumococcal disease in children: role of preceding respiratory viral infection. Pediatrics 2008;122(2): 229–37.
70. Finelli L, Fiore A, Dhara R, et al. Influenza-associated pediatric mortality in the United States: increase of *Staphylococcus aureus* coinfection. Pediatrics 2008; 122(4):805–11.
71. Cutts FT, Zaman SM, Enwere G, et al. Efficacy of nine-valent pneumococcal conjugate vaccine against pneumonia and invasive pneumococcal disease in The Gambia: randomised, double-blind, placebo-controlled trial. Lancet 2005; 365(9465):1139–46.
72. Klugman KP, Madhi SA, Huebner RE, et al. A trial of a 9-valent pneumococcal conjugate vaccine in children with and those without HIV infection. N Engl J Med 2003;349(14):1341–8.
73. Pilishvili T, Lexau C, Farley MM, et al. Sustained reductions in invasive pneumococcal disease in the era of conjugate vaccine. J Infect Dis 2010;201(1):32–41.
74. Kalaskar AS, Heresi GP, Wanger A, et al. Severe necrotizing pneumonia in children, Houston, Texas, USA. Emerg Infect Dis 2009;15(10):1696–8.
75. Obando I, Munoz-Almagro C, Arroyo LA, et al. Pediatric parapneumonic empyema, Spain. Emerg Infect Dis 2008;14(9):1390–7.
76. Black RE, Cousens S, Johnson HL, et al. Global, regional, and national causes of child mortality in 2008: a systematic analysis. Lancet 2010;375(9730):1969–87.
77. Woodhead M. Community-acquired pneumonia guidelines: much guidance, but not much evidence. Eur Respir J 2002;20(1):1–3.
78. Esposito S, Principi N. Unsolved problems in the approach to pediatric community-acquired pneumonia. Curr Opin Infect Dis 2012;25(3):286–91.
79. WHO guidelines on detecting pneumonia in children. Lancet 1991;338(8780): 1453–4.
80. World Health Organization. Technical bases for the WHO recommendations on the management of pneumonia in children at first-level health facilities. Geneva (Switzerland): WHO; 1991.
81. Kumar P, McKean MC. Evidence based paediatrics: review of BTS guidelines for the management of community acquired pneumonia in children. J Infect 2004; 48(2):134–8.
82. McIntosh K. Community-acquired pneumonia in children. N Engl J Med 2002; 346(6):429–37.

Rocky Mountain Spotted Fever in Children

Charles R. Woods, MD, MS

KEYWORDS

- Rocky mountain spotted fever • *Rickettsia rickettsii* • Rash
- Increased intracranial pressure • Sepsis • Doxycycline

KEY POINTS

- Rocky Mountain spotted fever (RMSF) is typically undifferentiated from many other infections in the first few days of illness.
- Treatment should not be delayed pending confirmation of infection when RMSF is suspected.
- Doxycycline is the drug of choice even for infants and children less than 8 years old.

INTRODUCTION

RMSF is caused by *Rickettsia rickettsii*, the prototypical member of the spotted fever subgroup of rickettsial species. RMSF was first recognized as a clinical entity in the 1890s in Idaho and Montana. In the past century, RMSF has been identified within 46 states in the United States. *R rickettsii* also causes disease in many parts of Central and South America, where the infection is given other names, such as Brazilian spotted fever or febre maculosa.[1,2]

The spotted fever subgroup of *Rickettsia* now consists of 20 known species that cause similar illnesses worldwide.[3–5] *R parkeri* and other related species are present among tick populations in the United States. Infection by these related species may account in part for the apparent increase in probable, but not confirmed, cases of RMSF in the United States in recent years.[6] RMSF remains a nationally notifiable disease, but reporting was changed in 2010 under the broader category of spotted fever rickettsiosis.[7]

The pathogenesis, clinical features, and management of infections caused by the various agents of spotted fever rickettsiosis are largely the same. Laboratory studies of *R conorii*, the cause of Mediterranean spotted fever, have provided many insights into *R rickettsii* infections.

Department of Pediatrics, University of Louisville School of Medicine, 571 South Floyd Street, Suite 321, Louisville, KY 40202, USA
E-mail address: charles.woods@louisville.edu

Pediatr Clin N Am 60 (2013) 455–470
http://dx.doi.org/10.1016/j.pcl.2012.12.001 **pediatric.theclinics.com**

MICROBIOLOGY

R rickettsii is an obligate intracellular bacterium that must invade eukaryotic cells for ongoing survival and replication. The microbes are pleomorphic, nonmotile coccobacilli that are approximately 0.3 μm by 1.0 μm in size and stain weakly gram negative. The species produces no known toxins.[8,9] The circular bacterial chromosome of *R rickettsii* is highly conserved and small (approximately 1.25 Mb) compared with most other bacterial species.[5,10,11] Whole-genome sequencing indicates a repertoire of approximately 1495 genes. The species lacks many genes that encode proteins necessary for carbohydrate metabolism or synthesis of lipids and nucleic acids and thus must scavenge multiple substrates from within the host cells it invades. It cannot use glucose but instead acquires adenosine triphosphate from host cells.[12] *R rickettsii* cannot be propagated in standard culture media; specific cell lines are required.[8,13]

VECTORS AND TRANSMISSION

Spotted fever rickettsia are zoonotic tick-borne microbes that are maintained in the wild by a cycle of transmission between ixodid (hard-bodied) ticks and small mammals. Humans are accidental hosts. Domesticated animals, primarily dogs, may serve to bring infected ticks into close proximity with humans. Dogs may develop illness with infection that is usually self-limited.[8] Once a tick is infected with one rickettsial species, it is resistant to infection by other rickettsia, a phenomenon labeled rickettsial interference.[14]

R rickettsii infection is maintained through all stages of the ixodid lifecycle, which takes a year or more to complete. The lifecycle requires 3 blood meals from mammalian hosts. Larvae emerge from eggs, feed, detach, and molt into nymphs. Nymphs feed, detach, and molt into adults. Adult females feed, detach, and lay eggs on the ground. *R rickettsii* is transmitted from adult females to eggs (transovarian) and during molting (trans-stadial). Transovarial transmission reduces survival and reproductive capacity of the tick hosts. Horizontal transmission, from tick to tick via blood of an infected mammal, occurs but plays a lesser role in maintaining the zoonosis.[15–18] Frequency of *R rickettsii* carriage by *Dermacentor variabilis* in the United States is less than 1%.[17,19]

RMSF is transmitted to humans only by adult ticks, which release microbes from their salivary glands after 6 to 10 hours of feeding.[1] At least 5 ixodid tick species may harbor *R rickettsii*[5,20,21]:

- *D andersoni* (Rocky Mountain wood tick)—predominant vector in the Eastern United States
- *D variabilis* (American dog tick)—predominant vector in the Western United States.
- *Rhipicephalus sanguineus* (brown dog tick)—recently recognized vector in Arizona and Mexico
- *Amblyomma cajennense* (the cayenne tick)—vector in Central and South America and in Texas
- *A aureolatum*—vector in Central and South America

The Lone Star tick, *A americanum*, also rarely may function as a vector for RMSF.[22,23] Tick vectors in the United States are shown in **Fig. 1**.

Tick hemolymph also harbors microbes. Transmission to humans can occur when ticks are crushed during attempted removal from the skin.[8] Infection has occurred via blood transfusion,[24] health care–associated needle-stick injury,[25] and laboratory accidents.[26,27]

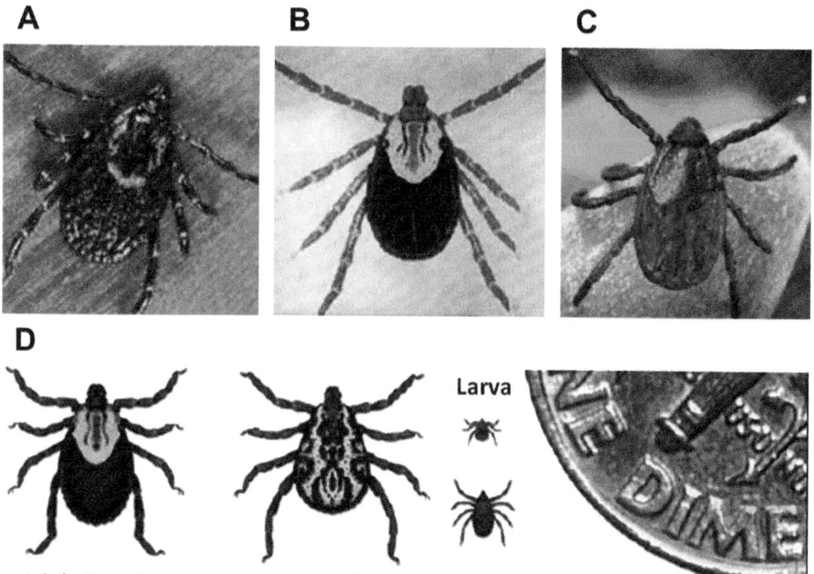

Fig. 1. Primary tick species responsible for transmission of RMSF in the United States. (*A*) Adult female *D variabilis*. (*B*) Adult female *D andersoni*. (*C*) Adult female *Rhipicephalus sanguineus*. (*D*) Relative sizes of adult female, adult male, nymph, and larval forms of *D variabilis*. (*Adapted from* Chapman AS, Bakken JS, Folk SM, et al. Diagnosis and management of tickborne rickettsial diseases: rocky mountain spotted fever, Ehrlichiosis, and Anaplasmosis—United States. A practical guide for physicians and other health-care and public health professionals. MMWR Morb Mortal Wkly Rep 2006;55(RR04):1–27.)

EPIDEMIOLOGY

The geographic distribution of RMSF correlates with presence of its tick vectors.[28] In the continental United States, only Vermont and Maine did not report cases from 2000 to 2007.[6,29] Geographic distribution of reported cases by counties in the United States in 2009 is shown in **Fig. 2**. The incidence of reported cases of RMSF in the United States since 1920 is shown in **Fig. 3**. The availability of effective antimicrobial agents in the 1950s was associated with a decline in reported cases that seemed to reverse in the 1960s. There seems to be a 30-year to 40-year cycle of disease for reasons that are unclear.[1]

Between 2000 and 2008, aggregate incidence was 2 to 4 per million among children ages 1 to 19 years old and 6 to 8 per million among adults over 40 years old.[7] Incidence in the United States rose from 1.7 per million persons (495 cases) in 2000 to 8 per million (2563 cases) in 2008. Explanations for this 4-fold increase include changes in diagnostic and surveillance practices in addition to potential increases in frequency, because most reported cases are probable rather than confirmed. Cross-reactivity of serologic tests for RMSF with other spotted fever rickettsia also may be a factor.[1,6,30]

The largest seroprevalence study in children showed a rate of 12% overall in convenience samples from 7 centers in endemic areas of the South and Midwest.[31] Seroprevalence rates were 10% to 16% among children in 2 communities in Arizona at the time of an outbreak of RMSF associated with the newly recognized brown dog tick vector in 2003 and 2004.[20,32]

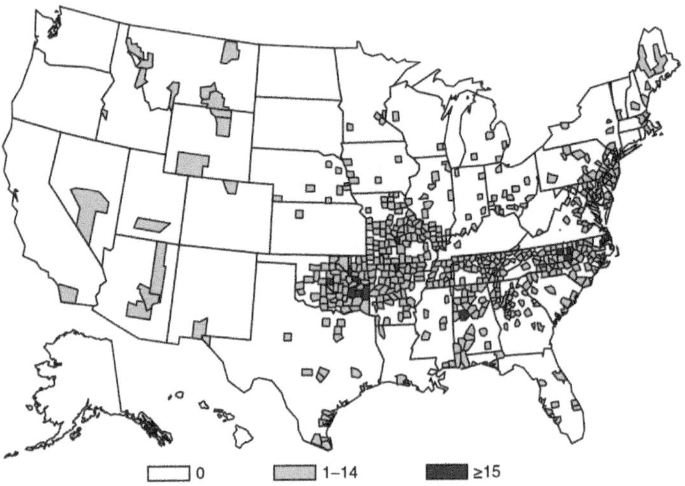

Fig. 2. Number of reported cases of RMSF by county, United States, 2009. RMSF is reported throughout most of the United States, reflecting the widespread distribution of the primary tick vectors responsible for transmission (*D variabilis* in the East, *D andersoni* in the West, and *Rhipicephalus sanguineus* in parts of the Southwest). (*From* the Centers for Disease Control and Prevention. Rocky mountain spotted fever (RMSF). Available at: http://www.cdc.gov/rmsf/stats/index.html. Accessed January 24, 2013.)

A great majority of cases in children and adults occur during April through September, but cases have been reported from all months of the year.[28,33] Male patients comprise approximately 57% of cases reported in recent years.[6] Cases are more common in rural and suburban areas due to increased opportunities for exposure to the tick vectors, but urban cases have been reported, even in New York City.[8,34] Clusters of cases among family members also have occurred.[35] Concurrent infections have been observed in humans and their dogs.[36]

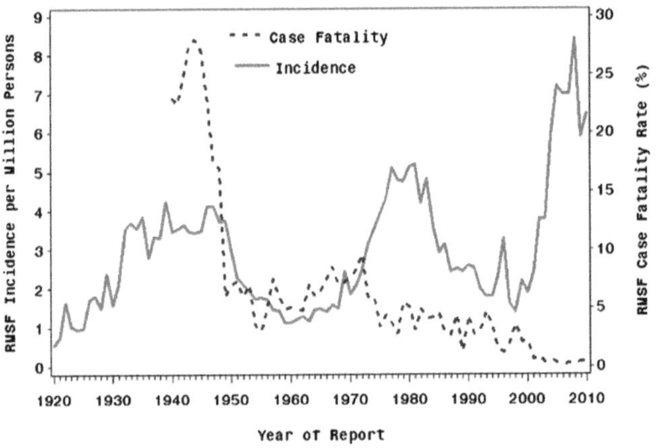

Fig. 3. Incidence and case-fatality of RMSF in the United States, 1920–2008. The recent increase in incidence and decrease in case fatality partially may reflect changes in reporting and diagnosis. Note the 30-year to 40-year cycle in incidence. (*From* the Centers for Disease Control and Prevention. Rocky mountain spotted fever (RMSF). Available at: http://www.cdc.gov/rmsf/stats/index.html. Accessed January 24, 2013.)

Host factors that may be associated with increased severity of RMSF include older age, male gender, and presence of glucose-6-phosphate dehydrogenase deficiency.[37–39] Greater severity also has been observed in African American patients. Issue of access to care, difficulties in recognizing the presence of rash, and delays in receipt of effective antimicrobial therapy may explain this racial disparity more than any host susceptibility or microbial virulence factors.[8,40]

PATHOGENESIS

R rickettsii has primary tropism for endothelial cells. As microbial replication progresses, blood vessels throughout the body, including the skin, brain, liver, spleen, lungs, and heart, become infected, with progressive focal disruptions of endothelial integrity. A distinctive perivascular infiltrate of lymphocytes and macrophages ensues. Most clinical features of RMSF derive from the resulting increased vascular permeability.[8]

Once *R rickettsii* is inoculated into the epidermis during adult tick feeding, microbes presumably spread to regional lymph nodes via lymphatic vessels.[26,41] *R rickettsii* then reach the bloodstream and begin to invade the endothelium of small and medium-sized blood vessels. Oxidative and peroxidative injury to endothelial membranes from the net effects of phospholipase, proteases, and free radical production leads to cell necrosis.[26,42–44]

Focal areas of vasculitis in the epidermis generate the erythematous spots of spotted fever. Capillaries, arterioles, and venules are involved.[45] Progressive endothelial injury can lead to microhemorrhages in addition to increased permeability. Leakage of fluid into organ tissues, such as in the lung or brain, which lack lymphatic vessels to drain interstitial fluid, can lead to pulmonary insufficiency and increased intracranial pressure, respectively.[26]

R rickettsii induces a procoagulant state, secondary to endothelial injury, with thrombin generation, platelet activation, increased fibrinolysis, and consumption of anticoagulants. Yet, development of actual disseminated intravascular coagulation is rare in RMSF. The multiorgan dysfunction that develops in some fatal cases seems more the result of vascular insufficiency than major hemorrhage or vaso-occlusive infarcts.[8,42,46,47]

At the molecular level, rickettsial outer membrane protein B (OmpB) and other microbial surface structures function as adhesins and bind microbes to endothelial cells. OmpB attaches to Ku70 molecules on the host cell surface and recruits additional Ku70 to the host cell membrane. Ku70 is a subunit of a DNA-dependent protein kinase ubiquitously expressed in mammalian cells and typically located in the nucleus and cytoplasm.[48,49] Localization of Ku70 to the cell membrane is restricted to endothelial cells and monocytes, the 2 main cellular targets in RMSF.

Attached microbes induce local rearrangement of the host cell cytoskeleton that leads to endocytosis.[26,49,50] This process is accomplished by microbial co-opting host cell actin nucleating protein complexes (Arp2/3) and various signaling processes, including those mediated by clathrin, caveolin 2, phosphoinositide 3-kinase, and other kinases.[13,51] After internalization, *R rickettsii* lyses its endosome using the enzymes phospholipase D and hemolysin C.[43] Rickettsia grow well in the high potassium concentration environs of the cytoplasm.[8]

Once free in the cytoplasm, *R rickettsii* migrate into adjacent cells by actin-based motility, which does not lyse the cells. Actin-based motility involves recruitment of host cell actin filaments, by expression of the microbial protein RickA, to form a filamentous comet tail. These actin structures propel organisms rapidly through the cytoplasm to the host cell surface, creating structures that invaginate membranes of adjacent cells. These protrusions are engulfed by the neighboring cell, resulting in local intercellular spread of infection.[8,43,52,53]

Disruption of endothelial intercellular adherens junction complexes occurs within 48 hours of infection and is associated with phosphorylation of vascular endothelial cadherin, a major component of junctional complexes.[54,55] This leads to the characteristic vascular hyperpermeability of RMSF.

Virulence of microbes that reside in tick salivary glands declines during the prolonged winter starvation period. Virulence is restored within 24 to 72 hours of either allowing ticks to take a blood meal or exposing them to a temperature of 37°C.[56,57] This likely reflects environmental regulation of microbial genes that facilitate virulence or simply replication or both.

Higher microbial inocula in prison volunteers, in a study subsequently criticized on ethical grounds, were associated with higher frequency of symptomatic infection, shorter incubation periods, and longer duration of fever.[8,58] Modeling studies suggest an inoculum of 23 organisms lead to symptomatic infection in 50% of those exposed. Risk of infection after intradermal inoculation of a single microbe is approximately 5%.[27]

HOST IMMUNE RESPONSE

Rickettsial infection of endothelial cells induces production of interleukin (IL)-6 and IL-8 and monocyte chemoattractant protein 1 via activation of nuclear factor-κB.[59,60] Natural killer cells are activated early in infection and produce interferon-γ, which can inhibit rickettsial growth. Infection also induces production of IL-1β and tumor necrosis factor α. Human endothelial cells can produce rickettsicidal amounts of nitric oxide (via inducible nitric oxide synthetase) and hydrogen peroxide in response to interferon-γ, IL-1β, and tumor necrosis factor α. Macrophages can kill rickettsia with hydrogen peroxide and tryptophan starvation in phagosomes by degradation of tryptophan by indoleamine 2,3-dioxygenase.[43,44]

Clearance of infection is associated with homing of CD4+ and CD8+ lymphocytes and macrophages to foci of infection in the microcirculation. These and dendritic cells are presumed the sources of proinflammatory cytokines that can activate killing within infected endothelial cells. CD8+ T-lymphocytes also may induce apoptosis of infected endothelial cells.[8,44,61]

Antibody responses directed against OmpA, OmpB, and Sca2 epitopes are protective against reinfection.[13,62,63] These antibodies typically are not produced in substantial quantities until a week or 2 after infection. Serologic response may be blunted by early treatment.[64]

CLINICAL FEATURES

The course of RMSF is variable, ranging from a mild to moderate, self-limited febrile illness to a severe life-threatening infection. A history of recent tick bite is reported in 50% to 66% of patients. Tick exposure can easily go unnoticed because the bites are painless and ticks may feed for several days without producing any irritation or discomfort. Ticks also often attach to the scalp, axillae, or perineum where they are not easily spotted. Eschars are rarely produced at the site of bite. The incubation period is typically 4 to 7 days but ranges from 2 to 14 days.[8,33,39,65–69]

Early symptoms and signs of infection are nonspecific. Fever is the earliest sign, occurs in at least 97% of children with RMSF, and often exceeds 102°F (38.9°C). Onset of illness is often abrupt but gradual onset occurs in approximately one-third of children and adults. Approximately 95% of children with RMSF have a rash at some point during the illness, compared with 80% of adults. In children, rash often appears on the first or second day of illness but may appear on the third or fourth day or beyond, which is more common in adults. The classic triad of fever, rash, and headache occurs in most but not all patients and often is not apparent early in the course.[8,33,39,65]

The typical exanthem consists of small, blanching pink macules on the ankles, wrists, or forearms (**Fig. 4**). The rash may become maculopapular and expand centripetally to involve proximal extremities and torso.[33,65,70] The spots of spotted fever are the end result of focal infection of small blood vessels in the skin. Palms and soles are involved in approximately half of cases, usually later in the course, and this is not pathognomonic for RMSF. The face is spared even when rash is diffuse. Rash may be evanescent or localized to a single area. A petechial component may develop in approximately 60% of children but usually not until 5 or more days into the illness. Patients with petechiae usually are severely ill. Skin lesions may progress to purpura or local areas of gangrene. Early skin findings may be difficult to appreciate in dark-skinned patients.[21,33,39,71]

Headache is present in 40% to 60% of children under 15 years old, more prominent in older children and adults, and often described as severe.[8,33,69] Headache is likely due to vasculitis-related increase in intracranial pressure, in addition to effects of circulating proinflammatory cytokines. Headache may manifest as irritability, inconsolability, or fussiness in infants and young children.

Malaise, myalgia, abdominal pain, nausea, vomiting, and/or diarrhea occur in at least 25% of children with RMSF.[33,69] Photophobia and conjunctival injection are sometimes seen. Lymphadenopathy, hepatomegaly, splenomegaly, and periorbital and peripheral edema are noted in approximately 20% to 25% of children. The constellation of symptoms and signs easily may be mistaken for common viral or bacterial infections that delay consideration of RMSF.

The central nervous system involvement occurs beyond headache. Altered mental status is seen in one-third or more of children ill enough to require hospitalization. Meningismus is noted in approximately 16%.[33,69] Seizures, cranial nerve palsies, coma, and hearing loss are not common but can occur. Significant neurologic manifestations are more common in older children and adults.[39] Death can result from cerebral herniation.

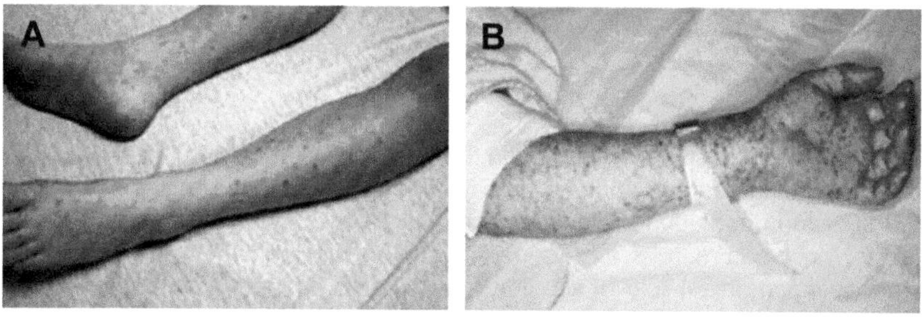

Fig. 4. Rash associated with RMSF. (*A*) Maculopapular rash on legs and feet. (*B*) Late petechial rash on forearm and hand. ([*A*] *Courtesy of* GS Marshall, University of Louisville School of Medicine, Louisville, KY; and [*B*] *From* Chapman AS, Bakken JS, Folk SM, et al. Diagnosis and management of tickborne rickettsial diseases: Rocky Mountain spotted fever, ehrlichioses, and anaplasmosis—United States: a practical guide for physicians and other health-care and public health professionals. MMWR Recomm Rep 2006;55(RR-4):1–27.)

Cough and sore throat occasionally occur. Pulmonary edema can develop in severe cases. Chest radiography within 48 hours of admission may show opacities suggestive of infiltrates or pneumonia in a third of hospitalized children.[33,72] Myocarditis can occur from vasculitis. Subclinical involvement may be common,[73] but heart failure, heart block, and other cardiac manifestations appear rare in children without advanced disease.

LABORATORY FINDINGS

Complete blood counts often are normal, especially early in the course. Thrombocytopenia, due to platelet sequestration and destruction in the microcirculation, occurs in approximately 60% of hospitalized children.[33,69] Fulminant disseminated intravascular coagulation is rare.[8] Leukocytosis is present in approximately 25% and leukopenia in approximately 10% of children.[33]

Hyponatremia occurs in up to half of patients, and 20% may have serum sodium concentrations below 130 mEq/L. This almost always reflects capillary leak from endothelial damage rather than secretion of inappropriate antidiuretic hormone. Mild to moderated elevations of hepatic transaminases are seen in approximately half of patients. Hyperbilirubinemia sufficient to produce jaundice is uncommon. Serum albumin concentrations may be low, consistent with increased vascular permeability.[33]

Serum creatinine and blood urea nitrogen concentrations may be elevated in advanced infection. Renal insufficiency is common in severe disease and may be caused by ischemia-related acute tubular necrosis, vasculitis of renal vessels, or microthrombosis. Creatine kinase concentrations may increase due to vasculitis-induced muscle injury.[8]

Cerebrospinal fluid obtained in 38 children hospitalized with RMSF showed mild pleocytosis in some, with an interquartile range of 3 to 38 white blood cells/mm^3. Mononuclear cell predominance is common. Cerebrospinal fluid protein concentrations are often mildly elevated, but hypoglycorrhachia is rare.[33,69]

CNS imaging is typically done only in severe cases of altered mental status. CT studies, when abnormal, have shown diffuse white matter changes, sulcal effacement from cerebral edema, and focal attenuations consistent with infarctions. MRI studies may demonstrate punctate areas of increased signal throughout the brain on T2-weighted images, consistent with perivascular inflammation, as well as arterial infarctions or meningeal enhancement.[74,75] Electroencephalography, when abnormal, usually demonstrates nonfocal cortical disturbances reflective of diffuse cerebral vasculitis.[8]

DIAGNOSIS

Serologic testing and skin biopsy remain the best means of confirming a diagnosis of RMSF. Immunofluorescent antibody assays are considered the best serologic tests for RMSF. Latex agglutination and enzyme-linked immunosorbent assays also are available. Most commercial assays measure both IgM and IgG. Demonstration of a seroconversion or a 4-fold or greater rise in serum antibody titers between acute and convalescent sera is considered confirmatory.[21] Antibodies against other spotted fever rickettsia, including *R parkeri*, can be cross-reactive in *R rickettsii* assays.[76]

IgM and IgG antibodies against *R rickettsii* typically increase concurrently during the second week of illness and usually are not detectable during the first 7 days of illness. Convalescent titers usually should be obtained 2 weeks after onset of illness, but seroconversion may take 4 weeks in some patients. A single immunofluorescent antibody assays titer greater than or equal to 1:64 or latex agglutination titer greater than or equal to 1:128 is suggestive of RMSF in compatible clinical settings. IgM concentrations wane after 3 to 4 months. IgG titers wane after 7 to 8 months but may persist at detectable levels for years.[21,65,77] Weil-Felix serologic tests, once a diagnostic mainstay, are not as reliable as current commercial assays.[78]

Skin biopsy (3–5 mm punch biopsy) of rash spots is useful in acute illness. Immunohistochemical staining is 100% specific and approximately 70% sensitive.[79] Polymerase chain reaction testing also can be done on skin specimens. Evaluation of skin biopsies for RMSF is not available in many locales. Health care providers can submit skin specimens to the Centers for Disease Control and Prevention for testing via their state health departments.[80]

Detection of *R rickettsii* by blood smears or polymerase chain reaction tests is insensitive due to low numbers of circulating bacteria. Culture of skin or other specimens using tissue culture methods is technically feasible but can be conducted only by laboratories, such as the Centers for Disease Control and Prevention, that can follow biosafety level 3 containment procedures.[21]

DIFFERENTIAL DIAGNOSIS

Other tick-borne infections caused by relatives of *R rickettsii* can be similar to RMSF. Human monocytic ehrlichiosis caused by *Ehrlichia chaffeensis* can be indistinguishable clinically from RMSF. In human monocytic ehrlichiosis, hepatic transaminase elevation is often more prominent, leukopenia more frequent, and rash less frequent than in RMSF.[21,81] Human granulocytic ehrlichiosis caused by *Anaplasma phagocytophilum* (and *E ewingii*) rarely has associated rash and may have more gradual onset of illness.[82] *R parkeri* and a newly recognized spotted fever group microbe, *Candidatus R andeanae*, can cause illness similar to mild RMSF. These microbes are transmitted by the Gulf Coast tick, *A maculatum*.[83]

Other infections that sometimes may mimic RMSF include human herpesvirus 6 (roseola), Epstein-Barr virus, enteroviruses, leptospirosis, human parvovirus, secondary syphilis, and *Mycoplasma pneumoniae*. Clinical courses of Kawasaki disease, drug reactions, erythema multiforme, and immune complex-mediated illnesses also can overlap substantially with RMSF. Petechial rashes can be seen with meningococcal infection, disseminated gonococcal infection, immune thrombotic thrombocytopenic purpura, and after group A streptococcal pharyngitis. Meningococcal infection usually progresses more rapidly than RMSF.[21]

Rash on palms and soles may be caused by drug hypersensitivity reactions, bacterial endocarditis, secondary syphilis, rate bite fever (*Streptobacillus moniliformis*), certain enteroviruses, ehrlichiosis, and meningococcal infection.[21]

TREATMENT

Doxycycline is the antimicrobial agent of choice for treatment of suspected RMSF in patients of all ages, even young infants.[65,84] Treatment should never be delayed while awaiting laboratory confirmation of the diagnosis.[29] When patients in endemic areas in spring and summer have fever and headache, providers should not wait for development of rash to initiate therapy.

Minimally ill febrile patients with epidemiologic risk but without other features indicative of RMSF can be observed during the first 3 days of illness, but such patients should be re-evaluated when illness continues beyond this time frame. A complete blood cell count and serum electrolyte concentrations may be helpful. Thrombocytopenia and/or hyponatremia should heighten suspicion for RMSF.[29,39]

Outpatient management is reasonable for patients who are only mildly ill. Hospitalized children generally require intravascular volume support. Intensive care monitoring and inotropic support may be necessary. Management of pulmonary edema or increased intracranial pressure may require mechanical ventilation. Dialysis may be needed for renal insufficiency develops.[65]

Because meningococcemia and RMSF can overlap substantially, a third-generation cephalosporin or other agent with activity against Neisseria *meningitidis* is usually administered when RMSF is suspected. β-Lactam antimicrobials are ineffective for RSMF.[21,65]

Doxycycline is administered at a dosage of 2.2 mg/kg per dose twice daily (every 12 hours when hospitalized) for children, up to the adult maximum dosage of 200 mg twice daily. Oral or intravenous routes may be used, depending on the degree of illness and the ability of patients to take oral medication. It is generally accepted to treat for 3 days after defervescence, which usually results in total course of 5 to 10 days. Patients initially treated intravenously can be switched to oral therapy when they can tolerate fluids or other oral therapies.[21,84]

The usual contraindication of age less than 8 years old for tetracyclines due to potential for dental discoloration does not apply when RMSF (or infections due to related microbes, including agents of human ehrlichiosis) is suspected. Short courses of doxycycline administered to young children at the dosage (indicated previously) for RMSF have not been associated with discoloration of permanent teeth.[65,85,86]

Chloramphenicol is the only other antimicrobial agent for which there is substantial clinical experience with treatment of RMSF. It is less effective for RMSF than doxycycline. Oral formulations of chloramphenicol are no longer available in the United States.[65,87]

Macrolides are not effective against *R rickettsii* and many related species and should not be prescribed for treatment of RMSF.[88] Sulfonamide antimicrobial agents also are inactive and anecdotal clinical experience and animal studies suggest that administration of these compounds may increase the severity of illness by mechanisms that are uncertain but potentially involve oxidative stress.[89,90]

PROGNOSIS

Most children with RMSF recover fully when treated. Serologic studies suggest subclinical or unrecognized symptomatic infections are somewhat common.[31] Case fatality among before availability of effective antimicrobials was usually 20% to 25%. Death can result from multiorgan system failure or cerebral herniation. Case fatality in the United States was approximately 2% in the early 1990s and decreased to 0.3% during 2003 to 2007. Children less than 10 years old (2.3%) and adults 70 years old or older (1.3%) have the highest case fatality. Patients with underlying immunosuppressive conditions have a 4.4-fold greater risk of death.[8,27,91]

Delay in therapy is associated with higher risk of death.[92,93] One large cohort study found case fatality of 5.3% among patients whose treatment was initiated on the fifth day of illness or beyond compared with 1.6% among those whose treatment was initiated earlier.[87] Delays in appropriate therapy more often result from clinician failure to consider RMSF than patient delay in seeking care.[65] In the most recent series of children hospitalized for RMSF in the United States, illness was present for a median of 6 days before admission, and 86% had at least 1 health care visit during that interval.[33] Factors associated with delay in therapy include presentation during winter or early spring; presentation with complaints other than fever, rash, and headache; and lack of history of tick bite.[39,87,93]

Neurologic deficits are the most common long-term sequelae. In the most recent pediatric series, 13 (15%) of 89 surviving patients had 1 or more neurologic deficits at the time of discharge. These included global encephalopathy, speech and/or swallowing dysfunction, ataxia or gait abnormality, and cortical blindness.[33] All had altered mental status and required initial intensive care. Other neurologic sequelae can include seizures, paresthesias, hearing loss, facial nerve palsy, and changes in personality.[94] Many neurologic deficits that occur during acute illness, including ataxia and cranial nerve palsies, improve or resolve over time.[33,69]

Avascular necrosis of digits, ear lobes, nose, and scrotum has been described.[33,69] This outcome occurs most commonly in patients who have progressed to septic shock.

PREVENTION

Tick exposure is more likely in wooded areas or areas with bushes and high grass or leaf litter. When working or recreating in such areas, wearing light-colored clothing that covers arms, legs, and other exposed areas and staying on the center of trails may be helpful. Locating play equipment in sunny, dry areas away from forest edges or creating a barrier of wood chips or gravel between recreation areas and forest may reduce likelihood of tick exposure. Permethrin-treated clothing can repel ticks and may be used by children of all ages and remains effective through approximately 20 washings. Maintaining tick-free pets also decreases tick exposure.[95,96]

For children older than 2 months of age, use of skin repellents that contain 20% to 30% diethyltoluamide on exposed skin can provide protection. Applications of newer microencapsulated formulations may be effective for 8 to 12 hours. Serious neurologic complications associated with use of diethyltoluamide in young children have been reported, but risk is low when products are used per manufacturer instructions.[65,95]

Children's bodies and clothing should be carefully inspected after possible tick exposure. Ticks often attach to exposed hairy regions, including the head, neck, and behind the ears. Risk of transmission increases the longer a tick is attached. Removal is best accomplished by grasping the tick close to the skin with fine tweezers, then gently pulling straight out without twisting.[95,96]

Because carriage of *R rickettsii* is 1% or less among its vectors, most tick bites do not result in infection. Antimicrobial prophylaxis for RMSF after tick exposure in endemic areas is not recommended. Formalin-fixed killed whole cell vaccines developed in past decades reduced disease severity but did not protect against infection. A live attenuated vaccine strain, *R rickettsii* Iowa, is protective in animal models but has not been studied in humans.[49,97]

REFERENCES

1. Lin L, Decker CF. Rocky mountain spotted fever. Dis Mon 2012;58(6):361–9.
2. Spencer RR. Rocky mountain spotted fever. J Infect Dis 1929;44:257–76.
3. Tamura A, Ohashi N, Urakami H, et al. Classification of Rickettsia tsutsugamushi in a new genus, Orientia gen. nov., as Orientia tsutsugamushi comb. nov. Int J Syst Bacteriol 1995;45(3):589–91.
4. Raoult D, Roux V. Rickettsioses as paradigms of new or emerging infectious diseases. Clin Microbiol Rev 1997;10(4):694–719.
5. Merhej V, Raoult D. Rickettsial evolution in the light of comparative genomics. Biol Rev Camb Philos Soc 2011;86(2):379–405.
6. Openshaw JJ, Swerdlow DL, Krebs JW, et al. Rocky Mountain Spotted Fever in the United States, 2000-2007: interpreting contemporary increases in incidence. Am J Trop Med Hyg 2010;83(1):174–82.

7. Centers for Disease Control and Prevention. Annual cases of RMSF in the United States. Available at: http://www.cdc.gov/rmsf/stats/index.html. Accessed October 1, 2012.
8. Chen LF, Sexton DJ. What's new in Rocky Mountain spotted fever. Infect Dis Clin North Am 2008;22(3):415–32.
9. Hayes SF, Burgdorfer W. Reactivation of Rickettsia rickettsii in Dermacentor andersonii ticks: an ultrastructural analysis. Infect Immun 1982;37(2):779–85.
10. Roux V, Drancourt M, Raoult D. Determination of genome sizes of Rickettsia spp. within the spotted fever group, using pulsed-field gel electrophoresis. J Bacteriol 1992;174(22):7455–7.
11. Andersson SG, Kruland CG. Reductive evolution of resident genomes. Trends Microbiol 1998;6(7):263–8.
12. Audia JP, Winkler HH. Study of the five Rickettsii prowazekii proteins annotated as ATP/ADP translocases (Tlc): only Tlc1 transports ATP/ADP, while Tlc4 and Tlc5 transport other ribonucleotides. J Bacteriol 2006;188(17):6261–8.
13. Riley SP, Goh KC, Hermanas TM, et al. The Rickettsia conorii autotransporter protein Sca1 promotes adherence to nonphagocytic mammalian cells. Infect Immun 2010;78(5):1895–904.
14. Carmichael JR, Fuerst PA. A rickettsial mixed infection in a Dermacentor variabilis tick from Ohio. Ann N Y Acad Sci 2006;1078:334–7.
15. McDade JE, Newhouse VF. Natural history of Rickettsia rickettsii. Annu Rev Microbiol 1986;40:287–309.
16. Allan SA. Ticks (Class Arachnida; Order Acarina). In: Samuel WM, Pybus MJ, Kocan AA, editors. Parasitic diseases of wild mammals. Ames (IA): Iowa State University Press; 2001. p. 72–106.
17. Stromdahl EY, Jiang J, Vince M, et al. Infrequency of Rickettsia rickettsii in Dermacentor variabilis removed from humans, with comments on the role of other human-biting ticks associated with spotted fever group Rickettsiae in the United States. Vector Borne Zoonotic Dis 2001;11(7):969–77.
18. Burgdorfer W, Brinton LP. Mechanisms of transovarial infection of spotted fever Rickettsiae in ticks. Ann N Y Acad Sci 1975;266:61–72.
19. Fritzen CM, Huang J, Westby K, et al. Infection prevalences of common tick-borne pathogens in adult lone star ticks (Amblyomma americanum) and American dog ticks (Dermacentor variabilis) in Kentucky. Am J Trop Med Hyg 2011;85(4):718–23.
20. Demma LJ, Traeger MS, Nicholson WL, et al. Rocky Mountain Spotted Fever from an unexpected tick vector in Arizona. N Engl J Med 2005;353(6):587–94.
21. Chapman AS, Bakken JS, Folk SM, et al. Diagnosis and management of tick-borne rickettsial diseases: rocky mountain spotted fever, Ehrlichiosis, and Anaplasmosis—United States. A practical guide for physicians and other health-care and public health professionals. MMWR Morb Mortal Wkly Rep 2006;55(RR04):1–27.
22. Breitschwerdt EB, Hegarty BC, Maggi RG, et al. Rickettsia rickettsii transmission by a lone star tick, North Carolina. Emerg Infect Dis 2011;17(5):873–5.
23. Smith MP, Ponnusamy L, Jiang J, et al. Bacterial pathogens in ixodid ticks from a piedmont county in North Carolina: prevalence of rickettsial organisms. Vector Borne Zoonotic Dis 2010;10(10):939–52.
24. Wells GM, Woodward TE, Fiset P, et al. Rocky mountain spotted fever caused by blood transfusion. JAMA 1978;239(26):2763–5.
25. Sexton DJ, Gallis HA, McRae JR, et al. Letter: possible needle-associated Rocky Mountain spotted fever. N Engl J Med 1975;292(12):645.

26. Walker DH, Valbuena GA, Olano JP. Pathogenic mechanisms of diseases caused by Rickettsia. Ann N Y Acad Sci 2003;990:1–11.
27. Tamrakar SB, Haas CN. Dose-response model of Rocky Mountain spotted fever (RMSF) for Human. Risk Anal 2011;31(10):1610–21.
28. D'Angelo LJ, Winkler WG, Bregman DJ. Rocky Mountain Spotted Fever in the United States: 1975-1977. J Infect Dis 1978;138(2):273–6.
29. Centers for Disease Control and Prevention. Consequences of delayed diagnosis of Rocky Mountain Spotted Fever in children—West Virginia, Michigan, Tennessee, and Oklahoma, May—July 2000. MMWR Morb Mortal Wkly Rep 2000; 49(39):885–8.
30. Centers for Disease Control and Prevention. Summary of notifiable diseases—United States, 2010. MMWR Morb Mortal Wkly Rep 2012;59(53):1–116.
31. Marshall GS, Stout GG, Jacobs RF, et al. Antibodies reactive to Rickettsia rickettsii among children in the southeast and south central regions of the United States. Arch Pediatr Adolesc Med 2003;157(5):443–8.
32. Demma LJ, Traeger M, Blau D, et al. Serologic evidence for exposure to Rickettsia rickettsii in eastern Arizona and recent emergence of Rocky Mountain spotted fever in this region. Vector Borne Zoonotic Dis 2006;6(4):432–9.
33. Buckingham SC, Marshall GS, Schutze GE, et al. Clinical and laboratory features, hospital course, and outcome of Rocky Mountain Spotted Fever in children. J Pediatr 2007;150(2):180–4.
34. Salgo MP, Telsak E, Currie B, et al. A focus of Rocky Mountain spotted fever within New York City. N Engl J Med 1988;318(21):1345–8.
35. Centers for Disease Control and Prevention. Fatal cases of Rocky Mountain Spotted Fever in family clusters—three states, 2003. MMWR Morb Mortal Wkly Rep 2004;53(19):407–10.
36. Paddock CD, Brenner O, Vaid C, et al. Short report: concurrent Rocky Mountain spotted fever in a dog and its owner. Am J Trop Med Hyg 2002;66(2):197–9.
37. Walker DH, Kirkman HN. Rocky Mountain spotted fever and deficiency in glucose-6-phosphate dehydrogenase. J Infect Dis 1980;142:771.
38. Walker DH. The role of host factors in the severity of spotted fever and typhus rickettsioses. Ann N Y Acad Sci 1990;590:10–9.
39. Helmick CG, Bernard KW, D'Angelo LJ. Rocky Mountain spotted fever: clinical, laboratory, and epidemiological features of 262 cases. J Infect Dis 1984; 150(4):480–8.
40. McDade JE. Diagnosis of rickettsial diseases: a perspective. Eur J Epidemiol 1991;7(3):270–5.
41. Mansueto P, Vitale G, Di Lorenzo G, et al. Immunology of human rickettsial diseases. J Biol Regul Homeost Agents 2008;22(2):131–9.
42. Rydkina E, Sahni SK, Santucci LA, et al. Selective modulation of antioxidant enzyme activities in host tissues during Rickettsia conorii infection. Microb Pathog 2004;36(6):293–301.
43. Walker DH. Rickettsiae and Rickettsial infections: the current state of knowledge. Clin Infect Dis 2007;45(Suppl 1):S39–44.
44. Valbuena G, Feng HM, Walker DH. Mechanisms of immunity against rickettsiae: new perspectives and opportunities offered by unusual intracellular parasite. Microbes Infect 2002;4(6):625–33.
45. Bradford WD, Hawkins HK. Rocky mountain spotted fever in childhood. Am J Dis Child 1977;131(11):1228–32.
46. Elgetany MT, Walker DH. Hemostatic changes in Rocky mountain spotted fever and Mediterranean spotted fever. Am J Clin Pathol 1999;112(2):159–68.

47. Schmaier AH, Srikanth S, Elghetany MT, et al. Hemostatic/fibrinolytic protein changes in C3H/HeN mice infected with Rickettsia conorii—a model for Rocky Mountain spotted fever. Thromb Haemost 2001;86(3):871–9.
48. Martinez JJ, Seveau S, Velga E, et al. Ku70, a component of DNA-dependent protein kinase, is a mammalian receptor for Rickettsia conorii. Cell 2005;123(6): 1013–23.
49. Chan YG, Riley SP, Martinez JJ. Adherence to and invasion of host cells by spotted fever group Rickettsia species. Front Microbiol 2010;1:139. http://dx.doi.org/10.3389/fmicb.2010.00139.
50. Martinez JJ, Cossart P. Early signaling events involved in the entry of Rickettsia conorii into mammalian cells. J Cell Sci 2004;117(Pt 21):5097–106.
51. Chan YG, Cardwell M, Hermanas TM, et al. Rickettsial outer-membrance protein B (rOmpB) mediates bacterial invasion through Ku70 in an actin, c-Cbl, clathrin and caveolin 2-dependent manner. Cell Microbiol 2009;11(4):629–44.
52. Heinzen RA. Rickettsial actin-based motility. Behavior and involvement of cytoskeletal regulators. Ann N Y Acad Sci 2003;990:535–47.
53. Gouin E, Welch MD, Cossart P. Actin-based motility of intracellular pathogens. Curr Opin Microbiol 2005;8:35–45.
54. Gong B, Ma L, Liu Y, et al. Rickettsiae induce microvascular hyperpermeability via phosphorylation of VE-cadherins: evidence from atomic force microscopy and biochemical studies. PLoS Negl Trop Dis 2012;6(6):e1699.
55. Woods ME, Olano JP. Host defenses to Rickettsia rickettsii infection contribute to increased microvascular permeability in human cerebral endothelial cells. J Clin Immunol 2008;28:174–85.
56. Spencer R, Parker R. Rocky Mountain spotted fever: infectivity of fasting and recently fed ticks. Public Health Rep 1923;38:333–9.
57. Thorner AR, Walker DH, Petri WA Jr. Rocky mountain spotted fever. Clin Infect Dis 1998;27(6):1353–9 [quiz: 60].
58. DuPont HL, Hornick RB, Dawkins AT, et al. Rocky Mountain spotted fever: a comparative study of the active immunity induced by inactivated and viable pathogenic Rickettsia rickettsii. J Infect Dis 1973;128(3):340–4.
59. Joshi SG, Francis CW, Silverman DJ, et al. NF-κB activation suppresses host cell apoptosis during Rickettsia rickettsii infection via regulatory effects on intracellular localization of levels of apoptogenic and anti-apoptogenic proteins. FEMS Microbiol Lett 2004;234(2):333–41.
60. Rydkina E, Turpin LC, Sahni SK. Rickettsia rickettsii infection of human macrovascular and microvascular endothelial cells reveals activation of both common and cell type-specific host response mechanisms. Infect Immun 2010;78(6):2599–606.
61. Walker DH, Olano JP, Feng HM. Critical role of cytotoxic T lymphocytes in immune clearance of rickettsial infection. Infect Immun 2001;69:1841–6.
62. Feng HM, Whitworth T, Olano JP, et al. Fc-dependent polyclonal antibodies and antibodies to outer membrane proteins A and B, but not to lipopolysaccharide, protect SCID mice against fatal Rickettsia conorii infection. Infect Immun 2004; 72(4):2222–8.
63. Chan YG, Riley SP, Chen E, et al. Molecular basis of immunity to rickettsial infection conferred through outer membrane protein B. Infect Immun 2011;79(6): 2303–13.
64. Carpenter CF, Gandhi TK, Kong LK, et al. The incidence of ehrlichial and rickettsial infection in patients with unexplained fever and recent history of tick bite in central North Carolina. J Infect Dis 1999;180(3):900–3.

65. Minninear TD, Buckingham SC. Managing Rocky Mountain spotted fever. Expert Rev Anti Infect Ther 2009;7(9):1131–7.
66. Dalton MJ, Clarke MJ, Holman RC, et al. National surveillance for Rocky Mountain spotted fever, 1981-1992: epidemiologic summary and evaluation of risk factors for fatal outcome. Am J Trop Med Hyg 1995;52(5):405–13.
67. Treadwell TA, Holman RC, Clarke MJ, et al. Rocky Mountain spotted fever in the United States, 1993-1996. Am J Trop Med Hyg 2000;63(1–2):21–6.
68. Kirk JL, Fine DP, Sexton DJ, et al. Rocky Mountain spotted fever. Clinical review based on 48 confirmed cases, 1943-1986. Medicine 1990;69(1):35–45.
69. Haynes RE, Sanders DY, Cramblett HG. Rocky Mountain spotted fever in children. J Pediatr 1970;76(5):685–93.
70. Davis AE, Bradford WD. Abdominal pain resembling acute appendicitis in Rocky Mountain spotted fever. JAMA 1982;247(20):2811–2.
71. Kirkland KB, Marcom PK, Sexton DJ, et al. Rocky Mountain spotted fever complicated by gangrene: report of six cases and review. Clin Infect Dis 1993;16(5):629–34.
72. Centers for Disease Control and Prevention. Rocky Mountain spotted fever. Symptoms, diagnosis and treatment. Available at: http://www.cdc.gov/rmsf/symptoms/index.html. Accessed October 1, 2012.
73. Bradford WD, Hackel DB. Myocardial involvement in Rocky Mountain spotted fever. Arch Pathol Lab Med 1978;102(7):357–9.
74. Maller VG, Agarwal AK, Choudhary AK. Diffusion imaging findings in Rocky Mountain spotted fever encephalitis: a case report. Emerg Radiol 2012;19(1):79–81.
75. Crapp S, Harrar D, Strother M, et al. Rocky Mountain spotted fever: 'starry sky' appearance with diffusion-weighted imaging in a child. Pediatr Radiol 2012;42(4):499–502.
76. Raoult D, Paddock CD. Rickettsia parkeri infection and other spotted fevers in the United States. N Engl J Med 2005;353(6):626–7.
77. Clements ML, Dumler JS, Fiset P, et al. Serodiagnosis of Rocky Mountain spotted fever: comparison of IgM and IgG enzyme-linked immunosorbent assay and indirect fluorescent antibody test. J Infect Dis 1983;148(5):876–80.
78. Kovacova E, Kazar J. Rickettsial diseases and their serological diagnosis. Clin Lab 2000;45(5–6):239–45.
79. Walker DH. Rocky Mountain spotted fever: a seasonal alert. Clin Infect Dis 1995;20(5):1111–7.
80. Centers for Disease Control and Prevention. In-depth information–Rocky Mountain Spotted Fever (RMSF). Available at: http://www.cdc.gov/rmsf/info/index.html. Accessed October 1, 2012.
81. Schutze GE, Buckingham SC, Marshall GS, et al. Human monocytic ehrlichiosis in children. Pediatr Infect Dis J 2007;26(6):475–9.
82. Jacobs RF, Schutze GE. Ehrlichiosis in children. J Pediatr 1997;131(2):184–92.
83. Ferrari FA, Goddard J, Paddock CD, et al. Rickettsia parkeri and Candidatus Rickettsia andeanae in Gulf Coast tics, Mississippi, USA. Emerg Infect Dis 2012;18(10):1705–7.
84. American Academy of Pediatrics. Rocky mountain spotted fever. In: Pickering LK, editor. Red book: 2012 report of the committee on infectious diseases. 29th edition. Elk Grove Village (IL): American Academy of Pediatrics; 2012. p. 623–5.
85. Lochary ME, Lockhart PB, Williams WT Jr. Doxycycline and staining of permanent teeth. Pediatr Infect Dis J 1998;17(5):429–31.

86. Volovitz B, Shkap R, Amir J, et al. Absence of tooth staining with doxycycline treatment in young children. Clin Pediatr 2007;46(2):121–6.
87. Holman RC, Paddock CD, Curns AT, et al. Analysis of risk factors for fatal Rocky Mountain spotted fever: evidence for superiority of tetracyclines for therapy. J Infect Dis 2001;184(11):1437–44.
88. Rolain JM, Maurin M, Vestris G, et al. In vitro susceptibilities of 27 rickettsiae to 13 antimicrobials. Antimicrob Agents Chemother 1998;42(7):1537–41.
89. Harrell GT. Rocky Mountain spotted fever. Medicine 1949;28(4):333–70.
90. Topping NH. Experimental Rocky Mountain spoted fever and endemic typhus treated with prontosil or sulfapyradine. Public Health Rep 1939;54:1143–7.
91. Dahlgren FS, Holman RC, Paddock CD, et al. Fatal Rocky Mountain spotted fever in the United States, 1999-2007. Am J Trop Med Hyg 2012;86(4):713–9.
92. Hattwick MA, Retailliau H, O'Brien RJ, et al. Fatal Rocky Mountain spotted fever. JAMA 1978;240(14):1499–503.
93. Kirkland KB, Wilkinson WE, Sexton DJ. Therapeutic delay and mortality in cases of Rocky Mountain spotted fever. Clin Infect Dis 1995;20(5):1118–21.
94. Archibald LK, Sexton DJ. Long-term sequelae of Rocky Mountain spotted fever. Clin Infect Dis 1995;20(5):1122–5.
95. American Academy of Pediatrics. Prevention of Tickborne Infections. In: Pickering LK, editor. Red book: 2012 report of the committee on infectious diseases. 29th edition. Elk Grove Village (IL): American Academy of Pediatrics; 2012. p. 207–9.
96. Centers for Disease Control and Prevention. Preventing tick bites. Available at: http://www.cdc.gov/ticks/avoid/on_people.html. Accessed October 1, 2012.
97. Ellison DW, Clark TR, Sturdevant DE, et al. Genomic comparison of virulent Rickettsia rickettsii Sheila Smith and avirulent Rickettsia rickettsii Iowa. Infect Immun 2008;76(2):542–50.

Childhood Parasitic Infections Endemic to the United States

Meagan A. Barry[a,b], Jill E. Weatherhead, MD[c,d], Peter J. Hotez, MD, PhD[a,d,e], Laila Woc-Colburn, MD[c,*]

KEYWORDS

• Chagas • Intestinal protozoa • Leishmania • Childhood • Toxoplasma • Toxocara

KEY POINTS

- Infections with the intestinal parasites *Cryptosporidium*, *Dientamoeba*, and *Giardia*, each of which can lead to differing forms of diarrheal disease, are common in children in the United States, particularly in northern states in the summer months.
- Chronic infection with *Trypanosoma cruzi*, the cause of Chagas disease, is present in hundreds of thousands of people in the United States, mostly in southern states.
- Local, vector-borne transmission of *T cruzi* has been reported in Texas, California, Tennessee, and Louisiana.
- Local, vector-borne transmission of *Leishmania* species, leading to cutaneous leishmaniasis, has been reported in Texas.
- *Toxocara* and *Toxoplasma* infections are endemic zoonotic infections in the United States and both are more frequent in African American populations and in individuals with lower socioeconomic status.
- Parasitic diseases endemic to the United States are not uncommon but are understudied. Further study is required to determine the true prevalence and morbidity from these diseases in the United States.

INTRODUCTION AND OVERVIEW OF CHILDHOOD PARASITIC INFECTIONS

Although parasitic infections are generally thought of as diseases of low- and middle-income countries, there is a rapidly expanding evidence base to indicate that these diseases also affect wealthy countries in North America, Europe, and Asia.[1] Most of

Disclosure statement: The authors have no conflict of interest.
[a] Interdepartmental Program in Translational Biology and Molecular Medicine, National School of Tropical Medicine, Baylor College of Medicine, One Baylor Plaza, Houston, TX 77030, USA; [b] BCM Medical Scientist Training Program, National School of Tropical Medicine, Baylor College of Medicine, One Baylor Plaza, Houston, TX 77030, USA; [c] Department of Medicine, National School of Tropical Medicine, Baylor College of Medicine, One Baylor Plaza, Houston, TX 77030, USA; [d] Department of Pediatrics, National School of Tropical Medicine, Baylor College of Medicine, One Baylor Plaza, Houston, TX 77030, USA; [e] Department of Molecular Virology and Microbiology, National School of Tropical Medicine, Baylor College of Medicine, One Baylor Plaza, Houston, TX 77030, USA
* Corresponding author.
E-mail address: woccolbu@bcm.edu

Pediatr Clin N Am 60 (2013) 471–485
http://dx.doi.org/10.1016/j.pcl.2012.12.011 pediatric.theclinics.com
0031-3955/13/$ – see front matter

the parasitic diseases endemic to the United States fall into 2 major categories (**Box 1**): (1) intestinal protozoan infections that disproportionately affect northern states during the summer months and are linked to recreational water use[2–4] and (2) neglected tropical diseases (NTDs) and related neglected infections that disproportionately affect people living in severe poverty.[5–7] The American South has the largest number of cases,[5–7] with Texas possibly representing the single most affected state in the nation.[7] Here the authors' provide an overview of the major parasitic infections affecting children in the United States, with an emphasis on new insights and developments reported in the biomedical literature over the last 5 years.

INTESTINAL PARASITIC INFECTIONS

Cryptosporidiosis

Cryptosporidiosis is an intestinal infection caused by a 4- to 6-μm protozoal coccidia. There are several species of *Cryptosporidium*, but the two of particular interest in children are *C hominis* and *C parvum*. Each year, approximately 10 000 to 12 000 cases of cryptosporidiosis are reported,[3] although the actual number of cases is probably much higher. Children aged 1 to 9 years are disproportionately affected, with the onset of infection peaking in the summer in association with communal swimming venues and recreational water use.[3] Overall, northern states have the highest incidence.[3] Cryptosporidiosis has been linked with large water-borne disease outbreaks in the United States,[2,8] which have been linked to zoonotic transmission in summer camps in some cases.[9,10] In addition to young children, immunosuppressed patients (human immunodeficiency virus [HIV]/AIDS and transplant) are particularly vulnerable to cryptosporidiosis.[11,12]

The intestinal parasitic infections described here (cryptosporidiosis, dientamoebiasis, and giardiasis) are all transmitted via the fecal-oral route, either through contaminated water or food. They also share a similar life cycle that begins with the ingestion of oocysts found in contaminated water or food or by autoinfection. Once the *Cryptosporidium* oocysts are excreted, they are highly contagious. The oocysts are also able to persist in the environment for a prolonged time, possibly up to 6 months.[3] The low infectious dose and prolonged infective capability of *Cryptosporidium* help explain why it is easily transmitted. Other factors influencing transmission are a prolonged incubation period and the lack of protective immunity in the host.[13]

The clinical presentation of cryptosporidiosis is large-volume watery diarrhea associated with nausea, vomiting, abdominal cramping, and anorexia. The diarrhea usually

Box 1
Major parasitic infections endemic in the United States

- Intestinal parasitic infections
  - Cryptosporidiosis
  - Dientamoebiasis
  - Giardiasis
- Parasitic neglected tropical diseases
  - Chagas disease
  - Cutaneous leishmaniasis
  - Toxocariasis
  - Toxoplasmosis

lasts between 5 and 10 days and is often self-limiting. In immunosuppressed patients, the diarrhea can last longer and results in malnutrition caused by poor absorption of nutrients and dehydration. Cryptosporidiosis can also present with extraintestinal manifestations, particularly in patients with HIV/AIDS and transplant patients,[14,15] which can lead to pancreatitis, biliary strictures, hepatitis, and pneumonia.[15]

Cryptosporidiosis can be diagnosed by oocyst visualization, antigen detection, or molecular testing. To visualize the oocyst, the stool is stained with trichrome or modified acid-fast stains or with a direct immunofluorescence stain (**Fig. 1**). Although the specificity of direct visualization of the oocyst is around 100%, the sensitivity can range from 37% to 97%.[13] In comparison, the antigen detection method gives a specificity and sensitivity of 90% and is the most widely use method today for the diagnosis of cryptosporidiosis. The antigen detection is a simple point-of-care testing method that is both economical and reliable.[16] Cryptosporidiosis antigen detection can be paired with the detection of antigens from other intestinal protozoan infections, such as giardiasis and amebiasis, for diagnosis in the field.

The drug used to treat cryptosporidiosis is nitazoxanide, a thiazole derivative.[13] Nitazoxanide has been has been approved by the Food and Drug Administration (FDA) since 2004 for use in children more than 1 year of age. See **Table 1** for pediatric dosing guidelines.[17] Nitazoxanide is a well-tolerated drug with few adverse side effects. In the immunosuppressed host, the reestablishment of the immune system

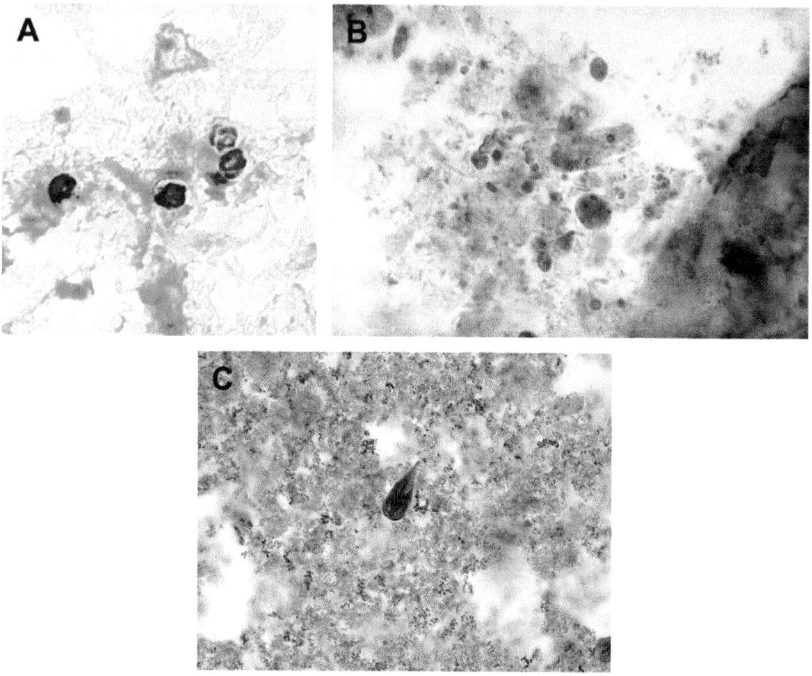

Fig. 1. (*A*) This photomicrograph revealed the morphologic details of *Cryptosporidium parvum* oocysts (ie, encapsulated zygotes) (modified acid-fast stain, original magnification × 1000). (*B*) *Dientamoeba fragilis* (trichrome stain, original magnification × 1000). (*C*) The morphologic characteristics of a blue-stained *Giardia intestinalis* protozoan trophozoite (*center*) (trichrome stain, original magnification × 1000). (*Courtesy of* The Public Health Image Library, Centers for Disease Control and Prevention; [*A*] CDC/DPDx [*B*] CDC [*C*] CDC/DPDx-Melanie Moser.)

Table 1
Dosing guidelines for cryptosporidiosis in the pediatric population

Drug		Nitazoxanide	
Age of patient	1–3 y	4–11 y	Older than 11 y
Dose	100 mg per dose	200 mg per dose	500 mg per dose
Frequency of doses	Twice daily	Twice daily	Twice daily
Duration of therapy	3 d	3 d	3 d

The nitazoxanide dose is based on the age of the patient.
Data from White Jr. CA. Nitazoxanide: a new broad spectrum antiparasitic agent. Expert Rev Anti Infect Ther 2004;2(1):43–9.

is critical, either by treating the HIV infection or by lowering the immunosuppressive medications, in addition to nitazoxanide therapy.[12]

Dientamoebiasis

Since the first report by Jepps and Dobell in 1918, dientamoebiasis has been involved in controversies ranging from the proper classification of the organism to the clinical significance of the syndrome. *Dientamoeba fragilis* is an intestinal protozoan of the trichomonadida family.[18] It can be found worldwide and is estimated to have a prevalence as high as 42% in some regions.[19] As opposed to other intestinal protozoans that are linked with poverty, dientamoebiasis is more prevalent in developed countries. Examples of prevalence rates in developed countries include 11.7% in the United States,[19] 11.5% in Canada,[20] and up to 16.9% in the United Kingdom.[19] The mode of transmission is thought to be fecal-oral; however, no cyst stage has been described for this pathogen.[18] There is some evidence that *Dientamoeba* may use the vector *Enterobious vermicularis* (pinworm) during transmission, although it is difficult to distinguish if the pinworm is a vector or simply a bystander.[18] Making this distinction more difficult to elucidate is that patients with dientamoebiasis often have polyparasitism with other intestinal protozoa, such as *Blastocystosis hominis, Giardia lamblia, Entamoeba histolytica*, and *Cryptosporidium spp.*[18–20]

Clinically, patients with dientamoebiasis present with abdominal pain, bloating, diarrhea, and loose stools, which lasts 3 to 7 days.[19] After this acute stage, patients can progress to the chronic stage, which can last from 1 month up to 2 years and may lead to irritable bowel syndrome (IBS).[21] The diagnosis of dientamoebiasis is challenging. Fresh or fixed stool, when examined under the light microscope, will show a rounded, amoeboidlike structure measuring 5 to 15 um (see **Fig. 1**).[18] The use of real-time polymerase chain reaction (PCR) that targets ribosomal RNA gives a sensitivity of 93.5% and specificity of 100%.[22]

The choice of drug in the treatment of dientamoebiasis is controversial because many therapeutic agents have been used successfully, including metronidazole, iodoquinol, erythromycin, paromomycin, and secnidazole.[18,23] The most commonly used treatment option is metronidazole, which has cure rates of up to 80%.[19] One study of 21 patients with a 2-month history of IBS who were found to have dientamoebiasis and were treated with iodoquinol and doxycycline found complete elimination of the *Dientamoeba* and 67% improvement in IBS symptoms.[24] Secnidazole, a nitroimidazole used to treat other intestinal protozoans, was recently shown to have good amebicidal properties when compared with other treatment options.[23] Advantages of secnidazole are that a single dose (30 mg/kg) can eliminate *Dientamoeba* with few adverse side effects.

Giardiasis

Giardia lamblia was one of the first protozoans to be seen in 1681 by Van Leewenhoek when examining stool under a microscope.[25] *G lamblia* is a flagellated protozoan with a global distribution. It is one of the causes of traveler's diarrhea and of diarrheal outbreaks from contaminated water.[4] It is also considered a zoonotic disease, first known as *beaver fever*. There are approximately 19 000 cases of giardiasis reported annually; as with cryptosporidiosis, infection is most common in children aged 1 to 9 years and occurs most frequently in the summer months in northern states.[4] Giardiasis and dientamoebiasis are also found commonly among internationally adopted children living in the United States.[26] Infection occurs via the fecal-oral route when contaminated food and water containing *Giardia* cysts is ingested. As mentioned previously, the life cycle is similar to that of cryptosporidiosis. *Giardia* predominantly infects cells of the duodenum and upper jejunum.[25]

Clinically, giardiasis presents as a mild to severe diarrheal disease, which can progress to a chronic form involving IBS. The incubation period of giardiasis is 9 to 15 days,[25] after which patients develop anorexia, abdominal cramping, bloating, and explosive foul-smelling diarrhea. This acute stage can be self-limiting. However, up to 50% of patients do not clear the *Giardia* and chronic disease can result.[25] During the chronic stage, patients experience weight loss, anorexia, malabsorption, and intermittent bouts of diarrhea, which can last for years.[25] In the pediatric population, this can lead to failure to thrive, stunned growth, lower IQ,[27] and urticaria.[25] Rarely the chronic stage can include arthritis, cholecystitis, and pancreatitis.[25] Giardiasis is diagnosed by direct observation of the stool (low diagnostic yield, see **Fig. 1**), serology using antigen detection kits (sensitivity and specificity >90%), and real-time PCR.[25,27]

Giardiasis is treated with nitroimidazole compounds, including metronidazole, tinidazole, secnidazole, and ornidazole.[25] See **Table 2** for dosing guidelines.[25,27] Metronidazole is very effective, with a cure rate of close to 95%.[25] Tinidazole is also very efficacious with few side effects and has the advantage of only requiring a single dose.[27] Nitazoxanide is an excellent alternative. It is FDA approved for the treatment of *Giardia* in children who are 1 year of age or older and has very few side effects. If patients do not respond to any of these medications, quinacrine is another highly efficacious option; however, this drug is associated with more adverse side effects.[25]

PARASITIC NTDS

Chagas Disease

Chagas disease is a chronic systemic infection caused by the parasite *Trypanosoma cruzi*. The disease is most commonly transmitted through defecation by *T cruzi*–infected triatomine insects after a blood meal. Chagas disease has long been known to be an important parasitic infection in Latin America, with 8 million people or more currently infected.[28] However, there is increasing attention to the presence of the disease in the United States. An estimated 300 000 cases of Chagas disease occur in the United States,[29] although there are very few programs of active surveillance for this disease and some estimates indicate that almost as many *T cruzi* infected individuals may live in Texas alone.[30] It is assumed that most of the Chagas disease cases in the United States result from immigration; however, new evidence documents at least 23 cases of autochthonous, vector-borne transmission within the United States,[31] and the disease is widespread among dogs living in Texas.[29] The triatomine vector can be found across the southern half of the country, with the largest species diversity in Texas, Arizona, and New Mexico.[29] Of increasing concern in the United States is maternal transmission of Chagas disease. Recently, the first case report of congenital

Table 2
Dosing guidelines for giardiasis in the pediatric population

Drug	Metronidazole			Tinidazole		Quinacrine		Nitazoxanide		
Age	Younger than 11 y	Older than 11 y	Older than 11 y	Younger than 11 y	Older than 11 y	Younger than 11 y	Older than 11 y	1–3 y	4–11 y	≥12 y
Dose	5 mg/kg	250 mg	2 g	30 mg/kg	2 g	2 mg/kg	100 mg	100 mg per dose	200 mg per dose	500 mg per dose
Frequency of doses	3 times daily	3 times daily	Once daily	Once	Once	3 times daily	3 times daily	Twice daily	Twice daily	Twice daily
Duration of therapy	10 d	10 d	3 d	Single dose	Single dose	7 d	7 d	3 d	3 d	3 d

Listed are alternative forms of therapy. Tinidazole or metronidazole are the preferred treatment options, with the best efficacy and fewest adverse side effects. Metronidazole can be given at a higher dose for a shorter duration of treatment or at a lower dose for a longer duration. Nitazoxanide is an excellent alternative, with high efficacy and few side effects. Quinacrine is also very effective and can be administered if either of these treatment options fail; however, it is associated with more adverse side effects.

Data from Wolfe MS. Giardiasis. Clin Microbiol Rev 1992;5(1):93–100; and Wright SG. Protozoan infections of the gastrointestinal tract. Infect Dis Clin North Am 2012;26(2):323–39.

Chagas disease in the United States confirmed by the Centers for Disease Control and Prevention (CDC) was published.[32] Reports suggest that vertical transmission occurs in 1% to 10% of pregnancies in infected women, which could indicate that there are as many as 638 cases of congenital Chagas annually in the United States.[32]

Chagas infection first presents as an acute illness that can either be asymptomatic or a self-limiting febrile illness.[28] After a decrease in parasitemia, patients enter the indeterminate chronic stage. Between 60% and 70% of patients in the indeterminate stage will never experience symptoms.[28] The remaining 30% to 40% of patients will develop chagasic cardiomyopathy or digestive symptoms, including megaesophagus or megacolon, often 10 to 30 years after the initial infection.[28] Congenital Chagas disease frequently has no specific symptoms, making recognition of the infection challenging for physicians.[32] Many infants are asymptomatic,[32] and the remaining 10% to 40% of infants present with features including low birth weight, low Apgar scores, respiratory distress, cardiac failure, anasarca, hepatosplenomegaly, and meningoencephalitis.[33] Severe congenital Chagas infection is associated with high neonatal mortality rates.[32]

Diagnosis of acute Chagas disease relies on detection of *T cruzi* trypomastigotes in blood by microscopic analysis.[28] Once parasitemia is low during the chronic infection phase, antibody-based tests are used for diagnosis, including enzyme-linked immunosorbent assay (ELISA), indirect immunofluorescence, or indirect haemagglutination.[28] Positive results from 2 of these tests are recommended for the diagnosis of Chagas disease in the chronic phase.[34] Although PCR is a more sensitive test, poor standardization and variable results across laboratories exclude it as a routine method of diagnosis.[34] PCR can be used to monitor treatment failure but should not be used to confirm treatment success because PCR cannot exclude the possibility of low levels of parasite in the tissue.[34] In neonates with suspected congenital Chagas disease, Giemsa-stained blood smears or buffy coat should be examined by light microscopy for trypomastigotes.[35] PCR should be used with caution and confirmed with a second specimen because low levels of *T cruzi* DNA can sometimes be found in uninfected neonates of women with Chagas disease.[32] Neonates with negative results should be retested at 4 to 6 weeks because parasitemia typically increases during the first month of life.[32] Antibody-based tests can be used after 9 to 12 months, when maternal antibodies have waned.[32]

There are 2 pharmacologic options for the treatment of Chagas disease. Neither of these drugs are FDA approved but may be obtained free of charge from the CDC under investigational protocols.[36] For questions regarding treatment or to obtain the medications contact the CDC Parasitic Diseases Public Inquiries (1-404-718-4745; e-mail chagas@cdc.gov). For after-hours emergencies contact the CDC Emergency Operations Center (770-488-7100) and ask for the on-call parasitic diseases physician. Benznidazole is the drug with the best safety profile and the highest efficacy rates and is recommended as the first-line therapy.[28] Alternatively, nifurtimox can be given. See **Table 3** for dosing guidelines.[28,33] All infected children less than 18 years of age should be treated.[28] Congenital Chagas disease should be treated promptly once a confirmatory diagnosis is obtained.[35] Cure rates are more than 90% when therapy is initiated within the first few weeks of life, and fewer adverse reactions occur than in the adult population if therapy occurs within the first year of life.[32,35] Recently, the nonprofit product development partnership Drugs for Neglected Diseases initiative registered a new pediatric formulation of benzimidazole in Brazil.[37] The formulation is comprised of a 12.5-mg tablet that is adapted for children less than 2 years of age (20 kg body weight), with the treatment comprised of 1, 2, or 3 tablets depending on weight (5–10 mg/kg/d).[37] Currently, the safety of benzimidazole and nifurtimox is

Table 3
Dosing guidelines for congenital Chagas infection or Chagas disease in the pediatric population

Drug	Benznidazole	Nifurtimox
Total daily dose	5–10 mg/kg daily	10–15 mg/kg daily
Dose divisions (total daily dose divided into doses per day)	2–3 doses	3 doses
Duration of therapy	60 d	60–90 d

Listed are the 2 alternative forms of therapy. Benznidazole has the best safety profile and the highest efficacy rates and is recommended as the first-line therapy.

Data from Rassi Jr. A, Rassi A, Marin-Neto JA. Chagas disease. Lancet 2010;375(9723):1388–402; and Oliveira I, Torrico F, Munoz J, et al. Congenital transmission of chagas disease: a clinical approach. Expert Rev Anti Infect Ther 2010;8(8):945–56.

unknown during pregnancy, so recommendations regarding the treatment of pregnant women suggest delaying therapy until after delivery and breastfeeding have concluded.[32] Targeted screening of pregnant women based on risk factors (history of living or having receiving a blood transfusion in a disease-endemic area) is recommended to identify pregnancies that could result in congenital Chagas disease as well as to prevent future possible congenital Chagas cases.[35]

Cutaneous Leishmaniasis

Leishmaniasis is a protozoan vector-borne zoonotic disease. *Leishmania*, the causative agent of Leishmaniasis, is transmitted to humans through the bite of the *Lutzomyia* sandfly.[38,39] The disease process is caused by more than 24 different species of *Leishmania*, most commonly *Leishmania braziliensis, panamensis, mexicana*, and *peruana* in North and South America.[40] These species lead to 4 distinct forms of disease, including mucosal leishmaniasis, chronic cutaneous leishmaniasis, diffuse cutaneous leishmaniasis, and visceral leishmaniasis with associated post-kala-azar dermal leishmaniasis.[41] Leishmaniasis is endemic in 88 countries around the world, putting approximately 350 million people at risk for disease. In the United States, leishmaniasis is typically isolated to foreign travelers, immigrants, and military personnel returning from endemic countries.[39] However, *L mexicana* is endemic in Texas; the Texas wood rat, *Neotoma micropus*, is a known mammalian reservoir. There have been a total of 30 autochthonous cases of cutaneous leishmaniasis in the United States, which have generally occurred in South Central Texas. The spread of disease in Texas is thought to be secondary to the habitat migration of the *N micropus* toward Northeast Texas.[39] In a recent case series, 9 autochthonous cases of cutaneous leishmaniasis were reported in North Texas around the Dallas–Fort Worth areas. Additionally, in the fall of 2012, a 2-year-old girl was diagnosed with cutaneous leishmaniasis at Texas Children's Hospital in Houston, Texas (Judith Campbell, MD, Houston, Texas, personal communication, October 2012). The patient had no travel history outside of Texas. The diagnosis was made through histology and molecular testing of tissue obtained via biopsy of her chronic cheek ulcerative lesion. She was treated for 6 weeks with oral ketoconazole.

Cutaneous leishmaniasis is a disfiguring disease process. Once inoculation occurs, symptoms may arise in approximately 1 week to 3 months. Typically, a small papule develops at the site of inoculation and subsequently forms a plaque or nodule on exposed skin surfaces. Eventually, these lesions can evolve into an ulcerating lesion leaving scars.[41,42] In diffuse cutaneous leishmaniasis, nodules are widespread and typically do not ulcerate.[41] In some cases of *L mexicana* infection, the lesions spontaneously resolve in 6 to 12 months. However, spontaneous resolution is far less likely and takes a more extended time period in other species, including *L braziliensis* and *L panamensis*.[39,41]

Cutaneous leishmaniasis is typically diagnosed by obtaining important epidemiologic information, including social history, travel history, military service, and biopsy of the lesion from the ulcer base with direct visualization of the amastigotes. Culture media, antileishmanial serologies, and PCR are available and allow for species identification.[40,41]

In the United States, there is no FDA-approved drug for cutaneous leishmaniasis. Proven successful treatment regimens are limited for cutaneous leishmaniasis because of species variation. Furthermore, medication regimens are outdated, toxic, expensive, and drug resistance is increasing.[38] Typically, observation alone for small lesions caused by *L mexicana* is recommended. For chronic lesions, disfiguring lesions, or to prevent dissemination to mucosal involvement, pentavalent antimonials, such as sodium stibogluconate, via an intravenous or intramuscular route are recommended despite inconsistent results. Other treatments, including intralesional antimonial medications, topical paromomycin, oral miltefosine, oral ketoconazole or fluconazole, and pentamidine, have undergone testing and have shown varying results depending on the species of *Leishmania* and disease burden.[40,41,43–45] Studies done at the Walter Reed Army Medical Center in Washington have shown success using liposomal amphotericin B instead of pentavalent antimonials for moderate to severe disease; however, the study did not include children.[45] The authors have also successfully treated adults with extensive cutaneous leishmaniasis with liposomal amphotericin B with excellent results. Other aims of treatment include accelerating self-cure with immunomodulators as adjuvant therapy.[43] After therapy, lesions are expected to decrease in size by 6 weeks, although complete resolution may not be observed for 6 to 12 months.[41]

Toxocariasis

Toxocariasis is a zoonotic helminth infection transmitted from either dogs (*Toxocara canis*) or cats (*Toxocariasis cati*). A large national study found a seroprevalence of 13.9% overall, with rates more than 20% in African Americans, especially in the southern United States.[46–48] Higher infection rates are associated with lower socioeconomic status.[49] Based on the high seroprevalence of toxocariasis, some investigators have suggested that this disease represents the most common helminth infection in the United States.[47] Transmission occurs with accidental oral ingestion of *Toxocara* eggs that have been shed in the feces of the dog or cat definitive host. Children are at particular risk of toxocariasis when they play in contaminated areas, such as playgrounds or sandboxes. Infection cannot be acquired from direct contact with an infected pet because the *Toxocara* eggs must embryonate in the environment before they are infectious.[36]

In the human gut, the *Toxocara* eggs hatch and disseminate hematogenously to the brain, heart, lungs, liver, muscle, and/or eyes. Once in the various human tissues, the larvae are unable to continue their normal life cycle, and a local inflammatory response to the dead larvae leads to the varied toxocara symptoms of the 2 classic clinical syndromes.[36] Visceral larva migrans, which occurs most frequently in young children, often presents as hepatitis and pneumonitis.[47] If the larvae penetrate the central nervous system (CNS), meningoencephalitis and cerebritis can occur with resulting seizures.[47] Recently, a correlation has been found between toxocariasis and epilepsy.[50] The second clinical syndrome, ocular larva migrans, which is most commonly seen in older children and adolescents, occurs when one or more larvae enter the eye.[47]

A granuloma or a granulomatous larval track results and vision loss is a common sequelae, with rates as high as 85% in one retrospective study,[47,51] although the reported number of cases annually in the United States is small.[52] A third nonclassic presentation, called covert toxocariasis, is actually much more common than the two classic presentations. Covert toxocariasis presents with some, but not all, of the visceral larva migrans symptoms, particularly wheezing, pulmonary infiltrates, and eosinophilia.[47] With this correlation between toxocara infection and wheezing, toxocariasis may be an important yet underappreciated environmental cause of childhood asthma.[47]

An ELISA-based antibody detection test is most commonly used to diagnose toxocariasis and can be obtained from the CDC. It should be noted that this test has limitations, including a sensitivity of only 78% and a high false positive rate caused by cross-reactivity with antibodies from other helminth infections.[36,53] As with any antibody-based test, a positive result cannot distinguish if the antibodies are from an active infection or if they remain from a resolved infection. Ocular larva migrans typically does not yield a positive ELISA test, so the diagnosis is a clinical one, based on granulomatous ophthalmologic examination findings.[54] Stool ova and parasite cannot be used diagnostically because *Toxocara* does not replicate in the human gut.[36]

Toxocariasis is often a self-limited illness that resolves once inflammation caused by the dead larvae dissipates. In these cases, no treatment is required. If patients are experiencing prolonged toxocariasis, sources of continual reinfection should be investigated.[36] In more severe cases, either albendazole or mebendazole can be given, although albendazole is preferred because of the limited CNS penetration of mebendazole.[55] Ivermectin has been shown by some to be an ineffective therapy.[56] Treatment of ocular larva migrans requires a longer duration of therapy[55] and concomitant prednisone.[57] See **Table 4** for pediatric dosing guidelines.[55,57] Surgical intervention may be necessary in complicated cases.[36] Prevention is paramount in reducing the toxocariasis disease burden. Household pets should be regularly dewormed and the fecal matter disposed of properly.[52] Children should be educated to wash their hands and to not ingest dirt (geophagy).[52]

Toxoplasmosis

Toxoplasmosis, caused by the obligate intracellular protozoa *Toxoplasma gondii*, occurs after consumption of raw or undercooked meat or ingestion of *T gondii* oocytes

Table 4
Dosing guidelines for toxocariasis in the pediatric population

	Severe Toxocariasis	Severe Toxocariasis	Ocular Larvae Migrans	
Drug	Albendazole	Mebendazole	Albendazole	Prednisone
Dose	400 mg per dose	100–200 mg per dose	400 mg per dose	1.0 mg/kg
Frequency of doses	Twice daily	Twice daily	Twice daily	Daily
Duration of therapy	5 d	5 d	14 d	Tapered over a few months

Mild symptoms will resolve without the need for therapy. More severe toxocariasis can be treated with either albendazole (the preferred therapy because of better CNS penetration) or mebendazole. Ocular larvae migrans requires a longer duration of therapy and concurrent prednisone therapy.

Data from Caumes E. Treatment of cutaneous larva migrans and toxocara infection. Fundam Clin Pharmacol 2003;17(2):213–6; and Barisani-Asenbauer T, Maca SM, Hauff W, et al. Treatment of ocular toxocariasis with albendazole. J Ocul Pharmacol Ther 2001;17(3):287–94.

from the environment (most commonly soil contaminated with feline feces).[58–60] Although cats are the definitive host, other mammals, including humans, can be infected. Toxocara and Toxoplasma coinfections are common, suggesting that cats may be an important reservoir for both infections.[61] Although toxoplasmosis is not ordinarily thought of as an NTD, in the United States, non-Hispanic blacks have the highest seroprevalence (more than 11% compared with 9% among white populations),[62] suggesting that it may be a health disparity. Furthermore, according to the *Morbidity and Mortality Weekly Report* in 2000, there are an estimated 400 to 4000 cases of congenital toxoplasmosis that occur each year in the United States.[58]

Primary infection is typically a self-limited illness. However, in 10% to 20% of immunocompetent hosts, an acute infection may present with isolated cervical or occipital lymphadenopathy. Even less frequently, acute infections can lead to ocular disease, such chorioretinitis or, rarely, myocarditis, polymyositis, pneumonitis, hepatitis, or encephalitits.[60] Primary infection can be more devastating if acquired during pregnancy. Women infected with *Toxoplasma* before conception rarely transmit the infection to their fetus. However, women infected with *Toxoplasma* after conception can transmit across the placenta to the fetus. Acquisition of *T gondii* between weeks 10 and 24 leads to the greatest risk of transmission to the fetus compared with later in pregnancy as well as to a greater disease burden to the fetus. An estimated one-half of untreated maternal infections are transmitted to the fetus.[63] Although the pregnant woman will typically be asymptomatic, an acute infection during pregnancy can lead to severe damage to the fetus, including the classic triad of symptoms: chorioretinitis, intracranial calcifications, and hydrocephalus. Despite these clinical signs of infection, many infants infected with *T gondii* prenatally are born visually normal and will not manifest additional clinical symptoms until later in childhood. If untreated, 85% of neonates with subclinical disease will develop signs and symptoms of active disease,[60,64] which can be developmentally devastating and include blindness, epilepsy, psychomotor or mental retardation, or death.[58–60,65] *Toxoplasma* is a cause of CNS disease in adults with HIV because of the reactivation of chronic infection but, for this reason, is less frequently a cause of CNS disease in children with HIV.

Diagnosis of toxoplasmosis can be obtained through indirect and direct methods. Organism-specific serologies (immunoglobulin A [IgA], IgM, and IgG) are useful in immunocompetent hosts, in early pregnancy to identify women at risk of acquiring infection during pregnancy, and in immunocompromised patients to identify patients at risk for reactivation of latent infection.[59] *T gondii* can also be directly visualized in fluids and tissues via microscopic examination or detected via DNA PCR of bronchoalveolar lavage fluid, blood, bone marrow aspirate, cerebrospinal fluid, and other tissue biopsy sites.[59,66,67]

Immunocompetent adults and children who are asymptomatic or with lymphadenitis are generally not treated. Others, including immunocompromised patients or immunocompetent patients with heavy disease burden, are treated with pyrimethamine, sulfadiazine, and folic acid for 4 to 6 weeks.[59,65] Women who become seropositive during pregnancy are treated throughout pregnancy with spiramycin and undergo both a fetal ultrasound to examine for clinical abnormalities in the fetus as well as amniotic fluid PCR at 18 weeks.[59,64,67] If amniotic fluid PCR is positive at 18 weeks, it is recommended to switch from spiramycin to folic acid, pyrimethamine, sulfadiazine, and folinic acid.[64] Postnatally, infants are treated with pyrimethamine and sulfadiazine for 12 months.

Public health measures for prevention have lead to an overall decreased incidence of toxoplasmosis infection around the world. Recommendations for continued reduction in infection include cooking meat to a safe temperature, peeling and washing fruits and vegetables, cleaning cooking surfaces and utensils after contact with raw foods, pregnant women avoiding cat litter, changing the litter box daily, not feeding raw or undercooked meat to cats, and keeping cats indoors.[58,67] Screening during pregnancy has also been considered to reduce fetal infection. Prenatal screening is controversial in the United States. Although the disease burden of vertically transmitted toxoplasmosis is high, screening in communities with a low incidence of disease is thought to lead to an increased risk of false-positive test results. Although screening programs are not universally practiced in the United States, seronegative women in other countries around the world, such as France, are recommended to have monthly serologic screening to detect for seroconversion early in pregnancy. If seroconversion is documented, the pregnant woman is treated and undergoes an ultrasound and PCR of amniotic fluid fetal.[64] As an alternative, states, such as New Hampshire and Massachusetts, have included toxoplasmosis screening in the state-mandated neonatal screening panels. According to the New England Newborn Screening Program, 40% of all children detected with toxoplasmosis on the newborn screen did not have clinical evidence of disease at birth. Although neonatal screening has been argued to be more cost-effective than prenatal screening, early detection in the mother can reduce vertical transmission to the fetus, and early detection in the fetus will allow for the early initiation of treatment of the newborn, resulting in a milder disease form.[68] Continuing education, determining serologic status, and early treatment of seropositive pregnant women is the only way to prevent transmission and infection in the neonate.[64] The debate between prenatal and neonatal screening is still being considered in the United States.

CONCLUDING REMARKS

Overall indications suggest that there is a significant disease burden that results from parasitic diseases in the United States. However, except for some large-scale studies produced from the National Health and Nutrition Survey and related surveys, we have limited precise information on the true prevalence and incidence of most of the parasitic disease infections in the United States. In part, this dearth of knowledge has resulted from inadequate funding to the CDC and state and local health agencies to more aggressively conduct active surveillance studies for parasitic infections. Increasingly, however, a new awareness is emerging of the impact of parasitic and NTDs in the United States but especially among the poorest populations living in the southern United States, which includes underrepresented minorities and people of color.[69]

REFERENCES

1. Hotez P. Neglected diseases amid wealth in the United States and Europe. Health Aff (Millwood) 2009;28(6):1720–5.
2. Hlavsa MC, Roberts VA, Anderson AR, et al. Surveillance for waterborne disease outbreaks and other health events associated with recreational water — United States, 2007–2008. MMWR Surveill Summ 2011;60(12):1–32.
3. Yoder JS, Harral C, Beach MJ. Cryptosporidiosis surveillance - United States, 2006-2008. MMWR Surveill Summ 2010;59(6):1–14.
4. Yoder JS, Harral C, Beach MJ. Giardiasis surveillance - United States, 2006-2008. MMWR Surveill Summ 2010;59(6):15–25.
5. Hotez PJ. Neglected infections of poverty in the United States of America. PLoS Negl Trop Dis 2008;2(6):e256.

6. Hotez PJ. America's most distressed areas and their neglected infections: the United States Gulf Coast and the District of Columbia. PLoS Negl Trop Dis 2011;5(3):e843.
7. Hotez PJ, Bottazzi ME, Dumonteil E, et al. Texas and Mexico: sharing a legacy of poverty and neglected tropical diseases. PLoS Negl Trop Dis 2012;6(3):e1497.
8. Polgreen PM, Sparks JD, Polgreen LA, et al. A statewide outbreak of Cryptosporidium and its association with the distribution of public swimming pools. Epidemiol Infect 2012;140(8):1439–45.
9. Centers for Disease Control, Prevention (CDC). Cryptosporidiosis outbreak at a summer camp–North Carolina, 2009. MMWR Morb Mortal Wkly Rep 2011; 60(27):918–22.
10. Hale CR, Scallan E, Cronquist AB, et al. Estimates of enteric illness attributable to contact with animals and their environments in the United States. Clin Infect Dis 2012;54(Suppl 5):S472–9.
11. Bandin F, Kwon T, Linas MD, et al. Cryptosporidiosis in paediatric renal transplantation. Pediatr Nephrol 2009;24(11):2245–55.
12. Krause I, Amir J, Cleper R, et al. Cryptosporidiosis in children following solid organ transplantation. Pediatr Infect Dis J 2012;31(11):1135–8.
13. Shirley DA, Moonah SN, Kotloff KL. Burden of disease from cryptosporidiosis. Curr Opin Infect Dis 2012;25(5):555–63.
14. Abubakar I, Aliyu SH, Arumugam C, et al. Treatment of cryptosporidiosis in immunocompromised individuals: systematic review and meta-analysis. Br J Clin Pharmacol 2007;63(4):387–93.
15. Wolska-Kusnierz B, Bajer A, Caccio S, et al. Cryptosporidium infection in patients with primary immunodeficiencies. J Pediatr Gastroenterol Nutr 2007;45(4): 458–64.
16. Minak J, Kabir M, Mahmud I, et al. Evaluation of rapid antigen point-of-care tests for detection of Giardia and Cryptosporidium species in human fecal specimens. J Clin Microbiol 2012;50(1):154–6.
17. White CA Jr. Nitazoxanide: a new broad spectrum antiparasitic agent. Expert Rev Anti Infect Ther 2004;2(1):43–9.
18. Johnson EH, Windsor JJ, Clark CG. Emerging from obscurity: biological, clinical, and diagnostic aspects of Dientamoeba fragilis. Clin Microbiol Rev 2004;17(3): 553–70 table of contents.
19. Stark D, Barratt J, Roberts T, et al. A review of the clinical presentation of dientamoebiasis. Am J Trop Med Hyg 2010;82(4):614–9.
20. Lagace-Wiens PR, VanCaeseele PG, Koschik C. Dientamoeba fragilis: an emerging role in intestinal disease. CMAJ 2006;175(5):468–9.
21. Stark D, van Hal S, Marriott D, et al. Irritable bowel syndrome: a review on the role of intestinal protozoa and the importance of their detection and diagnosis. Int J Parasitol 2007;37(1):11–20.
22. Stark D, Beebe N, Marriott D, et al. Detection of Dientamoeba fragilis in fresh stool specimens using PCR. Int J Parasitol 2005;35(1):57–62.
23. Nagata N, Marriott D, Harkness J, et al. In vitro susceptibility testing of Dientamoeba fragilis. Antimicrobial Agents Chemother 2012;56(1):487–94.
24. Borody T, Warren E, Wettstein A, et al. Eradication of Dientamoeba fragilis can resolve IBS-like symptoms. J Gastroenterol Hepatol 2002;17:A103.
25. Wolfe MS. Giardiasis. Clin Microbiol Rev 1992;5(1):93–100.
26. Staat MA, Rice M, Donauer S, et al. Intestinal parasite screening in internationally adopted children: importance of multiple stool specimens. Pediatrics 2011; 128(3):e613–22.

27. Wright SG. Protozoan infections of the gastrointestinal tract. Infect Dis Clin North Am 2012;26(2):323–39.
28. Rassi A Jr, Rassi A, Marin-Neto JA. Chagas disease. Lancet 2010;375(9723): 1388–402.
29. Bern C, Kjos S, Yabsley MJ, et al. Trypanosoma cruzi and Chagas' disease in the United States. Clin Microbiol Rev 2011;24(4):655–81.
30. Hanford EJ, Zhan FB, Lu Y, et al. Chagas disease in Texas: recognizing the significance and implications of evidence in the literature. Soc Sci Med 2007;65(1): 60–79.
31. Cantey PT, Stramer SL, Townsend RL, et al. The United States Trypanosoma cruzi Infection Study: evidence for vector-borne transmission of the parasite that causes Chagas disease among United States blood donors. Transfusion 2012; 52(9):1922–30.
32. Centers for Disease Control and Prevention (CDC). Congenital transmission of Chagas disease - Virginia, 2010. MMWR Morb Mortal Wkly Rep 2012;61(26): 477–9.
33. Oliveira I, Torrico F, Munoz J, et al. Congenital transmission of Chagas disease: a clinical approach. Expert Rev Anti Infect Ther 2010;8(8):945–56.
34. Rassi A Jr, Rassi A, Marcondes de Rezende J. American trypanosomiasis (Chagas disease). Infect Dis Clin North Am 2012;26(2):275–91.
35. Carlier Y, Torrico F, Sosa-Estani S, et al. Congenital Chagas disease: recommendations for diagnosis, treatment and control of newborns, siblings and pregnant women. PLoS Negl Trop Dis 2011;5(10):e1250.
36. Barry MA, Bezek S, Serpa JA, et al. Neglected infections of poverty in Texas and the rest of the United States: management and treatment options. Clin Pharmacol Ther 2012;92(2):170–81.
37. Paediatric dosage form of benznidazole (Chagas). Available at: http://www.dndi.org/portfolio/601.html. Accessed October 30, 2012.
38. Costa CH, Peters NC, Maruyama SR, et al. Vaccines for the leishmaniases: proposals for a research agenda. PLoS Negl Trop Dis 2011;5(3):e943.
39. Wright NA, Davis LE, Aftergut KS, et al. Cutaneous leishmaniasis in Texas: a northern spread of endemic areas. J Am Acad Dermatol 2008;58(4):650–2.
40. Tuon FF, Amato VS, Graf ME, et al. Treatment of New World cutaneous leishmaniasis–a systematic review with a meta-analysis. Int J Dermatol 2008;47(2):109–24.
41. Murray HW, Berman JD, Davies CR, et al. Advances in leishmaniasis. Lancet 2005;366(9496):1561–77.
42. Alvar J, Yactayo S, Bern C. Leishmaniasis and poverty. Trends Parasitol 2006; 22(12):552–7.
43. Croft SL, Olliaro P. Leishmaniasis chemotherapy–challenges and opportunities. Clin Microbiol Infect 2011;17(10):1478–83.
44. Sousa AQ, Frutuoso MS, Moraes EA, et al. High-dose oral fluconazole therapy effective for cutaneous leishmaniasis due to Leishmania (Vianna) braziliensis. Clin Infect Dis 2011;53(7):693–5.
45. Wortmann G, Zapor M, Ressner R, et al. Lipsosomal amphotericin B for treatment of cutaneous leishmaniasis. Am J Trop Med Hyg 2010;83(5):1028–33.
46. Congdon P, Lloyd P. Toxocara infection in the United States: the relevance of poverty, geography and demography as risk factors, and implications for estimating county prevalence. Int J Public Health 2011;56(1):15–24.
47. Hotez PJ, Wilkins PP. Toxocariasis: America's most common neglected infection of poverty and a helminthiasis of global importance? PLoS Negl Trop Dis 2009; 3(3):e400.

48. Won KY, Kruszon-Moran D, Schantz PM, et al. National seroprevalence and risk factors for Zoonotic Toxocara spp. infection. Am J Trop Med Hyg 2008;79(4): 552–7.
49. Herrmann N, Glickman LT, Schantz PM, et al. Seroprevalence of zoonotic toxocariasis in the United States: 1971-1973. Am J Epidemiol 1985;122(5):890–6.
50. Quattrocchi G, Nicoletti A, Marin B, et al. Toxocariasis and epilepsy: systematic review and meta-analysis. PLoS Negl Trop Dis 2012;6(8):e1775.
51. Woodhall D, Starr MC, Montgomery SP, et al. Ocular toxocariasis: epidemiologic, anatomic, and therapeutic variations based on a survey of ophthalmic subspecialists. Ophthalmology 2012;119(6):1211–7.
52. Centers for Disease Control, Prevention (CDC). Ocular toxocariasis–United States, 2009-2010. MMWR Morb Mortal Wkly Rep 2011;60(22):734–6.
53. Glickman L, Schantz P, Dombroske R, et al. Evaluation of serodiagnostic tests for visceral larva migrans. Am J Trop Med Hyg 1978;27(3):492–8.
54. Despommier D. Toxocariasis: clinical aspects, epidemiology, medical ecology, and molecular aspects. Clin Microbiol Rev 2003;16(2):265–72.
55. Caumes E. Treatment of cutaneous larva migrans and Toxocara infection. Fundam Clin Pharmacol 2003;17(2):213–6.
56. Magnaval JF. Apparent weak efficacy of ivermectin for treatment of human toxocariasis. Antimicrobial Agents Chemother 1998;42(10):2770.
57. Barisani-Asenbauer T, Maca SM, Hauff W, et al. Treatment of ocular toxocariasis with albendazole. J Ocul Pharmacol Ther 2001;17(3):287–94.
58. Lopez A, Dietz VJ, Wilson M, et al. Preventing congenital toxoplasmosis. MMWR Recomm Rep 2000;49(RR-2):59–68.
59. Montoya JG, Liesenfeld O. Toxoplasmosis. Lancet 2004;363(9425):1965–76.
60. Weiss LM, Dubey JP. Toxoplasmosis: a history of clinical observations. Int J Parasitol 2009;39(8):895–901.
61. Jones JL, Kruszon-Moran D, Won K, et al. Toxoplasma gondii and Toxocara spp. co-infection. Am J Trop Med Hyg 2008;78(1):35–9.
62. Jones JL, Kruszon-Moran D, Sanders-Lewis K, et al. Toxoplasma gondii infection in the United States, 1999 2004, decline from the prior decade. Am J Trop Med Hyg 2007;77(3):405–10.
63. Olariu TR, Remington JS, McLeod R, et al. Severe congenital toxoplasmosis in the United States: clinical and serologic findings in untreated infants. Pediatr Infect Dis J 2011;30(12):1056–61.
64. Montoya JG, Remington JS. Management of Toxoplasma gondii infection during pregnancy. Clin Infect Dis 2008;47(4):554–66.
65. McLeod R, Boyer K, Karrison T, et al. Outcome of treatment for congenital toxoplasmosis, 1981-2004: the National Collaborative Chicago-Based, Congenital Toxoplasmosis Study. Clin Infect Dis 2006;42(10):1383–94.
66. Montoya JG. Laboratory diagnosis of Toxoplasma gondii infection and toxoplasmosis. J Infect Dis 2002;185(Suppl 1):S73–82.
67. Robert-Gangneux F, Darde ML. Epidemiology of and diagnostic strategies for toxoplasmosis. Clin Microbiol Rev 2012;25(2):264–96.
68. Kim K. Time to screen for congenital toxoplasmosis? Clin Infect Dis 2006;42(10): 1395–7.
69. Hotez PJ. Fighting neglected tropical diseases in the southern United States. BMJ 2012;345:e6112.

Infections in Internationally Adopted Children

Judith K. Eckerle, MD[a], Cynthia R. Howard, MD, MPHTM[a], Chandy C. John, MD, MS[a,b,*]

KEYWORDS

- International adoptees • Screening • Multidisciplinary approach
- Latent tuberculosis infection

KEY POINTS

- The infectious and noninfectious health issues of international adoptees (IAs) are complex. Where possible, IAs should be evaluated at a clinic or a center specializing in international adoption, as specialized expertise and a multidisciplinary approach are often required for optimal evaluation and care of these children.
- IA children often have noninfectious health concerns, notably developmental delays and exposure to alcohol in utero, which require screening and evaluation by experts in these areas.
- Screening for specific infections for which IAs are at higher risk is important to prevent short- and long-term morbidity from these infections.
- Infections for which IAs are at higher risk and therefore require screening include viral (hepatitis A, B, and C and human immunodeficiency virus [HIV]), bacterial (syphilis and tuberculosis), and parasitic (stool helminths and *Giardia*) infections.
- All persons who will be in close contact with IAs should be vaccinated with hepatitis A vaccine or documented as immune to hepatitis A before the adoption of the IA child.
- Latent tuberculosis infection (LTBI) occurs in 21% to 28% of IAs. All IAs should be tested for tuberculosis on arrival and again 6 months after arrival (tuberculin skin test [TST] in children <5 years of age, TST or interferon-gamma release assay (IGRA) in children ≥5 years of age).
- It is critical to follow up on the results of tuberculosis screening and to treat children with LTBI with appropriate therapy, as children younger than 4 years with LTBI have the greatest risk of developing tuberculosis (TB) disease.
- Other infectious disease testing depends on specific risk factors.
  - If history or physical findings are suggestive of sexual abuse, test for gonorrhea and chlamydia.
  - If the child lived in a malaria endemic area, perform a blood smear for malaria.
  - If the child has eosinophilia that persists after successful treatment of helminth infection, test for *Toxocara canis* and *Strongyloides* and, if from a schistosomiasis endemic area, for schistosomiasis.

Conflicts of Interest: None.

[a] Division of Global Pediatrics, Department of Pediatrics, University of Minnesota Medical School, 717 Delaware Street Southeast, 3rd Floor, Minneapolis, MN 55414, USA; [b] Department of Medicine, University of Minnesota Medical School, 717 Delaware Street Southeast, Minneapolis, MN 55414, USA

* Corresponding author. Division of Global Pediatrics, University of Minnesota Medical School, 717 Delaware Street Southeast, Room 366, Minneapolis, MN 55414.

E-mail address: ccj@umn.edu

Pediatr Clin N Am 60 (2013) 487–505
http://dx.doi.org/10.1016/j.pcl.2012.12.010 pediatric.theclinics.com
0031-3955/13/$ – see front matter

INTRODUCTION

The number of international adoptions in the United States approached 16,000 in 1998, peaked at almost 23,000 in 2005, and was 9319 in 2011. For more than 30 years, until 1995, South Korea had been the leading country for international adoption in the United States. As of 2011, the 5 main countries of origin for adoptions to the United States are China, Ethiopia, Russia, South Korea, and Ukraine.[1]

In the 1980s, physicians began to research and understand the increased risks infectious diseases present in the internationally adopted population. Poor or absent prenatal care and low socioeconomic resources are common among IAs. Prenatal risk factors such as maternal illness, malnutrition, and exposures to maternal infectious diseases or drug or alcohol exposures, as well as orphanage and institutional care, all contribute to the increased potential for medical and infectious diseases in IAs. The first American Academy of Pediatrics (AAP) recommendations regarding universal screening for infectious and noninfectious diseases were issued in 1991[2] given low rates of complete IA screening after arrival to the United States at that time.[3]

IAs often have complex medical and psychosocial health problems that go beyond infectious disease issues. These health problems are beyond the scope of this article but have been summarized in other recent reviews.[4–6] IAs should ideally be evaluated at a clinic specializing in international adoption, because of the medical complexity of many of the health problems in these children and the need for a multidisciplinary team with expertise and experience in these health problems. Health screening of IAs should be done within the first 2 to 3 weeks postadoption to allow the children to first settle in with their adoptive family and then be seen for a comprehensive examination by an adoption provider or general pediatrician.

Evaluation of the IA child should start with a detailed history and physical examination, followed by routine screening for specific infectious diseases, micronutrient deficiencies, developmental delays, and tailored additional screening based on risk factors elicited from the history and physical examination.

MEDICAL HISTORY AND PHYSICAL EXAMINATION

All IAs require a thorough history and physical examination, as many have medical, social, or behavioral issues that require investigation in addition to infectious issues. With regards to infectious disease, key findings to be assessed in IAs by medical history and physical examination are summarized in **Tables 1** and **2**.

INFECTIOUS DISEASE SCREENING

Recent guidelines for IA health screening tests were published in the Yellow Book in 2010 and in the Red Book in 2012.[7,8] **Fig. 1** summarizes the routine infectious disease and other screening tests performed on all IA children seen at the University of Minnesota International Adoption Clinic (IAC), and **Table 3** summarizes the screening done if prompted by specific findings on history taking or physical examination.

Vaccine Preventable Infections

Immunization practices for IAs vary widely in the countries of origin, as well as in what is done for adoptees once they join their families in the United States. Vaccines vary by country, and availability of vaccines is variable depending on the country of birth. Rarely do vaccine schedules meet US standards, due to cost and other factors (**Table 4**).

Table 1
Key medical history findings to assess in internationally adopted child that may relate to acute or chronic infections

History	Comments
Care before adoption	Evaluate for risk of abuse, sexually transmitted diseases
Time spent in institution	Prolonged time in institution is related to increased risk of diarrhea, tuberculosis, and other infectious diseases
Growth chart, if available	May see stunting with infectious diseases such as repeated episodes of diarrhea or recurrent malaria
Maternal infection history, including syphilis and HIV testing	Often not known
Immunization records, including BCG	See section on immunization; records often unreliable
Country of origin	Institutional care and poor country resources can increase risk of infectious diseases

Abbreviation: BCG, bacille Calmette-Guérin.

Studies of IAs have shown wide variation in the response rate to vaccinations, with as low as a 56% response rate to the mumps vaccine in children from China.[9] Inaccurate documentation, poorly stored vaccines, stressed immune systems, and timing issues can all contribute to the lack of response. For this reason, 2 options exist for IAs as recommended by the AAP. First, in any age but especially in children younger than 6 months, it is acceptable to choose to start over and fully reimmunize. Alternatively, titers can be sent to demonstrate immunity to given/documented vaccinations or illnesses reported (eg, hepatitis A and varicella).

Measles/mumps/rubella (MMR), hepatitis A and B, polio, diphtheria/tetanus, *Haemophilus influenzae* type b, and varicella are all vaccination titers that can be verified by serology. Although pertussis titers do not correlate well with immunity, if immunity is demonstrated to diphtheria and tetanus, pertussis immunity is assumed. If protective titers are documented for a vaccine, the IA child does not need to be revaccinated,

Table 2
Key physical examination findings to assess in the internationally adopted child that may relate to acute or chronic infections

Examination Area	Specific Signs
Height, weight	—
Skin	Look for birthmarks, signs of abuse (eg, bruises), signs of infection (eg, scabies and tinea)
Face	Signs of fetal alcohol spectrum disorder or other syndromes
Abdomen	Hepatosplenomegaly (could indicate several infectious and noninfectious diseases, including malaria, schistosomiasis, sickle cell disease)
Genitalia	Signs of abuse, sexually transmitted diseases, ritual or other circumcision, precocious puberty
Head circumference (OFC)	Microcephaly or macrocephaly are clues to cognitive issues, prenatal infections, and other medical issues (eg, hydrocephalus and rickets)

Abbreviation: OFC, occipital-frontal circumference.

Viral

- ❑ Hepatitis A total Ig (with reflex testing for IgM if total Ig positive)
- ❑ Hepatitis B (SAg, SAb, Core Ab)**
- ❑ Hepatitis C Ab*
- ❑ HIV Ab*

Bacterial

- ❑ Syphilis screening (Anti-treponemal Ab, RPR, VDRL)
- ❑ Tuberculin skin test (TST) if <5yo *
- ❑ TST or Quantiferon Gold blood test if ≥5yo*

Parasitic

- ❑ Stool examination for ova and parasites x 3
- ❑ Giardia Stool antigen

Vaccine Preventable Infections

- ❑ Measles, Mumps and Rubella Ab
- ❑ Diphtheria and Tetanus Ab
- ❑ Haemophilus influenzae type b Ab
- ❑ Polio Types 1 and 2 Ab
- ❑ Varicella Ab

General Health Screening

- ❑ Complete blood count, including a peripheral eosinophil count and red blood cell indices*
- ❑ Vitamin D total*
- ❑ Iron panel including C-reactive protein*
- ❑ Thyroid stimulating hormone (TSH) and free thyroxine (free T4)

* Retest at 6 mo
** Retest at 6 mo if test results negative on initial testing

Fig. 1. Recommended infectious disease and general health screening for all newly arrived international adoptees.

Table 3
Screening to consider in internationally adopted children, based on history and clinical findings

Indication	Test
Infectious Disease Screening	
Suspected sexual abuse	*Neisseria gonorrhea* and *Chlamydia trachomatis* PCR
Resided in malaria endemic area	Thick and thin blood smear for malaria
Diarrhea with fever, especially if bloody diarrhea is present	Stool cultures
Eosinophilia	Depending on area and risk factors, consider testing for antibodies to *Schistosoma* species, *Strongyloides stercoralis*, and *T. canis*[a]
Other Screening	
Clinical findings consistent with disorders assessed in newborn screen	Newborn screen for congenital metabolic and other disorders

Abbreviation: PCR, polymerase chain reaction.
[a] Recommend sending to the Centers for Disease Control and Prevention laboratories.

Table 4
Immunization schedules from top 5 countries that participate in international adoption

	Ukraine	Ethiopia	South Korea	Russia	China
MMR	M12, Y6	(Measles only, W6)	M12–15, Y4–6	Y1, Y6	M18
DTaP	M3, M4, M5	W6, W10, W14	M2, M4, M6, M15–18, Y6	M3, M4.5, M6, M18, Y6	M3, M4, M5, M18
DT	Y6		Y11–12	Y6–7, Y14	Y6
Hib	M3, M4, M18	W6, W10, W14		M6, M7	M6, M7
HepB	B, M1, M6	W6, W10, W14	B, M1, M6	B, M1, M6	B, M1, M6
BCG	D3, Y7	B	B-W4, variable	D3, Y7, Y14	B
IPV/OPV	IPV: M5, M18, Y6, Y14,	OPV: W6, W10, W14	IPV: M2, M4, M6, Y4–6	IPV: M3, M4.5, then OPV M6, M18, M20, Y14	OPV: M2, M3, M4, Y4
PCV		W6, W10, W14			
VZV			M12–15		
HepA			M12–15		M18

Abbreviations: B, birth; BCG, bacille Calmette-Guérin; DT, diphtheria-tetanus toxoid; DTaP, diphtheria, tetanus, and pertussis; HepA, hepatitis A; HepB, hepatitis B; Hib, *Haemophilus influenzae* type B; IPV, injectible polio vaccination; M, month; MMR, measles/mumps/rubella; OPV, oral polio vaccine; PCV, pneumococcal conjugate vaccine, VZV, Varicella zoster virus; W, week; Y, year.

and families can proceed with vaccinations that were not available/given at the typical schedule for age. However, if protective titers are not found for a specific vaccine, then the primary care physician should restart vaccinations on the catch-up schedule available online at http://www.cdc.gov/vaccines/schedules/downloads/child/catchup-schedule-pr.pdf.

Vaccinations such as the pneumococcal conjugate, hepatitis A, MMR, and varicella vaccines are frequently not available before adoption and should be tested for with titer or restarted.

Bacterial Infections

Tuberculosis

TB is caused by *Mycobacterium tuberculosis* complex organisms. One-third of the world is estimated to have infection with *M. tuberculosis*, and every year, 9 million people develop clinical disease caused by the infection. Approximately 1 million cases of TB (11%) occur in children younger than 15 years[10,11] Twenty-two high-prevalence countries have been identified as having 80% of the TB cases worldwide. All 10 countries with the highest numbers of adoptees to the United States, including Russia, Ethiopia, Vietnam, China, and India, are on this list.[12] LTBI is defined as a positive result on IGRA, for example, the QuantiFERON-GOLD blood test, or a positive result on TST, with no clinical evidence of active pulmonary disease by radiographic imaging.[7] LTBI was present in 21% to 28% of all IAs in 2 recent surveys.[13–15]

The bacille Calmette-Guérin (BCG) vaccine is given to newborns in 157 countries. A comprehensive database of countries that administer BCG vaccination is available at http://www.bcgatlas.org/.[16] Although BCG vaccination within 6 months of a TST may result in a false-positive TST result,[17] the AAP and Centers for Disease Control (CDC) recommend that TST results be interpreted according to standard guidelines, regardless of BCG vaccination history. The vast majority of IAs are older than 6 months, and therefore, it has been more than 6 months since their BCG vaccination, which is typically done at birth. For the small percentage of IAs who have a still-healing BCG scar or known BCG immunization within the past 6 months, some clinicians would defer a TST in children until greater than 6 months after the immunization, but care should be taken that testing is done on follow-up and not missed. BCG administration does not affect IGRA testing.

The AAP recommends screening for TB (TST in children <5 years of age; TST or IGRA in children ≥5 years of age) in all internationally adopted children. Children in the international adoption system are seen and examined by panel physicians in their country of origin. Panel physicians are doctors who have been selected and trained for standardization by their respective governmental Department of State. They perform examinations for children who are applying for visas, before travel. Panel examinations are generally limited to major or serious communicable disease and/or mental health defects. However, panel examinations do include evaluation for LTBI or TB in children 2 to 14 years of age by TST, with chest radiograph testing in those with a positive TST result, and screening for TB in children 15 years or older.[18] Children younger than 2 years do not have any screening for LTBI or TB unless they have symptoms of TB.

Because many IAs are younger than 2 years and the quality of TST administration can vary among sites, the authors recommend that all IAs be screened for TB when seen in the United States, regardless of prior testing. IA children should be screened by TST if younger than 5 years and may be screened by TST or IGRA if 5 years or older.[19] In IA children, without other major risk factors for TB, a positive TST result is 10 mm of induration. Children should be retested by TST or IGRA 6 months after adoption, as up to 20% may be negative on initial testing but positive on testing 6 months later.[15] All children with a positive TST or IGRA result must have a chest radiograph and repeat physical examination to assess for evidence of tuberculous disease. An algorithm for evaluation and treatment of TB and LTBI is outlined in **Fig. 2**.

LTBI is common in IAs, and TB disease, although rare, has also been reported in IAs. It is critical that a clear system is in place for follow-up of a child's TB screening test results and that all children with LTBI or TB disease are treated appropriately, particularly because children younger than 4 years with LTBI have the highest risk of disease activation. Children with LTBI can usually be treated with isoniazid (INH) for 9 months. The primary physician should see the child monthly to monitor for side effects, medication compliance, and any sign of tuberculous disease (**Box 1**).

Congenital syphilis

Syphilis is a sexually transmitted illness caused by the bacterial spirochete *Treponema pallidum*. Transmission rate from an infected birth mother to her fetus depends on the stage of syphilis in the mother. Transmission ranges from 60% to 100% in mothers with primary and secondary syphilis and is about 40% in mothers with early latent syphilis and 8% in mothers with late latent syphilis.[7] Transmission can occur via hematogenous spread in utero and/or by direct contact through the birth process.[20]

Worldwide, there have been rising trends in syphilis infection.[21–23] A contributing factor in South Korea may be the passing of legislation that made prostitution illegal and thus took away the routine screening and treatment of sex workers in the country.[22] China has experienced a rapidly growing syphilis epidemic since the early 1990s, with the reported incidence of congenital syphilis increasing from 0.01 cases per 100,000 live births in 1991 to 19.7 cases per 100,000 live births in 2005.[24] Syphilis remains a rare infection in internationally adopted children but one that has the potential for severe complications if not treated, so screening and treatment where indicated for this infection is critical in internationally adopted children.

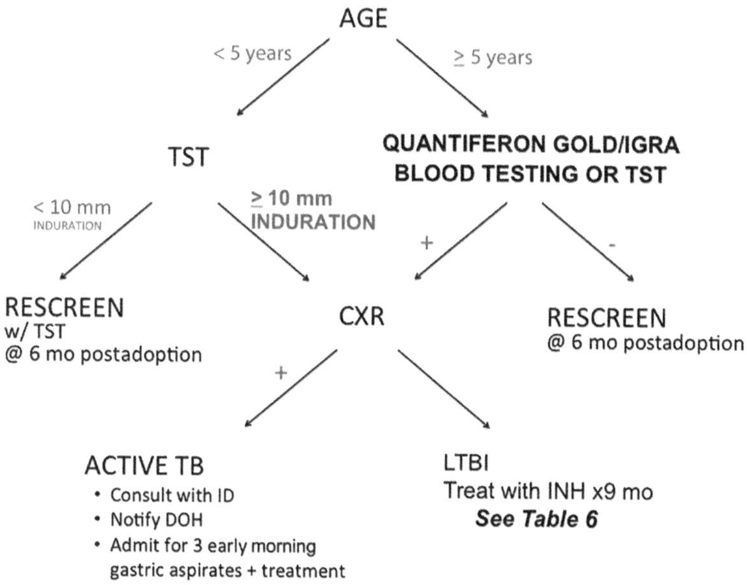

Fig. 2. Evaluation and treatment of tuberculosis in the internationally adopted child. ID, infectious diseases specialist.

Box 1
Treatment recommendations for LTBI

1. Treatment of LTBI: INH 10 to 15 mg/kg once daily × 9 months (maximum dose 300 mg/d).[a]
2. INH crushed or swallowed tablets help prevent the osmotic diarrhea that is seen in treatment with the liquid form of INH.
3. In children without known liver disease, liver function test monitoring is not needed unless clinical symptoms arise.
4. Children should be seen by their primary care physician once a month during treatment to monitor compliance as well as clinical symptom check.
5. In malnourished children, supplementation with pyridoxine should be considered during INH treatment.
6. Alternative therapy in children older than 12 years consists of one weekly dosing of INH and rifapentine given by directly observed therapy by the health department, total 12-week therapy.

[a] For suspected drug-resistant TB, consult with an infectious diseases specialist.

Untreated maternal syphilis can lead to stillbirth, abortion, perinatal death, or hydrops in up to half of affected fetuses. Numerous other complications can result from congenital syphilis in the surviving neonate. Some complications of congenital syphilis manifest at birth or within the first month of life, whereas others manifest much later in life. **Table 5** lists the findings associated with congenital syphilis and their time of appearance. Although sexual abuse can potentially lead to syphilis in an internationally adopted child, all cases of syphilis seen at the University of Minnesota IAC have been presumed to be congenital syphilis. All cases seen to date at the IAC have also been picked up by screening testing and not because of clinical abnormalities.

Syphilis is among the few screening tests that are done before adoption in children from nearly every participating country, but screening should be repeated to verify results. The CDC recommends screening with nontreponemal tests (Venereal disease research laboratory [VDRL] or rapid plasma reagin [RPR]) and then confirming with a treponemal test (fluorescent treponemal antibody absorption [FTA-ABS], treponema pallidum particle agglutination [TP-PA], microhemagglutination assay [MHA-TP], treponema pallidum enzyme immunoassay [TP-EIA]), but for cost and personnel reasons,

Table 5
Clinical manifestations of congenital syphilis

Age	Clinical Symptom
Birth	Stillbirth, hydrops fetalis, preterm birth, asymptomatic
Infancy	Hepatosplenomegaly, snuffles (copious nasal secretions), lymphadenopathy, mucocutaneous lesions, pneumonia, osteochondritis, pseudoparalysis, edema, rash, hemolytic anemia, thrombocytopenia
>2 y	Central nervous system, bone, joint, teeth, eye, skin issues
5–20 y	Interstitial keratitis, Hutchinson teeth, anterior bowing of shins, frontal bossing, mulberry molars, saddle nose, rhagades, Clutton joints
10–40 y	Eighth cranial nerve deafness

Data from American Academy of Pediatrics. Red Book: 2012 Report of the Committee on Infectious Diseases. In: Pickering LK, editor. 29th edition. Elk Grove Village (IL): American Academy of Pediatrics; 2012.

many laboratories now screen with the treponemal test and then confirm with the non-treponemal test. This reverse screening approach results in a larger number of initial false-positive test results. Treponemal tests remain positive for life and cannot be used to follow success of treatment.

The reader is referred to the Red Book: 2012 Committee on Infectious Diseases of the AAP[7] for guidelines on diagnosis and treatment of congenital syphilis, as both diagnosis and treatment are complex. Some children may come from areas where other diseases caused by spirochetes (yaws, frambesia, pinta, and bejel) may lead to a positive treponemal antibody test. Treatment of these children, especially if the nontreponemal test result is negative or equivocal, is not clear-cut. Consultation with a pediatric infectious diseases clinician familiar with syphilis is advised for any child with suspected congenital syphilis. Long-term outcomes of children with asymptomatic congenital syphilis have not been well studied, and this is an area that requires further research.

Viral Infections

Hepatitis A

Infection with the hepatitis A virus can lead to diarrhea and liver inflammation. Risk of contracting hepatitis A is through fecal-oral transmission and is increased with crowding, in certain ethnic populations and in low-income communities and communities with limited access to sanitation.[25] All these risks are common for orphanage populations abroad, and many adoptees come from countries with a high prevalence of hepatitis A (**Fig. 3**).

From 80% to 95% of acutely infected children younger than 5 years are asymptomatic with hepatitis A infection,[26] but they are able to spread infection to other family and community members who are more likely to develop disease. Symptoms when present can include nonspecific gastrointestinal (GI) complaints (nausea, vomiting, and diarrhea), muscle or joint pain, and jaundice. Supportive care is recommended. Illness in symptomatic children is usually self-limited, but hepatitis A infection is severe in older adults or immunocompromised individuals. In 2007 and 2008, multiple cases of internationally adopted children who infected members of their adoptive families or community were reported.[27,28] Based on these case reports, the Advisory Committee on Immunization Practices issued a new recommendation in 2009 of "routine hepatitis A vaccination for household members and other close personal contacts (eg, regular babysitters) of adopted children newly arriving from countries with high or intermediate hepatitis A endemicity."[29] Hepatitis A is not currently part of the AAP recommendations for universal screening of IAs, but because of the recent cases of asymptomatic infection and spread to family members, the University of Minnesota IAC conducts routine screening of all IA children for hepatitis A. This screening permits evaluation of asymptomatic infection in children from endemic areas and of the immune status and need for vaccination with the hepatitis A vaccine. Testing of total antibodies to hepatitis A, with automatic testing of positive samples for hepatitis A IgM antibodies, identifies those who are hepatitis A immune (positive total antibodies, negative IgM), those who are acutely infected (positive total antibodies, positive IgM), and those who are nonimmune (negative total antibodies). Alternatively, routine testing for IgG and IgM to hepatitis A can be performed. Catch-up vaccination should be performed on IA children who do not have IgG or total antibodies to hepatitis A. Children who have acute hepatitis A infection do not need subsequent vaccination, but all close contacts and family members need urgent hepatitis A vaccination if not already vaccinated or immune.

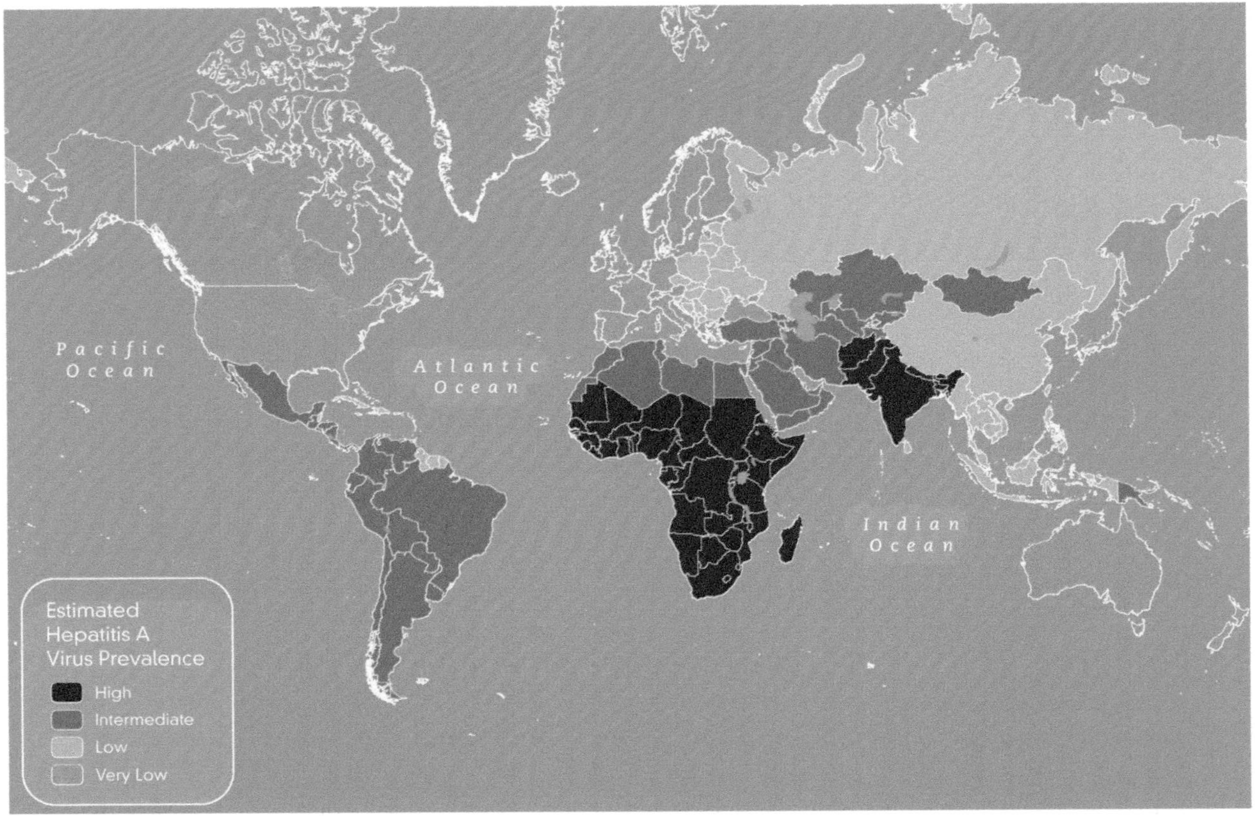

Fig. 3. Prevalence of hepatitis A virus infection worldwide. (*From* Centers for Disease Control and Prevention. CDC Health Information for International Travel 2012. New York: Oxford University Press; 2012.)

Hepatitis B

Hepatitis B is caused by the hepatitis B virus (HBV) and can cause liver inflammation and chronic liver damage. Perinatal transmission results in greater than 90% lifelong or chronic infection. Later infection at age 1 to 5 years creates a 25% to 50% chronic disease rate.[7]

Only about 5% to 15% of children who are younger than 5 years are symptomatic, whereas symptoms increase with increasing age at the time of HBV infection. The most serious consequence from HBV is liver damage in approximately 25% of untreated, chronic infections that can result in cirrhosis (scarring) and/or primary hepatocellular carcinoma that rarely occurs in childhood but peaks in incidence at around 50 years of age.[30] Hepatitis B immune globulin (HBIG) and hepatitis B vaccine are about 95% effective in preventing transmission[31] and are available domestically but are not widely available in most countries that participate in intercountry adoption. South Korea is currently the only country that actively provides HBIG to infants of HBV seropositive birth mothers. However, hepatitis B testing is done from virtually all countries before referral. If testing is done before 6 months of age and results are found to be negative, screening should be repeated to ensure accurate detection.

For families who adopt a child with hepatitis B, close contacts should ensure that they have had HBV vaccination, which is the most effective way to prevent transmission. The United States offers universal vaccination for hepatitis B, and because of vaccination programs, the incidence of HBV infection has decreased dramatically in the United States.[32] Likewise, hepatitis B was common in Asia, but since vaccination programs started 18 years ago, the prevalence in 2008 in China was 1% for children with hepatitis B younger than 5 years and 4% for those aged 5 to 14 years, with similar results in South Korea.[33] Hepatitis B testing should be done as part of the panel for newly arrived adoptees and includes HepBSag, HepBSab, and HepBCoreAb (**Fig. 4**). If HepBSab result is negative, then catch-up vaccinations should be initiated and repeat HepBSag and HepBSab should be performed with the 6-month follow-up laboratory testing. If the hepatitis BSAg test result is found to be positive, further testing is required in consultation with a pediatric gastroenterology liver specialist.

Hepatitis C

Hepatitis C (Hep C) infection is caused by the hepatitis C virus (HCV) and is a major worldwide cause of liver disease (**Fig. 5**). It is estimated that there are approximately 170 million HCV carriers worldwide.[34] Perinatal transmission is the most common method of transmission in the internationally adopted population, although only 2.7% to 5.6% of children born to HCV-positive women contract the virus. HCV transmission to the newborn is higher from birthmothers coinfected with HIV.[35] If perinatal transmission occurs, it results in about 80% of affected children having chronic infection.[7] The virus was transmitted by infected needles (estimated 68% of all Hep C infections)[36] or transfusions before 1992, when screening for Hep C was instituted.

Symptoms vary, but most children with HCV have few symptoms. Children with Hep C infection should be evaluated and followed up by a pediatric gastroenterologist, and liver function tests should be checked regularly. Factors that can worsen liver function in patients with HCV infection include other infectious diseases such as HIV, medications, alcohol consumption, and obesity. The most serious issue from HCV is liver damage (cirrhosis), which is rare in children (estimated at <5% in the first 20 years of life) but increases in frequency in adults (25% incidence, lifelong).[37] Ethiopia and some countries in Eastern Europe intermittently test for hepatitis C virus antibody (HCVAb), depending on maternal risk factors as well as availability of resources. In the vast majority of cases, if a child is positive for HCVAb, it is from maternal antibody

Interpretation of Hepatitis B Serologic Test Results

Hepatitis B serologic testing involves measurement of several hepatitis B virus (HBV)-specific antigens and antibodies. Different serologic "markers" or combinations of markers are used to identify different phases of HBV infection and to determine whether a patient has acute or chronic HBV infection, is immune to HBV as a result of prior infection or vaccination, or is susceptible to infection.

HBsAg **anti-HBc** **anti-HBs**	negative negative negative	Susceptible
HBsAg **anti-HBc** **anti-HBs**	negative positive positive	Immune due to natural infection
HBsAg **anti-HBc** **anti-HBs**	negative negative positive	Immune due to hepatitis B vaccination
HBsAg **anti-HBc** **IgM anti-HBc** **anti-HBs**	positive positive positive negative	Acutely infected
HBsAg **anti-HBc** **IgM anti-HBc** **anti-HBs**	positive positive negative negative	Chronically infected
HBsAg **anti-HBc** **anti-HBs**	negative positive negative	Interpretation unclear; four possibilities: 1. Resolved infection (most common) 2. False-positive anti-HBc, thus susceptible 3. "Low level" chronic infection 4. Resolving acute infection

Adapted from: A Comprehensive Immunization Strategy to Eliminate Transmission of Hepatitis B Virus Infection in the United States: Recommendations of the Advisory Committee on Immunization Practices. Part I: Immunization of Infants, Children, and Adolescents. MMWR 2005;54(No. RR-16).

DEPARTMENT OF HEALTH & HUMAN SERVICES
Centers for Disease Control and Prevention
Division of Viral Hepatitis

www.cdc.gov/hepatitis

- **Hepatitis B surface antigen (HBsAg):** A protein on the surface of hepatitis B virus; it can be detected in high levels in serum during acute or chronic hepatitis B virus infection. The presence of HBsAg indicates that the person is infectious. The body normally produces antibodies to HBsAg as part of the normal immune response to infection. HBsAg is the antigen used to make hepatitis B vaccine.
- **Hepatitis B surface antibody (anti-HBs):** The presence of anti-HBs is generally interpreted as indicating recovery and immunity from hepatitis B virus infection. Anti-HBs also develops in a person who has been successfully vaccinated against hepatitis B.
- **Total hepatitis B core antibody (anti-HBc):** Appears at the onset of symptoms in acute hepatitis B and persists for life. The presence of anti-HBc indicates previous or ongoing infection with hepatitis B virus in an undefined time frame.
- **IgM antibody to hepatitis B core antigen (IgM anti-HBc):** Positivity indicates recent infection with hepatitis B virus (≤6 mos). Its presence indicates acute infection.

Fig. 4. Interpretation of hepatitis B serologic test results. (*From* Centers for Disease Control and Prevention. Hepatitis B information for health professionals. Available at: http://www.cdc.gov/hepatitis/hbv/#. Accessed Feb 20, 2013.)

and does not represent current infection. Maternal antibody can take up to 18 months to disappear in a noninfected child. HCVAb should be tested for in the newly arrived IA given that risk factors for Hep C infection may not be known in the history and many adoptees are now being adopted from higher-prevalence countries of origin.[7] Hep C polymerase chain reaction (PCR) should also be sent for if the child is younger than 18 months and has a known history of exposure or prior positive antibody testing.

There are no current cures for Hep C infection, but antiviral and other medications may decrease risk of liver disease from chronic Hep C infection.

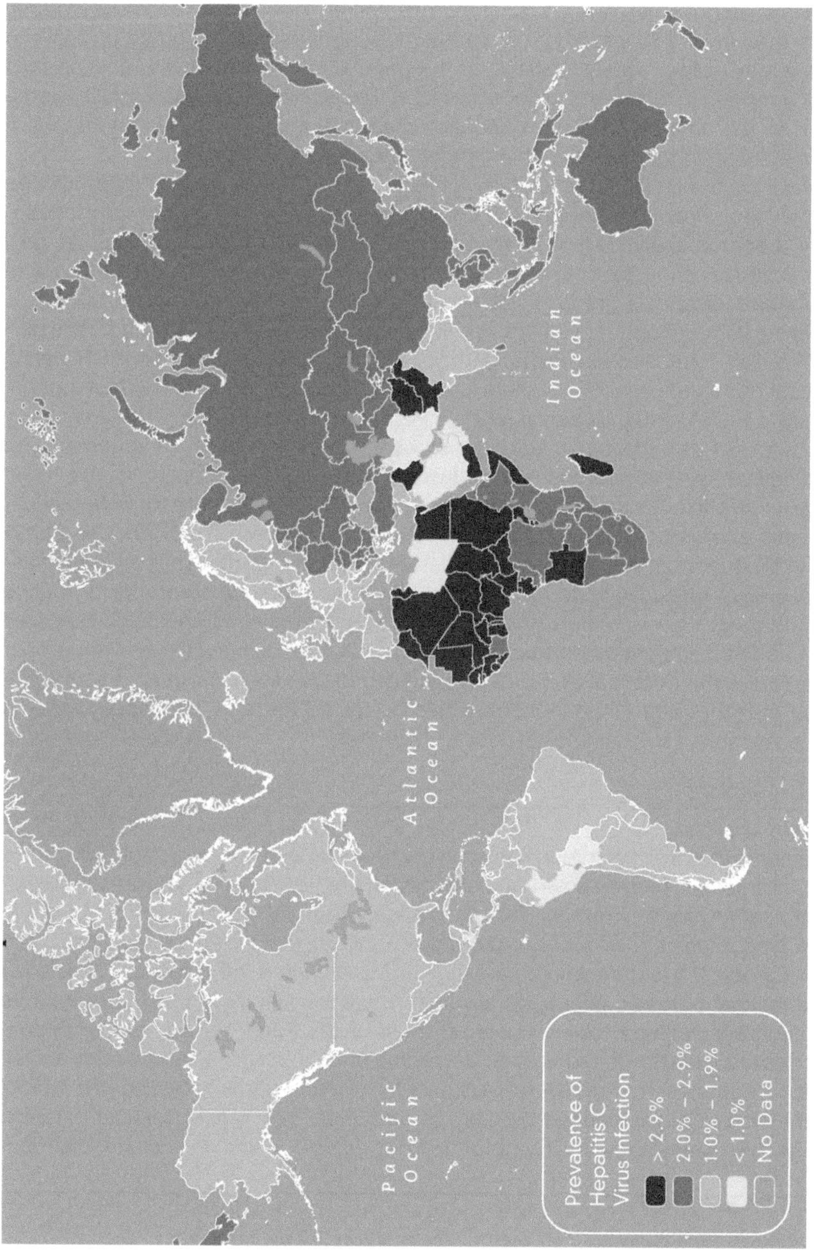

Fig. 5. Prevalence of hepatitis C virus infection worldwide. (*From* Centers for Disease Control and Prevention. CDC Health Information for International Travel 2012. New York: Oxford University Press; 2012.)

HIV

HIV can cause a wide range of symptoms. Perinatal transmission is the most common mode of infection in the internationally adopted population, although HIV infection is rare in children adopted to the United States (<1% of IA have HIV infection). Without prophylaxis, approximately 12% to 40% of children born to HIV-positive women contract the virus.[7] HIV prophylaxis is now available in some countries of origin of IAs, but it may not be widely available to the population of women who give up their child for adoption. Breastfeeding accounts for a third to half of the cases of HIV transmission, so the time that the child was admitted into a care center is an important factor in estimating the last probable time of HIV exposure for the child.

Especially in the first 6 months of life, children with HIV may be asymptomatic. As they grow older, they typically develop symptoms that may include fevers, lymphadenopathy, hepatomegaly, failure to thrive, and recurrent infections. In orphanages, other infections and institutional neglect can also cause poor growth, so it may be difficult to make a diagnosis of HIV on purely clinical grounds in some cases.

Screening with HIV antibody or enzyme-linked immunosorbent assay (ELISA) is performed from all current countries that participate in international adoption. PCR testing is available from most countries if there is a history of exposure, high-risk background, or a positive ELISA result. However, all new IAs should have HIV 1 and HIV 2 antibody testing by ELISA as part of their standard screening, as the reliability and accuracy of HIV testing in outside laboratories is not always known, and this infection should never be missed in a child. About 93% of HIV-infected children test positive for DNA by PCR by 2 weeks after exposure, and 95% are positive by 1 month old.[38] Positive ELISA results in IAs are most frequently a reflection of passive maternal antibody transmission and are not reflective of active infection. However, there are programs for waiting children that have documented HIV infection. HIV-infected children should be cared for by a pediatric infectious diseases specialist with expertise in HIV, as with proper care they have the potential to live active and productive lives. Children arriving with a history of HIV and/or HIV exposure should be tested for other infectious diseases including hepatitis as recommended for all new IAs.

Parasitic Infections

Intestinal parasites

Intestinal parasites are a common finding in the newly arrived adoptee. Multiple studies of parasitic infections have shown varying rates and types of ova or parasites identified on stool examinations (**Table 6**). This rate ranges from 9% in Chinese[6,13] to 53% in Ethiopian adoptees.[5] Giardiasis is particularly prevalent in children adopted from Eastern Europe.[13] Most intestinal parasites are transmitted via fecal-oral transfer of cysts. Intestinal parasitic infections are seen more frequently in child care centers and institutional settings, which make up most of the living conditions for children being adopted into the United States. Screening should be done shortly after arrival, with 3 stool samples from separate days sent for ova and parasite testing and 1 stool examination for *Giardia* antigen by enzyme immunoassay. Most intestinal parasitic infections are asymptomatic. Symptoms from *Giardia* infection include diarrhea,

Table 6
Most common stool parasitic infections of internationally adopted children

Frequency	Parasites
Frequent	*Giardia intestinalis, Blastocystis hominis, Dientamoeba fragilis*
Occasional	*Trichuris trichiura, Ascaris lumbricoides, Strongyloides stercoralis*

bloating, and abdominal distention, whereas symptoms of intestinal helminths are highly variable. IA children rarely have complaints specific to intestinal helminths. Abdominal pain is a common complaint among IAs, but it is as common in those without helminth infection as those with helminth infection. Bacterial infection of the GI tract is not common in IAs, and stool cultures should be done only if there are bloody stools, fever, or other signs of *Salmonella*, *Shigella*, or *Campylobacter* infection.

Treatment of Giardia is recommended for the internationally adopted population. Although some cases of pediatric giardiasis resolve without treatment, IAs may have other risk factors such as growth stunting, malnutrition, stress of multiple transitions, or other medical issues that compromise the immune system and make it more difficult to clear the parasite. Given additional risk of transmission to family members during the time needed for bonding and attachment, treatment is indicated and typically curative with oral metronidazole. Drug resistance is uncommon, and retesting for *Giardia* is not recommended unless the child has persistent symptoms. Treatment of the 3 most common intestinal parasitic infections in IAs is outlined in **Table 7**.

Malaria

Malaria is caused by the genus *Plasmodium*, which includes *P. falciparum, P. vivax, P. ovale, P. malariae*, and *P. knowlesi*. It is transmitted through the bite of an infected mosquito or, more rarely, by perinatal transmission from an infected birth mother.

Symptoms are often nonspecific but almost always include high fevers. Other symptoms may include sweating, nausea, vomiting, cough, and diarrhea. Severe anemia may be a presenting sign in young children or infants. Central nervous system involvement

Table 7
Drug treatment of the 3 most common stool parasitic infections in internationally adopted children

Infection	Drug of Choice	Adult Dosage	Pediatric Dosage
Blastocystis hominis	Metronidazole[a]	750 mg PO tid 10 d	35–50 mg/kg/d (max 2 g) PO in 3 doses × 10 d
Dientamoeba fragilis	Iodoquinol[b,c]	650 mg PO tid × 20 d	30–40 mg/kg/d (max 2 g) PO in 3 doses × 7 d
	OR		
	Paromomycin[c,d]	25–35 mg/kg/d PO in 3 doses × 7 d	25–35 mg/kg/d PO in 3 doses × 7 d
	OR		
	Metronidazole[c]	500–750 mg PO tid × 10 d	35–50 mg/kg/d PO in 3 doses × 10 d
Giardia intestinalis	Metronidazole[c]	250 mg PO tid × 5–7 d	15 mg/kg/d PO in 3 doses × 5–7 d
	OR		
	Tinidazole	2 g PO once	≥3 y: 50 mg/kg PO once (max 2 g)
	OR		
	Nitazoxanide	500 mg PO bid × 3 d	1–3 y: 100 mg PO bid × 3 d 4–11 y: 200 mg PO bid × 3 d >12 y: 500 mg PO bid × 3 d

Abbreviations: bid, 2 times per day; PO, oral; tid, 3 times per day.

[a] Clinical significance of these organisms and therefore indication for treatment is controversial. Metronidazole resistance may be common in some areas.

[b] Taken after meals.

[c] Not FDA approved for this indication.

[d] Take paromomycin with food.

Data from American Academy of Pediatrics. Red Book: 2012 Report of the Committee on Infectious Diseases. In: Pickering LK, editor. 29th edition. Elk Grove Village (IL): American Academy of Pediatrics; 2012.

may manifest as seizures, impaired consciousness, or coma. Children with coma due to *P. falciparum* (cerebral malaria) have a high mortality rate (15–20%).[39,40]

Adoption from sub-Saharan African countries, notably Ethiopia, has increased in the past decade, so malaria testing is a more frequent concern, but countries in Asia, Latin America, and the Caribbean (Haiti) may also have malaria endemic regions. Malaria screening by microscopy should be performed on IAs newly arrived from a malaria endemic region because children can be asymptomatically infected and later develop clinical symptoms. Parasite testing with thick and thin blood smears should be performed. Any febrile child from a malaria endemic area should have 3 smears done, each separated by at least 12 hours to rule out malaria as the cause.[8] Treatment of malaria is complex and beyond the scope of this article, but further guidance on treatment can be found in the AAP Red Book. For severe cases of malaria, the CDC Malaria Hotline (770-488-7788) is available for consultation.

Children with uncomplicated malaria typically recover well. Cerebral malaria is linked to increased rates of seizures[40] and permanent cognitive deficits in working memory and attention skills[41] and may need further evaluation by neurology, psychology, and/or neuropsychology if deficits persist after settling into their adoptive home.

Scabies

Scabies is a contagious skin disease caused by adult female *Sarcoptes scabei* mite that burrows under the skin and causes intense pruritus. Because children are in such close proximity to each other in care centers and orphanages, scabies is a common infestation and is seen in as many as 10% of new IAs to the United States.[42]

The incubation period is up to 4 to 6 weeks after exposure, so it is common for parents or other family members to develop bumps a few weeks after visiting their child or after introducing their child into their household.

The treatment of choice is topical scabies treatment cream (insecticide) permethrin, 5%. Scabies is a slow-moving bug and therefore unlikely to infect remote contacts, but family contacts should all be treated. Treatment is application of topical permethrin from hairline to toes for 4 hours (for children 2–6 months old) and for 8 to 14 hours for older children and adults, then shower or bathe.[7] For babies or toddlers, mittens on their hands are recommended to prevent them from licking or ingesting the medication. Environmental decontamination is also recommended with washing all clothing and linens in hot water and drying in a hot dryer. If hot water is not available, it is acceptable to place all linen and clothing in plastic bags and store the bags away from the family for 7 days, as the mite cannot survive for more than 4 days without skin contact. Hypersensitivity to the proteins can persist for weeks, despite successful treatment of the mite, and so retreatment is only recommended if symptoms continue to persist for many weeks after initial therapy or if new lesions develop despite treatment. Pets do not need treatment.

EOSINOPHILIA IN THE INTERNATIONALLY ADOPTED CHILD

Eosinophilia can be found in the laboratory testing of new adoptees. Estimates of eosinophilia in IAs range from 4% to 19%.[43,44] Stool should first be examined for helminth infection, with 3 stool specimens tested. If stool test shows negative results, then further antibody testing is recommended for schistosomiasis, *T. canis*, and *Strongyloides*, if the child comes from an area where one or more of these infections is endemic.[45] Further testing for schistosomiasis can be done with stool or urine (noon to 3 PM is the highest shedding time in urine).[7] Consideration of lymphatic filariasis should also be given for children older than 2 years whose country of origin is considered endemic for the disease.[7]

SUMMARY

The infectious and noninfectious health issues of IAs are complex. Where possible, IAs should be evaluated at a clinic or center specializing in international adoption, as specialized expertise and a multidisciplinary approach are often required for optimal evaluation and care of these children. Infections for which IAs are at higher risk and therefore require screening include viral (hepatitis A, B, and C and HIV), bacterial (syphilis, TB), and parasitic (stool helminths, *Giardia*). LTBI is frequent in IAs and all IAs should be tested for TB on arrival and again 6 months after arrival. Children with LTBI must be treated with INH for 9 months, as children younger than 4 years with LTBI have the greatest risk of developing TB disease. Other infectious disease testing depends on specific risk factors in the IA child. Appropriate infectious and noninfectious disease screening and treatment provide IA children the best chance to thrive in their new environment.

REFERENCES

1. Intercountry Adoption Statistics. Bureau of Consular Affairs USDoS Web site. Available at: http://adoption.state.gov/about_us/statistics.php. Accessed October 2, 2012.
2. Committee on Early Childhood, Adoption & Dependent Care. Initial medical evaluation of an adopted child. Pediatrics 1991;88(3):642–4.
3. Hostetter MK, Iverson S, Dole K, et al. Unsuspected infectious diseases and other medical diagnoses in the evaluation of internationally adopted children. Pediatrics 1989;83(4):559–64.
4. Jones VF, High PC, Donoghue E, et al. Comprehensive health evaluation of the newly adopted child. Pediatrics 2012;129(1):e214–23.
5. Miller LC, Tseng B, Tirella LG, et al. Health of children adopted from Ethiopia. Matern Child Health J 2008;12(5):599–605.
6. Miller LC, Hendrie NW. Health of children adopted from China. Pediatrics 2000; 105(6):e76.
7. Pickering L, Baker C, Kimberlin D, et al, editors. Red Book: 2012 report of the Committee on Infectious Diseases. Elk Grove Village (IL): American Academy of Pediatrics; 2012.
8. Howard CR, John CC. International travel with infants and children: international adoptions. Traveler's health (Yellow Book). Atlanta (GA): Centers for Disease Control and Prevention; 2011. Available at: http://wwwnc.cdc.gov/travel/yellowbook/2012/chapter-7-international-travel-infants-children/international-adoption.htm.
9. Viviano E, Cataldo F, Accomando S, et al. Immunization status of internationally adopted children in Italy. Vaccine 2006;24(19):4138–43.
10. Nelson L, Wells C. Global epidemiology of childhood tuberculosis childhood TB. Int J Tuberc Lung Dis 2004;8(5):636–47.
11. CDC. Available at: www.cdc.gov/tb/publications/ltbi/pdf/TargetedLTBI.pdf. Accessed November 21, 2012.
12. WHO. Global tuberculosis control 2011 (Annex 2). Geneva (Switzerland): WHO; 2011.
13. Saiman L, Aronson J, Zhou J, et al. Prevalence of infectious diseases among internationally adopted children. Pediatrics 2001;108(3):608.
14. Staat DD, Klepser ME. International adoption: issues in infectious diseases. Pharmacotherapy 2006;26(9):1207–20.
15. Trehan I, Meinzen-Derr JK, Jamison L, et al. Tuberculosis screening in internationally adopted children: the need for initial and repeat testing. Pediatrics 2008; 122(1):e7–14.

16. Zwerling A, Behr MA, Verma A, et al. The BCG World Atlas: a database of global BCG vaccination policies and practices. PLoS Med 2011;8(3):e1001012.
17. Burl S, Adetifa UJ, Cox M, et al. The tuberculin skin test (TST) is affected by recent BCG vaccination but not by exposure to non-tuberculosis mycobacteria (NTM) during early life. PLoS One 2010;5(8):e12287.
18. Immigrant, Refugee, and Migrant Health Branch of the Division of Global Migration and Quarantine (DGMQ), Centers for Disease Control and Prevention (CDC). Tuberculosis Screening and Treatment Technical Instructions (TB TIs) using Cultures and Directly Observed Therapy (DOT) for Panel Physicians. October 1, 2009. Available at: http://www.cdc.gov/immigrantrefugeehealth/pdf/tuberculosis-ti-2009.pdf. Accessed October 10, 2012.
19. Mazurek G, Jereb J, LoBue P, et al. Guidelines for using the QuantiFERON®-TB gold test for detecting *Mycobacterium tuberculosis* infection, United States. December 16, 2005. Available at: http://www.cdc.gov/mmwr/preview/mmwrhtml/rr5415a4.htm. Accessed October 10, 2012.
20. Berman SM. Maternal syphilis: pathophysiology and treatment. Bull World Health Organ 2004;82(6):433–8.
21. Baek JO, Jee HJ, Kim TK, et al. Recent trends of syphilis prevalence in normal population in Korea: a single center study in Seoul. Korean J Derm 2011;49(2):106–10.
22. Lee V, Jung Y. The correlation between the new prostitution acts and sexually transmitted diseases in Korea. Korean J Policy Studies 2009;24(1):111–25.
23. Lee J, Park KT, Kim JS, et al. Clinico-serologic manifestation and serologic response to treatment of syphilis. Korean J Derm 2011;49(2):111–8.
24. Zhou H, Chen XS, Hong FC, et al. Risk factors for syphilis infection among pregnant women: results of a case-control study in Shenzhen, China. Sex Transm Infect 2007;83(6):476–80.
25. Jacobsen K, Koopman J. Declining hepatitis A seroprevalence: a global review and analysis. Epidemiol Infect 2004;132(6):1005–22.
26. Jacobsen K. The global prevalence of hepatitis A virus infection and susceptibility: a systematic review. Geneva (Switzerland): World Health Organization; 2009.
27. Fischer GE, Teshale EH, Miller C, et al. Hepatitis A among international adoptees and their contacts. Clin Infect Dis 2008;47(6):812–4.
28. Pelletier AR, Mehta PJ, Burgess DR, et al. An outbreak of hepatitis A among primary and secondary contacts of an international adoptee. Public Health Rep 2010;125(5):642.
29. Centers for Disease Control and Prevention (CDC). Updated recommendations from the Advisory Committee on Immunization Practices (ACIP) for use of hepatitis A vaccine in close contacts of newly arriving international adoptees. MMWR Morb Mortal Wkly Rep 2009;58(36):1006–7.
30. American Academy of Pediatrics. Pickering LK, Kimberlin DW, Long SS, editors. Red Book: 2009 report of the Committee on Infectious Diseases. Elk Grove Village (IL): American Academy of Pediatrics; 2002.
31. Mast EE, Margolis HS, Fiore AE, et al. A comprehensive immunization strategy to eliminate transmission of hepatitis B virus infection in the United States. MMWR Recomm Rep 2005;54(RR16):1–31.
32. Barker L, Santoli J, McCauley M. National, state, and urban area vaccination coverage among children aged 19-35 months–United States, 2003. MMWR Morb Mortal Wkly Rep 2009;53(29):658–61.
33. Liang X, Bi S, Yang W, et al. Epidemiological serosurvey of hepatitis B in China–declining HBV prevalence due to hepatitis B vaccination. Vaccine 2009;27(47):6550–7.

34. WHO. Hepatitis C. 2004. Available at: http://www.who.int/csr/disease/hepatitis/whocdscsrlyo2003/en/index4.html#incidence. Accessed October 10, 2012.
35. Ferrero S, Lungaro P, Bruzzone BM, et al. Prospective study of mother-to-infant transmission of hepatitis C virus: a 10-year survey (1990–2000). Acta Obstet Gynecol Scand 2003;82(3):229–34.
36. Alter MJ. Prevention of spread of hepatitis C. Hepatology 2002;36(5B):s93–8.
37. Global Burden Of Hepatitis C Working Group. Global burden of disease (GBD) for hepatitis C. J Clin Pharmacol 2004;44:20–9.
38. Dunn DT, Brandt CD, Krivinet A, et al. The sensitivity of HIV-1 DNA polymerase chain reaction in the neonatal period and the relative contributions of intra-uterine and intra-partum transmission. AIDS 1995;9(9):F7.
39. Murphy SC, Breman JG. Gaps in the childhood malaria burden in Africa: cerebral malaria, neurological sequelae, anemia, respiratory distress, hypoglycemia, and complications of pregnancy. Am J Trop Med Hyg 2001;64(Suppl 1):57–67.
40. Idro R, Jenkins NE, Newton CR. Pathogenesis, clinical features, and neurological outcome of cerebral malaria. Lancet Neurol 2005;4(12):827–40.
41. Boivin MJ, Bangirana P, Byarugaba J, et al. Cognitive impairment after cerebral malaria in children: a prospective study. Pediatrics 2007;119(2):e360–6.
42. Miller LC. The handbook of international adoption medicine: a guide for physicians, parents, and providers. New York: Oxford University Press; 2004.
43. Miller LC. International adoption: infectious diseases issues. Clin Infect Dis 2005;40(2):286–93.
44. Valentini P, Gargiullo L, Ceccarelli M, et al. Health status of internationally adopted children. The experience of an Italian "GLNBI" paediatric centre. Ital J Public Health 2012;9(3):e7527.
45. Looke D, Robson J. 9: Infections in the returned traveller. Med J Aust 2002;177(4):212.

Travel-Related Infections in Children

Thomas G. Fox, MD, John J. Manaloor, MD,
John C. Christenson, MD*

KEYWORDS

• Travel • Infections • Children • Malaria • Diarrhea

KEY POINTS

- An increasing number of children are traveling to developing countries placing them at risk for malaria and traveler's diarrhea.
- Children visiting friends and relatives are at a greater risk of acquiring a travel-related infection, such as malaria and typhoid fever.
- Travel-related infections are preventable through adherence to preventive measures such as insect bite protection, antimalarial prophylaxis, vaccination, and consumption of safe food and water.
- Clinicians must be familiar with the epidemiology and clinical manifestations of travel-related infections to assure prompt recognition and treatment.

INTRODUCTION

In 2011, international tourism arrivals increased by more than 4% to 982 million. An additional increase of 3%–4% was expected in 2012. Although much of the growth represents increased travel to Europe, travel to Southeast and South Asia, South America, and Africa has also increased.[1] Fifty-one percent of travel was by air for leisure and recreation. Another 27% was for visiting friends and relatives (VFR), health, or religion. Some increases were to regions considered remote or exotic, which could pose different risks to travelers. Clinicians are expected to encounter pediatric travelers with malaria, travel-associated diarrhea, enteric fevers, and dermatoses such as cutaneous larva migrans. Although preventive measures are effective, certain at-risk populations, such as VFR travelers, are frequently unprepared and become ill.

In the assessment of the ill pediatric traveler, physicians must consider geographic, seasonal, and environmental factors and assess compliance to pretravel advice. A traveler taking an appropriate antimalarial agent as instructed is less likely to have

Ryan White Center for Pediatric Infectious Disease, Riley Hospital for Children, Indiana University School of Medicine, 705 Riley Hospital Drive, ROC-4380, Indianapolis, IN 46202, USA
* Corresponding author.
E-mail address: jcchrist@iupui.edu

Pediatr Clin N Am 60 (2013) 507–527
http://dx.doi.org/10.1016/j.pcl.2012.12.004 **pediatric.theclinics.com**
0031-3955/13/$ – see front matter

malaria. Travelers to certain regions, such as Southeast Asia, are more likely to have dengue as the cause of their febrile illness. Travel to certain regions of southern Africa poses no risk for malaria or yellow fever.

VFR children pose a significant challenge. They tend to be younger and stay longer in high-risk and at times remote areas of developing countries. Children frequently become ill during or after travel.[2] Children with malaria and typhoid fever are often hospitalized. A perception of low risk, a lack of access to a travel clinic or someone knowledgeable in travel medicine, refusal of medical insurance to cover pretravel care, and a lack of financial resources to purchase vaccines and prophylactic medications are among the reasons why most lack appropriate pretravel advice, antimalarial prophylaxis, or vaccinations. Many stay in family homes, which may increase their risk for acquiring certain diseases such as enteric infections. Many regions are endemic with dengue fever, yellow fever, typhoid fever, and malaria. A younger age places the child at greater risk of severe disease. In one study, 46% of VFR children were less than 5 years of age.[3]

In a group of children whose family had visited a travel clinic for pretravel advice, diarrhea, abdominal pain, and fever were the most frequent posttravel complaints.[4] Most episodes of illness occurred in the first 10 days of travel. In a large study of ill pediatric travelers, most had been tourists to Asia and sub-Saharan Africa or Latin America.[5] Diarrhea (28%), dermatologic conditions, systemic febrile illnesses (23%), and respiratory conditions were most commonly reported. Travelers to sub-Saharan Africa were more likely to have malaria. Dermatologic conditions such as cutaneous larva migrans were more likely in children returning from Latin America.

This review addresses the most common infectious conditions observed among pediatric travelers. Discussion will be categorized according to presenting clinical features such as fever, diarrhea, and cutaneous conditions.

FEVER

Fever is a frequent manifestation of infection in children. Fortunately, most are mild and self-limiting and require no medical intervention. However, in a child returning from an endemic region, fever may be the initial presentation of a serious infection such as malaria, dengue, or enteric fever. Among hospitalized children returning from the tropics with febrile illnesses, diarrhea and malaria were the most common. A treatable cause was identified in only 46% of children.[6] Eight percent of ill children returning from international travel were found to have malaria; 69% of these children required hospitalization.[5] Most cases were caused by *Plasmodium falciparum* after travel to sub-Saharan Africa.

Because morbidity and mortality associated with travel to the tropics is significant, recognition and early treatment is imperative. Clinicians must differentiate between minor, self-limiting illnesses and diseases such as malaria, enteric fever, and infectious gastroenteritis. In most instances, fever will not be the only manifestation of disease. Chills, sweats, headaches, fatigue, neck pain, malaise, vomiting, diarrhea, and abdominal pain may be present and help with the clinical diagnosis. At times, clinical presentations in children will differ from those observed in adults. The well-described classical fever patterns associated with malaria in adults are rarely observed in children, in whom patterns are more erratic.

The etiologic diagnosis of a febrile illness is easier when the person traveled to an endemic area and returns to a nonendemic area. Specific incubation periods are helpful in determining a possible etiology. A too-short or too-long incubation period could eliminate some conditions. **Box 1** lists diseases according to incubation period.

Box 1
Incubation periods for common infections that cause fever

Incubation Period Less Than 14 Days

Malaria, dengue fever, rickettsial infections, leptospirosis, enteric fevers, diarrheal illnesses, viral respiratory infections, yellow fever, meningococcal and pneumococcal sepsis and meningitis

Incubation Period 2–6 Weeks

Malaria, enteric fevers, hepatitis A and E, acute schistosomiasis, leptospirosis, amoebic liver abscess, infectious mononucleosis, toxoplasmosis

Incubation Period Greater Than 6 Weeks

Malaria, tuberculosis, hepatitis B, visceral leishmaniasis, schistosomiasis, amoebic liver abscess, brucellosis, visceral larva migrans

Incubation periods of less than 14 days would support the diagnosis of malaria, dengue, and typhoid fever. Incubation periods greater than 14 days would rule out dengue. Known exposures to individuals with an infectious condition, such as measles or chickenpox, may help the clinician by providing a precise incubation period.

Plasmodium falciparum is the most common species of malaria acquired in West Africa. It has the highest morbidity and mortality. If suspected, prompt effective treatment is required.

In travelers to Southeast Asia and South and Central America, leptospirosis and dengue fever have become more common causes of undifferentiated fevers than malaria. Dengue fever was responsible for 6% of systemic febrile illnesses among ill-returning children.[5] In the Amazon basin of Ecuador, leptospirosis was the most common cause of acute undifferentiated fever (13.2%), followed by malaria (mostly *Plasmodium vivax*) at 12.5%.[7] Rickettsial infections were also seen. Many of these conditions are indistinguishable, requiring molecular or serologic diagnostic testing.

Enteric fevers caused by *Salmonella typhi* or *Salmonella paratyphi* are rarely acquired in developed countries. Although foodborne outbreaks of typhoid fever have been reported in the United States in recent years, most cases are acquired from travel to developing countries, especially India and Pakistan. Overall, typhoid fever was responsible for only 1% of febrile illnesses among returning pediatric travelers seeking medical care.[5] VFR children represent a large number of reported infections.

In diarrheal infections caused by nontyphoidal *Salmonella* spp. and *Shigella* spp., fever can be an associated feature. Most travel-related diarrheal infections occur in children less than 2 years, most while the person is still traveling. Prolonged disease was common, and many required hospitalization. Among ill-returned pediatric travelers, diarrheal infections represented 28% of all pediatric illnesses.[5]

More than 30% of febrile illnesses are caused by more cosmopolitan-type infections, such as acute otitis media, pharyngitis, infectious mononucleosis, and soft tissue and urinary tract infections.

Clinical syndromes or examination findings may lead to a diagnosis. A child with a sepsis-like presentation may have a life-threatening infection like typhoid fever, meningitis, leptospirosis, or malaria. Coughing and tachypnea may represent a pneumonic process. Fever and jaundice may represent leptospirosis or hepatitis A or E. Meningismus, headache, vomiting, and photophobia, all suggest a central nervous system infection. Purpura may suggest meningococcal disease, whereas eschars and chagomas may support the diagnosis of rickettsioses or Chagas disease, respectively. The presence of lymphadenopathy, tonsillitis, and hepatosplenomegaly would suggest infectious mononucleosis. A person with fever and polyarthropathy arriving from northern Australia may have Ross River fever, but a traveler returning from an island in the Indian Ocean with the same symptoms may have Chikungunya. **Box 2** provides differential diagnoses according to syndromic features.

Box 2
Febrile syndromes

Fever and Hepatitis

Hepatitis A, B, and E; leptospirosis, infectious mononucleosis, amebiasis (eg, liver abscess)

Fever and Eosinophilia

Schistosomiasis (eg, Katayama fever), ascariasis, strongyloidiasis

Fever and Lymphadenopathies

Toxoplasmosis, Epstein-Barr virus (mononucleosis-like), cytomegalovirus, tularemia, human immunodeficiency virus (eg, acute retroviral syndrome), brucellosis

Fever and Arthropathies

Ross River virus, Chikungunya virus, dengue fever, pyogenic septic arthritis, acute rheumatic fever, human parvovirus B19

Fever and Diarrhea

Shigellosis, salmonellosis, amebiasis, Campylobacteriosis, *Clostridium difficile* enteritis, diarrheagenic *Escherichia coli*, rotavirus

Fever—Chronic, Relapsing, Recurrent

Malaria, relapsing fever, enteric fever, brucellosis, Q fever, leptospirosis, Familial Mediterranean fever

Fever and Hemorrhagic Manifestations

Dengue fever, yellow fever, Lassa fever, Rift Valley fever, viral hemorrhagic fevers (eg, Machupo, Marburg, Ebola), meningococcal

Fever and Exanthem (Type)

Dengue fever (maculopapular), Chikungunya (maculopapular), measles (maculopapular), rubella (maculopapular), rickettsial (maculopapular, eschar, petechial, vesiculopustular), *Neisseria meningitidis* (petechial, purpura), enterovirus (maculopapular), drug reactions (erythema multiforme), varicella-zoster virus (vesicular), tuberculosis (erythema nodosum, papulonecrotic tuberculids), yellow fever (maculopapular)

Fever and Central Nervous System Disease

N meningitidis meningitis, *Streptococcus pneumoniae* meningitis, enterovirus, malaria, arboviral meningoencephalitis, rabies, Japanese encephalitis virus, West Nile virus, tuberculosis, *Angiostrongylus* (eg, eosinophilic meningitis)

Fever and Abdominal Pain

Enteric fevers (eg, typhoid, paratyphoid), yersiniosis, adenovirus, liver abscess

Fever, Respiratory Symptoms, and Pneumonia

Pneumococcal, influenza, respiratory syncytial virus, tuberculosis, histoplasmosis, coccidioidomycosis, adenovirus, legionellosis, Q fever, plague, tularemia, diphtheria, anthrax, hantavirus

An initial workup for fever in a returning pediatric traveler may consist of a complete blood count and differential, liver function tests, blood cultures, stool culture, urinalysis, and thick and thin smears for malaria. Serologic testing is needed to confirm dengue. Patients with a cough may require a chest film, and evidence of pneumonic infiltrates may require respiratory viral testing or sputum for gram stain and culture. Tuberculin skin testing or interferon-γ release assays may be required to confirm the diagnosis of tuberculosis in a young child with an atypical or complex disease. A stool culture may be useful in patients with diarrhea, as determined by the duration and type of symptoms; some may require testing for *Clostridium difficile* toxin. Examination for ova and parasites may be useful in persons with chronic diarrhea. Antigen assays for *Cryptosporidium* and *Giardia* are particularly sensitive. Individuals with complaints of pharyngitis and evidence of exudative disease would benefit from rapid streptococcal antigen assay with a backup throat culture (or polymerase chain reaction [PCR]) if necessary. Patients with symptoms suggestive of meningitis require a lumbar puncture. Some individuals may require diagnostic imaging with a computed tomography scan or magnetic resonance imaging. Joint aspiration is required for patients with suspected pyogenic septic arthritis.

MALARIA

Epidemiology

Malaria is a mosquito-borne protozoa infection caused by erythrocyte-infecting *Plasmodium* species. The most important species infecting humans are *P falciparum, P vivax, Plasmodium ovale, Plasmodium malariae,* and *Plasmodium knowlesi*. The major vector is the *Anopheles* mosquito, which is endemic in many regions of the world, including the United States. Regions of the world with the most malarial transmission are sub-Saharan Africa, Southeast Asia-Pacific, Amazonian South America, and parts of Central America. *P knowlesi* is widely distributed in Malaysian Borneo, Peninsular Malaysia, and the Philippines.

Resistance to antimalarial agents in *P falciparum* contributed to its uncontrolled prevalence in Africa. Outside Central America, most *P falciparum* strains are resistant to chloroquine. *P falciparum* is resistant to mefloquine in some Asian countries (ie, regions bordering Thailand, Myanmar, Laos, and Cambodia). *P vivax* is the most prominent species outside Africa, especially in Asia where better diagnosis and antimalarial treatments are available, resulting in less *P falciparum*. However, resistance does not escape *P vivax*. Chloroquine resistance is reported in areas of Indonesia and Malaysia. *Plasmodium ovale* is rarely observed outside Africa. Recently, resistance to artemisinin compounds has been reported in Southeast Asia.

Clinical Manifestations

Nonspecific clinical features are usually observed in children. Fever, vomiting, headaches, chills, myalgias, and anorexia are common. Gastrointestinal symptoms, such as diarrhea, abdominal pain, and distension are also observed. Thrombocytopenia is frequently seen.

Severe malaria may result from cerebral involvement, acute respiratory distress syndrome, severe malarial anemia, or multiorgan involvement. Most children with severe malaria will die unless they are hospitalized and promptly treated with effective support and antimalarial medications. Coma, seizures, metabolic acidosis, profound hypoglycemia, and shock are associated with high mortality.[8] Although most of the serious complications are observed with *P falciparum,* severe malarial anemia in young infants is seen frequently with *P vivax.*

Diagnosis

Visualization of the parasite on blood smears has been the method of choice for malaria diagnosis for decades. Unfortunately, there is great variability of practitioners' ability to perform proper microscopy. The use of rapid diagnostic tests (RDTs) is becoming more widespread. In a laboratory-based study, RDT performed better than the Giemsa-stained blood smears (GS). Rapid antigen capture assay (BinaxNOW Malaria test; Alere, Waltham, MA) had a sensitivity of 97% compared with 85% of GS with a negative predictive value of 99.6% versus 98.2% with GS for all malaria. The sensitivity was 100% for *P falciparum.*[9] Most RDTs are less effective in the diagnosis of *P malariae, P ovale* or *P knowlesi* than *P falciparum* or *P vivax*. In addition, they cannot quantify parasitemia level, which is important when following a patient's response to therapy. For this reason, in centers in which high-quality microscopy is available, it remains the test of choice for diagnosis of malaria. RDTs can be used adjunctively or in centers in which high-quality microscopy is not available. PCR has the highest sensitivity for detection of infection and can be used to detect all 5 species that infect humans. However, its availability is still limited, and it typically cannot be run immediately in the way that microscopy can. In a study from Thailand, loop-mediated isothermal amplification was compared with nested PCR and microscopy.[10] Loop-mediated isothermal amplification is a molecular method that compares favorably with PCR but is cheaper, simpler, and faster. Using PCR as a gold standard, loop-mediated isothermal amplification detected 100% of blood specimens with *P falciparum* with 100% specificity. Microscopy showed 92% sensitivity and 93% specificity. Loop-mediated isothermal amplification performed just as well with specimens containing *P vivax,* whereas microscopy detected only 68% of positive specimens. The new fluorescent assay, Partec Rapid Malaria Test, may be easier to perform and provides quicker results compared with GS.[11]

Management

Recently, the World Health Organization updated its guidelines for malaria treatment.[12] Treatment recommendations for uncomplicated and severe malaria are briefly summarized below, but the reader is referred to the Centers for Disease Control (CDC) Web site for full guidelines for the treatment of severe and uncomplicated malaria (http://www.cdc.gov/malaria/diagnosis_treatment/clinicians2.html).

Artemisinin-based combinations are the recommended treatment for uncomplicated chloroquine-resistant *P falciparum* malaria. Artemether-lumefantrine, artesunate plus amodiaquine, artesunate plus mefloquine, and artesunate plus sulfadoxine-pyrimethamine are being used throughout the world. Of these, only artemether-lumefantrine (Coartem, Novartis Pharmaceuticals Corporation, Basel, Switzerland) is licensed in the United States. Artemether-lumefantrine therapy is given for 3 days.[13] Other effective treatments available in the United States for uncomplicated malaria include atovaquone-proguanil, or quinine plus tetracycline or doxycycline or clindamycin. Uncomplicated malaria caused by chloroquine susceptible *P falciparum* (generally limited to Haiti and Central America west of the Panama Canal) can be treated with chloroquine.

Severe malaria is always a medical emergency. Parenteral antimalarial treatment should be started immediately. Therapy should be started with whichever effective antimalarial is first available. Parenteral antimalarials are usually administered intravenously for a minimum of 24 hours and then switched to an oral regimen. In the United States, parenteral quinine is not available, so intravenous quinidine is the current drug of choice for severe malaria. Artesunate is superior to quinine in the treatment of severe malaria but is not yet US Food and Drug Administration approved for treatment of severe malaria in the United States and is not widely available. It is available from the CDC for patients who cannot tolerate quinidine or have a contraindication to quinine. The CDC malaria hotline can be reached at 770-488-7788 or 855-856-4713 (toll free), Monday through Friday, 9 AM–5 PM, and emergency consultation after hours can be obtained by calling 770-488-7100 and requesting to speak to the Malaria Branch clinician. Although a 3-case series of adults with severe *P falciparum* malaria who were treated successfully with oral artemether-lumefantrine alone has been reported, these patients had laboratory and not clinical criteria for severe malaria.[14] Oral therapy is not appropriate in any case of severe pediatric malaria, but if quinidine is not immediately available and oral therapy is available, it should be given while awaiting the quinidine therapy.

Chloroquine combined with primaquine is the treatment of choice for chloroquine-susceptible *P vivax* infections. An artemisinin-based combination regimen is recommended for infections suspected to be caused by chloroquine-resistant *P vivax.* Primaquine is recommended for 14 days to eliminate the hepatic hypnozoite stage and prevent relapses. Severe *P vivax* or *P knowlesi* infections should be treated with artemisinin combination regimens. To avoid medication-induced hemolysis, testing to rule out glucose-6-phosphate dehydrogenase deficiency is advised before treating with primaquine. There is currently a shortage of primaquine in the United States. Full details on appropriate medication for treatment of all *Plasmodium* species that infect humans are available on the CDC Web site noted above.

Children with severe malaria presenting with respiratory distress and metabolic acidosis benefit from blood transfusions. Close monitoring for hypoglycemia is imperative. Seizures can be a complication of cerebral malaria or profound hypoglycemia.

ENTERIC FEVER

Epidemiology

Enteric fever, an infection caused by *Salmonella enterica* serotype Typhi (typhoid fever) or *S enterica* serotype Paratyphi A, B, C (paratyphoid fever), is a frequent cause of morbidity and mortality in many parts of the world. Most infections occur in Southern and Southeast Asia. Parts of Africa and Latin America are affected but at a lower frequency. It is estimated that 22 million cases occur worldwide each year, with more than 200,000 deaths.[15] Infections from *S paratyphi* A are becoming more frequent than those from *S typhi* among travelers.[16]

The major factor responsible for the magnitude of this problem is poor sanitary infrastructure resulting in substandard drinking water and contaminated food. Person-to-person transmission from chronic asymptomatic infections among inhabitants also contributes to the infection of susceptible individuals.

Clinical Manifestations

Although fever, gastrointestinal symptoms (eg, vomiting, severe diarrhea, abdominal distension, pain), cough, relative bradycardia, rose spots, and splenomegaly are frequently regarded as features of typhoid and paratyphoid fever, many patients lack these, making diagnosis difficult if solely based on clinical features. Jaundice is frequently observed among children. In a study of travelers with enteric fever, clinical and laboratory features were indistinguishable between *S typhi* and *S paratyphi,* which suggests that milder disease is not always observed with *S paratyphi* as originally thought.[17] Unfortunately, early features of enteric fever mimic other conditions such as pneumonia, malaria, sepsis, dengue, acute hepatitis, and rickettsial infections.

Children younger than 5 years had more severe disease. More than 95% of these children had fever, 20%–41% hepatomegaly, 5%–20% splenomegaly, 19%–28% abdominal pain, and 8%–35% diarrhea.[18,19] Intestinal perforation was a rare complication. Cough was observed in approximately 15% of patients.[18] Thrombocytopenia and disseminated intravascular coagulation are markers of severe disease.[15]

Relative bradycardia and rose spots are seldom observed in children. Febrile convulsions have been reported in children with enteric fever and may be the presenting symptom. Because typhoid fever vaccines are only approximately 50% effective, the diagnosis needs to be considered even in vaccinated children.

Diagnosis

Blood cultures are frequently positive, stool, less so, but both should be obtained, as this increases the likelihood of detection of infection. Repeated blood cultures yield a sensitivity of approximately 80% for detection of enteric fever. Although liver enzymes are frequently elevated, leukocytosis is not always observed. However, leukocytosis is more frequently observed in children than adults.[18] Leukopenia and anemia are frequently associated with enteric fevers. Many suggest that bone marrow cultures have a higher sensitivity. However, obtaining this type of specimen is invasive and impractical under most circumstances.

The Widal test, a classical test that measures antibodies against O and H antigens of *S typhi,* was used in the past to diagnose typhoid fever and is still used frequently in low- and middle-income countries for this purpose, but it lacks sensitivity and specificity and should not be used as a diagnostic test for typhoid fever.[15,20] Newer pathogen-specific serologic are an improvement on the Widal test but still lack acceptable sensitivity and specificity. Multiplex PCR assays show promise, but are not yet widely tested to fully assess sensitivity and specificity and are not commercially available.

Management

Amoxicillin and trimethoprim-sulfamethoxazole are no longer recommended as first-line agents because of a high frequency of treatment failures, resistance, and relapse. Relapse rates in children are 2%–4% after therapy, whereas carrier rates occur in fewer than 2% of infected children.[15] Antimicrobial resistance observed in many countries has influenced the choice of agent for treating typhoid and paratyphoid fevers. Ceftriaxone is the recommended agent in severe cases when parenteral therapy is indicated. Azithromycin is an oral alternative for nonsevere cases. Although fluoroquinolones are generally associated with high cure rates, defervescence within a week, and lowered relapse and fecal carriage rates, isolates from many Asian countries show resistance, rendering them ineffective.

Proper hydration, perfusion, and fever control are integral components of treating enteric fever. Mixed infections with multiple pathogens can occur. Treatment against enteric fever should be considered for children with unremitting fevers after completing adequate antimalarial therapy.[21]

LEPTOSPIROSIS

Epidemiology

Leptospirosis is becoming an important cause of febrile disease in urban communities within developing countries. Urine from wild and domestic animals is the source of human infection. Contact with infected animals, poor sanitation and water quality, flash flooding, and overcrowding are contributing factors. Approximately

268 pathogenic serovars of *Leptospira* have been identified. *Leptospira interrogans* is the primary pathogenic species.[22] In a low-income region of Dhaka, Bangladesh, leptospirosis accounted for 2%–8% of acute outpatient febrile episodes.[23] Eighteen percent of dengue-negative individuals were found to have leptospirosis during a dengue outbreak in the same region in 2001.

Clinical Manifestations

Jaundice and renal failure, known as *hepatorenal syndrome* or *Weil disease*, is the stereotypical presentation associated with leptospirosis; however, this condition represents just a smaller number of cases. *Leptospira* causes a nonspecific febrile illness in most cases. It mimics other diseases such as malaria and dengue.[24,25] Hemorrhagic pneumonia and meningitis are also described with infection and are associated with high mortality.

Diagnosis

Visualization of leptospires by dark field microscopy, detection of specific antibody in serum, or DNA by PCR are the most frequently used methods for diagnosis.

Management

Penicillin for 5 days is the agent of choice for treatment. Erythromycin (5 days) and doxycycline (10 days) are alternative agents.

DENGUE

Epidemiology

Dengue is an acute febrile illness caused by a flavivirus transmitted by the mosquitoes *Aedes aegypti* and *Aedes albopictus*. Dengue remains a common cause of hospitalizations in Southeast Asia. In Vietnam, dengue was responsible for one-third of febrile illnesses presenting to a public primary care clinic. Areas of the Caribbean, Central America, and Africa have experienced epidemics.

Clinical Manifestations

Initial clinical features are highly nonspecific; most episodes are not suspected clinically. Approximately 32% of the cases without a clinical diagnosis are positive by serologies; this is mostly among young children less than 15 years. In patients with acute dengue, other diseases are suspected clinically, such as pharyngitis, typhoid fever, tonsillitis, leptospirosis, and hepatitis.[26] Dengue is frequently characterized by acute onset of fever and 2 of the following: retro-orbital pain, rash, headaches, myalgias, arthralgias, leukopenia, or hemorrhagic manifestations, such as positive tourniquet test, bleeding gums, thrombocytopenia, petechiae, or purpura or ecchymoses.[27] Febrile seizures have been observed. Asymptomatic infections are common.[28]

Disease is frequently associated with high fever and intense joint and muscle pain. Dengue hemorrhagic fever (DHF) and dengue shock syndrome (DSS) are frequent severe complications. Promptly recognizing signs of DHF and DSS and initiating appropriate treatment is critical for reducing fatalities. Massive capillary leak is usually observed after the child becomes afebrile (days 3–6). Close monitoring is appropriate at this stage of the illness. A drop in platelet count accompanied by increasing hematocrit usually precedes shock. Persistent vomiting along with abdominal pain are signs of impending shock.

Diagnosis

Acute and convalescent serologic tests are necessary for the diagnosis. PCR assay is also available through the Dengue Branch of the CDC.

Management

Treatment is supportive. No effective antiviral therapy is available at this time. The use of crystalloid oral and intravenous fluids and colloids are critical components of the management of DHF and DSS.[29] Aspirin and nonsteroidal anti-inflammatory agents should be avoided.

OTHER CONDITIONS WITH FEVER

Clinicians should not forget that common infections, such as acute otitis media and bacterial pneumonia, can cause fever in young children returning from the tropics.[30] Hospitalized febrile children with a history of travel to the tropics are frequently found to have nonspecific fever. Although rare among travelers, pyogenic arthritis, pyomyositis, osteomyelitis, rheumatic fever, and meningitis have been reported.

Respiratory infections are common among travelers. Influenza and parainfluenza viruses are among the most common pathogens. In a GeoSentinel study of travelers, influenza was reported frequently during the months of December through February in the Northern Hemisphere.[31] Travel duration of greater than 30 days increased the risk of influenza infection and lower respiratory tract involvement. VFR persons are 6 times more likely to acquire influenza.

Tuberculosis is a rarely reported travel-related infection. Acquiring this infection is not easy. It is greatly influenced by duration of contact with the contagious individual and the degree of contagiousness of that individual because those with cavitary lung disease are more likely to infect others. In the United States, a large number of pediatric infections are observed among refugees, immigrants, and contacts of foreign-born individuals. In one report, more than 80% of pediatric tuberculosis infections were related to travel.[32] Staying with parents and relatives in high-prevalence regions was the major risk factor for these pediatric travelers.

DIARRHEAL ILLNESS

Epidemiology

Traveler's diarrhea (TD) is common during or immediately after return from international destinations and is the most frequent travel-related disease in children and adults, with rates approaching 60% for travel to certain areas.[33] TD is responsible for considerable morbidity for the child and accompanying family.[34,35] Compared with older children and adults, TD in infants and young children is more severe and prolonged.[35] Food and water are common sources of infection, and person-to-person transmission is not typical.

Bacterial pathogens cause most diarrheal illnesses in travelers to developing countries, whereas viruses predominate in industrialized nations.[36] Data on TD in adults and gastrointestinal infection in native children are extrapolated to the child traveler, but, in reality, little is known about the etiologies specific to pediatric TD.[36] Diarrheagenic strains of *Escherichia coli* cause most TD, with Enterotoxigenic *E coli* (ETEC) playing the predominant role.[37]

The bacterial species responsible for invasive diarrhea in developed countries are also important causes of TD. These pathogens frequently cause dysentery (fever and bloody stools) and are especially prevalent in Southeast Asia. The most common etiologies include species of *Shigella*, nontyphoidal *Salmonella*, and *Campylobacter*. Less frequent bacterial agents include *Aeromonas*, *Plesiomonas*, and *Vibrio* species (including *Vibrio cholerae* and noncholera species).[37] Viruses cause a significant proportion of TD, whereas parasitic disease is uncommon.

Enteroaggregative *E coli* (EAEC) is a newly recognized pathogen and a common cause of TD.[38] Infection with EAEC is indistinguishable from that of ETEC, but unlike ETEC, a significant proportion of patients infected with EAEC will have bloody diarrhea.[39] EAEC is an important cause of persistent diarrhea and causes disease in both developing and industrialized nations.[39]

In the United States and other developed countries, antibiotics are often withheld in pediatric patients with bloody diarrhea because of the potentially increased risk of hemolytic uremic syndrome (HUS) in patients receiving antibiotics for enterohemorrhagic *E coli* (usually *E coli* O157:H7) infection.[40] Infection with *E coli* O157:H7 is uncommon in developing countries, and HUS has been reported on only rare occasions in travelers.[37] However, a recent outbreak of HUS in Germany related to the foodborne transmission of a hypervirulent strain of Shiga toxin-producing EAEC (O104:H4) highlights the potential for emerging pathogens in TD, especially during an epidemic.[41]

Norovirus and rotavirus are the most important viral causes of diarrheal disease in travelers. Norovirus may be responsible for a larger proportion of TD cases than previously recognized and is often present in the gastrointestinal tract as a copathogen with ETEC.[42,43] Rotavirus remains the most important viral cause of diarrhea worldwide.[44] Countries instituting rotavirus vaccine have seen a substantial decline in the incidence of disease.

Parasites play an important role in chronic diarrhea after travel.[45] *Giardia lamblia* infection is among the most frequent pathogens isolated from adults with traveler's diarrhea and may lead to protracted diarrhea with malabsorption necessitating therapy. Parasitic infections in individuals with human immunodeficiency virus (HIV) can result in prolonged illness with malnutrition and wasting. In the absence of HIV, infection with certain pathogens—*Cryptosporidium*, *Cyclospora*, and *Isospora*—may results in a self-limited illness that resolves without antimicrobial therapy, but patients with persistent symptoms should be treated. *Entamoeba histolytica* requires treatment because of the risk of extraintestinal dissemination.[45]

Arcobacter species and Enterotoxigenic *Bacteroides fragilis* are newly emerging pathogens in traveler's diarrhea. These pathogens can be difficult to detect and are often resistant to standard treatment.[46]

Clinical Manifestations

Most cases of TD are mild and self-limited. Typical symptoms include watery diarrhea, urgency, nausea, and crampy abdominal pain.[47] Young children may have a more severe and prolonged course. Pitzinger and colleagues[35] in 1991 provided the best study on the clinical epidemiology of childhood TD in a series of 363 pediatric patients. The average time to diarrhea onset was 8 days after departure. Interestingly, the duration of symptoms was longer in children less than age 3 and adolescents. Young children were more likely to present with fever and bloody stools and have prolonged symptoms.[35]

Diarrheal illness is rarely life threatening, but children are more susceptible to the effects of gastrointestinal fluid losses. TD may result in clinically significant hypovolemia requiring intravenous fluids or hospitalization. Infection with invasive pathogens (eg, *Salmonella*, *Shigella*, and *Campylobacter*) can lead to sepsis and intestinal perforation.[36]

Diagnosis

Stool culture can detect various enteric bacteria causing TD. However, standard laboratory methods cannot distinguish most diarrheagenic *E coli*, including ETEC and EAEC, from nonpathogenic species of *E coli* that normally colonize the human bowel. Identification of ETEC requires molecular techniques like PCR or DNA probe,[48] and EAEC is isolated using cell culture based methods.[38] These methods may not be available in all clinical laboratories. Stool culture should be obtained in patients with severe symptoms or signs of infection with invasive pathogens, such as bloody stool, fever, or severe abdominal pain, as these organisms (ie, *Salmonella, Campylobacter* and *Shigella*) are readily detected by standard stool culture, and antibiotic susceptibility data can help guide therapy.

Diagnostic testing for rotavirus (by detection of viral antigen by enzyme immunoassay) is available in many laboratories.

In cases of chronic diarrhea, stool examination for ova and parasites as well as stool antigen testing for select pathogens (eg, *Giardia, Cryptosporidium*) is important. A serum enzyme immunoassay for *Entamoeba histolytica* is positive in approximately 95% of patients with extraintestinal amebiasis, 70% of patients with active intestinal infection, and 10% of asymptomatic individuals who are passing *E histolytica* cysts. It is a useful adjunctive test but does not replace the testing of multiple stool samples for *E histolytica* trophozoites and cysts.

Management

Fluid resuscitation

Correcting dehydration and electrolyte imbalances and repleting ongoing volume losses are paramount in the management of gastrointestinal infections in children. Children are more susceptible to dehydration. Oral rehydration solutions containing appropriate amounts of glucose and electrolytes are an important component in the management of the child with TD and dehydration.[49,50] Small and frequent administration is critical in the vomiting child.[50] Failure to correct dehydration with oral therapy may necessitate intravenous fluids. If possible, breastfeeding should continue during the illness, and the child's regular diet can be resumed with resolution of significant vomiting.[36]

Antimicrobial therapy

Antibiotics are effective in the treatment of adults with TD.[51] However, controversy exists in the treatment of children, and no studies on the treatment of pediatric TD are available. The World Health Organization does not recommend the routine treatment of infectious diarrhea in children but instead suggests targeted therapy in patients with suspected shigellosis (ie, dysentery), cholera, or giardiasis.[50] Treatment of TD decreases the duration and severity of illness, which could reduce the need for supportive measures, such as inpatient hospitalization and intravenous fluids. Antibiotic therapy should not be withheld from children for fear of HUS. Pediatric travelers with severe gastrointestinal disease, specifically those with bloody diarrhea, are unlikely to be infected with Shiga toxin–producing *E coli* and should receive antimicrobial therapy.[52]

The preferred agents for TD are azithromycin, ciprofloxacin, and rifaximin, with azithromycin the drug of first choice in children. Historically used agents (eg, ampicillin, trimethoprim-sulfamethoxazole, and doxycycline) have become obsolete in the treatment of TD because of high rates of antibiotic resistance; however, resistance to newer agents is emerging.[33] The selection of an antimicrobial agent should be based in part on geography. For example, ciprofloxacin is not recommended for therapy for TD in visitors to South and Southeast Asia because of widespread quinolone-resistant *Campylobacter.*[33] Rifaximin is a nonabsorbable oral antibiotic that has emerged as a safe and effective therapy for adults with TD caused by noninvasive enteropathogens.[51] It has been used safely for conditions other than TD in children, but there are little data on its utility in TD in children. Azithromycin is the drug of choice for childhood TD because it is well tolerated in children, is conveniently dosed once per day, and is effective against bacterial pathogens of TD, including ciprofloxacin-resistant *Campylobacter.*[52] Patient-directed therapy should be considered in families traveling with children. It is reasonable to dispense short courses of antibiotic therapy for children before travel for parent-directed administration on the onset of diarrheal illness.[36]

Antidiarrheal agents

These agents work by decreasing gut motility, decreasing intraluminal fluid secretion, or both. The most widely used agent, loperamide, is well tolerated in adults and is effective in reducing the quantity of passed stools.[51] Loperamide has not been studied specifically in childhood TD.[53] Its use could be considered in children $\geq$12 years of age and should be limited to 2 days. Serious potential side effects include central nervous system depression and toxic megacolon, especially with overdoses.[36] It should not be administered to patients with fever or bloody stools.

Bismuth subsalicylate is an antisecretory agent with antimicrobial properties that can have a modest effect on the reduction of diarrheal stools in adults with TD.[54] Limited data exist suggesting potential benefits in childhood diarrhea.[55] Its use in children is usually not recommended, however, because of the risk of salicylate intoxication at high doses.[56]

DERMATOLOGIC CONDITIONS

Epidemiology

Dermatologic conditions are a frequent complication of foreign travel and the third most common reason for physician consultation in returning visitors.[57,58] While usually representing self-limited illnesses, skin symptoms can be the superficial manifestations of a life-threatening systemic infection.[59] Tropical skin infections are common in travelers to exotic locales, but the so-called cosmopolitan skin disorders are in reality more common.[57,60] Travelers to tropical island destinations are more likely to acquire skin infections than those who voyage to cooler inland areas.[60] Exposure to disease vectors, usually insects, increases the odds of many travel-acquired skin infections.

Clinical Manifestations

Dermatologic manifestations are common in several life-threatening infections acquired during travel. Therefore, the first objective of the medical provider is to decide whether the child's skin complaint could represent a serious infection. The presence of fever significantly increases the chances of severe disease. Patients presenting with rash and fever after return from foreign travel require expedited evaluation and possibly hospital admission for diagnostic workup and empiric antimicrobial therapy. A detailed exposure history should be taken and include specific destinations of travel and all exposures to animals and insects. It is important to characterize the rash in terms of its appearance and distribution and whether it is itchy, tender, or painless.[61]

Fever and Rash

Children with benign viral infections often present with rash, but the presence of fever with rash can signal a more severe underlying infection. Dengue fever may cause fever and rash in returning foreign visitors. A variety of rashes can be present, but most commonly diffuse erythema with "islands of pallor" is seen during fever defervescence.[62] Petechiae and purpura can be seen in the hemorrhagic form of this viral infection and in patients with meningococcemia. A variety of other arboviruses can cause fever and rash, including West Nile and Chikungunya.[57] The clinician should have a heightened suspicion for measles in the unvaccinated child who has traveled abroad. Infection with *S typhi* (typhoid fever) can result in a red macular rash known as *rose spots*.

Cosmopolitan Infections

Bacterial infection

Pyoderma is a broad term for any suppurative infection of the skin and is one of the most common skin infections in travelers.[63] As in the United States, *Staphylococcus aureus* is the most common causative agent. Impetiginous infections are more likely the result of *Streptococcus pyogenes*. The prevalence of community-associated methicillin-resistant *S aureus* and Panton-Valentin leukocidin-positive methicillin-susceptible *S aureus* is increasing worldwide, and travel has been associated with the acquisition of virulent bacterial strains.[64]

Scabies

The human mite *Sarcoptes scabiei* is a common cause of diffuse pruritis in the traveler. Infestation is characterized by intense itching that is worse at night and usually spares the head and face. Microscopic examination of skin scrapings can be diagnostic, and most patients respond to treatment with 5% permethrin.[57]

Parasitic Infections

Cutaneous larva migrans

Hookworm infection of the skin causes cutaneous larva migrans, the most common skin disease of tropical origin.[65] The adult hookworms reside in the intestinal tracts of dogs and cats, where eggs are shed in the feces. Exposure is common in resource-poor communities with large feral animal populations.[65] The traveler encounters larvae through contact with sand and dirt, often during trips to beaches. Young children can acquire infection in various parts of the body, but the feet are the most common anatomic site affected. The period from infestation to clinical symptoms is short, and patients present with a characteristic red serpiginous tract that ascends the affected body part and causes intense pruritis.[57] Vesicles and bullae are occasionally seen, and secondary bacterial infection can result.[65] Cutaneous larva migrans is a clinical diagnosis, and although the infection is eventually self-resolving, ivermectin or albendazole is recommended to decrease the intensity and duration of symptoms.

Leishmaniasis

Various species of the vector-borne parasite *Leishmania* cause skin infections in travelers to tropical and subtropical destinations. Travel-related infections may be on the increase, and infection is more common in men and in those spending more than 8 weeks abroad.[66] The protozoan is spread to humans through the bite of the sand fly, where a papular lesion develops. This bite progresses to a nodule and finally an ulcerative but painless lesion results. Symptoms of infection develop a median of 15 days following return from travel, but the diagnosis is often made much later because it is not initially recognized as a possibility.[67] Any patient presenting with a nonhealing ulcerative lesion who has traveled to an endemic country deserves a diagnostic evaluation for leishmaniasis. Biopsy of the lesion is required for visualization of amastigotes, which can be seen within macrophages. Tissue PCR is also available for diagnosis. The treatment of Old World (eastern hemisphere) disease is controversial, because most cases resolve spontaneously. New World infection has a higher likelihood of leading to tissue destruction or visceral involvement and warrants therapy. Antimony-containing compounds have been the mainstay of therapy, although they may be less effective in pediatrics because of their unique pharmacokinetic properties in children.[68] Miltefosine is a new antiparasitic agent with promising efficacy.[69]

Myiasis and tungiasis

Less common than hookworm infection, myiasis and tungiasis are notable parasitic diseases that plague the tropical traveler. Myiasis is defined as infestation with the larvae of various fly species. In travelers to Central and South America, most infestations are caused by the human botfly (*Dermatobia hominis*), whereas the Tumbu fly (*Cordylobia anthropophaga*) causes most disease in Africa. Botfly adults deposit their eggs on mosquitoes, where they hatch into larvae and are delivered to their human host when the mosquito lands to take a blood meal. The larva burrows into the skin of its unknowing host, where a fully developed larva develops in 5–10 weeks.[57] The Tumbu fly lays its eggs on moist linens and clothing, where they hatch and invade their host on contact.

Myiasis is recognized by the characteristic furuncular lesion with a central pore that the parasite uses to breathe. Definitive treatment of myiasis is larva removal.[70] An occlusive substance like petroleum jelly is applied to the lesion to obstruct the breathing pore, which leads to emergence of the larva within 24 hours. Tweezers are used to extract the parasite, taking care not to rupture its body. The wound is thoroughly cleansed to prevent secondary infection.

Tungiasis (known as jiggers) results from skin penetration of the gravid female sand flea (*Tunga penetrans*). This parasite is endemic in many countries, but infection is most common in visitors to poor communities where intimate animal contact is commonplace.[70] The characteristic white papules with central black dots develop almost exclusively on the feet and are often found in the periungual areas. Young children can get lesions on the hands. Intense itching and pain with typical lesions clues the clinician in to the diagnosis, and extruded eggs, visible to the naked eye, can aid in diagnosis. Surgical excision of larvae is recommended.[70]

Rickettsioses

Species of *Rickettsiae* are significant causes of zoonotic infection and are increasingly recognized as pathogens in travelers[71] *Rickettsia rickettsiae* is a tick-borne bacteria that causes Rocky Mountain spotted fever and is endemic in North America and parts of South America. Patients with Rocky Mountain spotted fever typically present with fever, petechial rash, and headache with evidence of systemic inflammation. However, they rarely have any evidence of a prior tick bite. In contrast, many rickettsioses acquired abroad present with a systemic illness and inoculation eschars at sites of previous tick bites.[71] A patient presenting with a systemic illness, eschars with regional lymphadenopathy, and rash is likely infected with a species of *Rickettsiae*.

African tick bite fever caused by *Rickettsia africae* seems to be the most common rickettsial disease in travelers. The bacterium is transmitted from the bite of the cattle tick, and the typical presentation consisting of fever, headache, and eschars with lymphadenopathy. Vesicular rash with blisters in the mouth may also be seen. Travelers engaging in wild game safaris are at elevated risk of infection.[71]

Mediterranean spotted fever is acquired in Europe, Africa, and Asia and presents similarly to African tick bite fever. Murine typhus (*Rickettsia typhi*) is transmitted from its rodent host to humans via fleas, and coastal regions are the most frequently infested areas. No eschar develops after flea bite, and the clinical course is often a benign nonspecific febrile illness.

Contact with the larvae of certain species of mites (chiggers) in Southeast Asia can lead to infection with *Orientia tsutsugamushi* and the clinical disease scrub typhus. An inoculation eschar is common along with fever and regional lymphadenitis. Treatment is required for this potentially fatal disease.

The diagnosis of rickettsial infection can be difficult, and the best option is acute and convalescent antibody serology. It should be recognized, however, that cross-reaction between rickettsial species is common. Doxycycline therapy should be given in suspected cases.

Miscellaneous causes of dermatitis

Arthropod-related dermatitis is common in foreign and domestic locales and is a common reason for seeking medical care after travel.[59] The bite of any arthropod can lead to a local inflammatory response. Mosquitos, chiggers, sand flies, and scabies mites are common offenders. Local wound care is suggested to prevent secondary infection. Cercarial dermatitis, or "swimmer's itch," is caused by fresh water exposure to any of several varieties of nonhuman schistosomes. Cercariae burrow into the skin and cause intense itchy red papular lesions. Disease is self-limited, and no specific therapy is required.[72] In contrast, patients infected with human schistosomes (schistosomiasis) require treatment. The patient presenting with diffuse urticarial rash and peripheral eosinophilia should be evaluated for schistosomiasis along with other systemic helminthic infections like ascariasis and strongyloidiasis.[63]

PEDIATRIC TRAVELER WITH EOSINOPHILIA

Epidemiology

Eosinophilia is an uncommon problem among returning pediatric travelers. The evaluation of the returned traveler with eosinophilia must include the geographic region traveled and the presence of symptoms and physical findings. Although the immigrant, refugee, or internationally adopted child deserves evaluation, the extent of the problem in the pediatric traveler is unclear. Eosinophilia (absolute eosinophil count $\geq$500 cells/mm^3), although still uncommon in the traveler, is increasing, as is the frequency of travel.

Eosinophilia develops in approximately 10% of asymptomatic children returning from travel to the tropics, among whom a helminth (parasitic worm) infection is ultimately diagnosed. In a study of Israeli travelers, 8.6% had eosinophilia. Schistosomiasis was found in 4.4% of travelers.[73] Only 23.7% of the remaining 4.2% had a parasitic infection identified. Of interest, an empiric course of albendazole was found to be effective in resolving the eosinophilia.

Eosinophilia is more common in the traveler with a history of prolonged stay in the tropics. In the presence of cutaneous lesions, eosinophilia may indicate infections such as cutaneous larva migrans or *Ascaris* infestation. High fevers, urticarial, and eosinophilia several weeks after returning from the tropics may represent a form of schistosomiasis called *Katayama fever*. Noninfectious conditions can cause eosinophilia: asthma, eczema, allergic rhinitis, and drug reactions.

The likelihood of acquiring parasitic disease and eosinophilia is directly associated with the duration of time spent in endemic areas.[74–76] Even though some helminthic infections are self-limited, as many as 75% of returning travelers with eosinophilia have infections that result in sequelae for other family members.[77,78]

Infection with unicellular protozoa and amoebic parasites does not routinely result in eosinophilia.[79] However, helminthic infections are often associated with eosinophilia, particularly when the pathogen invades or migrates through tissues.[80,81]

Diagnosis

Symptoms such as rash, swelling, and fever, in addition to geography and other risk factors during travel, can differentiate certain helminthic infections from others.

Direct visualization of parasites in the stool (usually ova or larvae) is often attempted in the diagnosis of helminth infection in the traveler with eosinophilia.[82] However, ova are produced only by mature adult worms; therefore, and in the absence of detectable ova or larval forms, the cause of the observed eosinophilia may not be readily discernable.

Serology is a pivotal diagnostic modality in circumstances in which visualization is not possible, but is plagued by cross-reactivity. Additionally, antibody responses may only be detectable during the convalescent phase.

Management

Although most diagnostic algorithms are based on the patient's geographic exposure, some experts suggest empiric use of anthelmintics such as albendazole.[73,83] Others, when assessing pediatric refugees with eosinophilia, suggest specific serologic tests for *Strongyloides* and *Schistosoma* species. Practically, a short course of albendazole is routinely effective against roundworms (Ascariasis), and hookworms (*Ancylostoma* spp). However, albendazole has limited activity against many important and eosinophilia-inducing pathogens such as filaria, tapeworms, flukes, *Schistosoma*, *Strongyloides*, and *Trichinella* among others. Therefore, in cases of persistent eosinophilia that do not resolve with empiric therapy, it is critical to continue to pursue a diagnosis.

TRAVELER WITH JAUNDICE AND HEPATITIS

In years past, hepatitis A (HAV) was a frequent cause of hepatitis and jaundice among travelers. The widespread use of vaccination has greatly diminished its incidence. In the United States, HAV vaccination is routinely initiated at 1 year of age. However, many countries do not have a routine vaccination program against HAV. Jaundice as a sign of HAV infection has always been an infrequent finding in young children less than 5 years of age in whom the infection frequently is subclinical. Although VFR parents may be immune to HAV, the non-VFR unvaccinated adult may not be protected. However, their unvaccinated parents would become jaundiced and clinically ill.

With the declining incidence of traveler-associated HAV, hepatitis and jaundice may be more likely to be related to infections such as leptospirosis, especially in those traveling to Southeast Asia. Hepatitis E infections may be acquired from travel to this region, especially if the traveler has contact with swine and rice paddies in farming communities.[84] When initially presenting with fever, hepatitis E infection may not be distinguishable from malaria, dengue, or leptospirosis.

REFERENCES

1. World Tourism Organization. UNTWO Tourism Highlights 2012 edition; Madrid (Spain): 2012.

2. Bacaner N, Stauffer B, Boulware DR, et al. Travel medicine considerations for North American immigrants visiting friends and relatives. JAMA 2004;291:2856–64.
3. Han P, Yanni E, Jentes ES, et al. Health challenges of young travelers visiting friends and relatives compared with those traveling for other purposes. Pediatr Infect Dis J 2012;31:915–9.
4. Newman-Klee C, D'Acremont V, Newman CJ, et al. Incidence and types of illness when traveling to the tropics: a prospective controlled study of children and their parents. Am J Trop Med Hyg 2007;77:764–9.
5. Hagmann S, Neugebauer R, Schwartz E, et al. Illness in children after international travel: analysis from the GeoSentinel Surveillance Network. Pediatrics 2010;125:e1072–80.
6. West NS, Riordan FA. Fever in returned travellers: a prospective review of hospital admissions for a 2(1/2) year period. Arch Dis Child 2003;88:432–4.
7. Manock SR, Jacobsen KH, de Bravo NB, et al. Etiology of acute undifferentiated febrile illness in the Amazon basin of Ecuador. Am J Trop Med Hyg 2009;81:146–51.
8. Tripathy R, Parida S, Das L, et al. Clinical manifestations and predictors of severe malaria in Indian children. Pediatrics 2007;120:e454–60.
9. Stauffer WM, Cartwright CP, Olson DA, et al. Diagnostic performance of rapid diagnostic tests versus blood smears for malaria in US clinical practice. Clin Infect Dis 2009;49:908–13.
10. Poschl B, Waneesorn J, Thekisoe O, et al. Comparative diagnosis of malaria infections by microscopy, nested PCR, and LAMP in northern Thailand. Am J Trop Med Hyg 2010;83:56–60.
11. Nkrumah B, Agyekum A, Acquah SE, et al. Comparison of the novel Partec rapid malaria test to the conventional Giemsa stain and the gold standard real-time PCR. J Clin Microbiol 2010;48:2925–8.
12. World Health Organization. Guidelines for the treatment of malaria. 2nd edition. Geneva (Switzerland): World Health Organization; 2010.
13. Stover KR, King ST, Robinson J. Artemether-lumefantrine: an option for malaria. Ann Pharmacother 2012;46:567–77.
14. Kopel E, Marhoom E, Sidi Y, et al. Successful oral therapy for severe falciparum malaria: the World Health Organization criteria revisited. Am J Trop Med Hyg 2012;86:409–11.
15. Bhutta ZA. Current concepts in the diagnosis and treatment of typhoid fever. BMJ 2006;333:78–82.
16. Meltzer E, Sadik C, Schwartz E. Enteric fever in Israeli travelers: a nationwide study. J Travel Med 2005;12:275–81.
17. Patel TA, Armstrong M, Morris-Jones SD, et al. Imported enteric fever: case series from the hospital for tropical diseases, London, United Kingdom. Am J Trop Med Hyg 2010;82:1121–6.
18. Siddiqui FJ, Rabbani F, Hasan R, et al. Typhoid fever in children: some epidemiological considerations from Karachi, Pakistan. Int J Infect Dis 2006;10:215–22.
19. Bhutta ZA. Impact of age and drug resistance on mortality in typhoid fever. Arch Dis Child 1996;75:214–7.
20. Adeleke SI, Nwokedi EE. Diagnostic value of Widal test in febrile children. Afr Scient 2008;9:5–8.
21. Uneke CJ. Concurrent malaria and typhoid fever in the tropics: the diagnostic challenges and public health implications. J Vector Borne Dis 2008;45:133–42.
22. Vijayachari P, Sugunan AP, Shriram AN. Leptospirosis: an emerging global public health problem. J Biosci 2008;33:557–69.

23. Kendall EA, LaRocque RC, Bui DM, et al. Leptospirosis as a cause of fever in urban Bangladesh. Am J Trop Med Hyg 2010;82:1127–30.
24. Bruce MG, Sanders EJ, Leake JA, et al. Leptospirosis among patients presenting with dengue-like illness in Puerto Rico. Acta Trop 2005;96:36–46.
25. LaRocque RC, Breiman RF, Ari MD, et al. Leptospirosis during dengue outbreak, Bangladesh. Emerg Infect Dis 2005;11:766–9.
26. Phuong HL, de Vries PJ, Nga TT, et al. Dengue as a cause of acute undifferentiated fever in Vietnam. BMC Infect Dis 2006;6:123.
27. Gregory CJ, Santiago LM, Arguello DF, et al. Clinical and laboratory features that differentiate dengue from other febrile illnesses in an endemic area–Puerto Rico, 2007-2008. Am J Trop Med Hyg 2010;82:922–9.
28. Capeding RZ, Brion JD, Caponpon MM, et al. The incidence, characteristics, and presentation of dengue virus infections during infancy. Am J Trop Med Hyg 2010; 82:330–6.
29. Rocha C, Silva S, Gordon A, et al. Improvement in hospital indicators after changes in dengue case management in Nicaragua. Am J Trop Med Hyg 2009;81:287–92.
30. Alabi BS, Abdulkarim AA, Olatoke F, et al. Acute otitis media–a common diagnosis among febrile children in the tropics. Trop Doct 2006;36:31–2.
31. Leder K, Sundararajan V, Weld L, et al. Respiratory tract infections in travelers: a review of the GeoSentinel surveillance network. Clin Infect Dis 2003;36: 399–406.
32. Lobato MN, Hopewell PC. Mycobacterium tuberculosis infection after travel to or contact with visitors from countries with a high prevalence of tuberculosis. Am J Respir Crit Care Med 1998;158:1871–5.
33. Ouyang-Latimer J, Jafri S, VanTassel A, et al. In vitro antimicrobial susceptibility of bacterial enteropathogens isolated from international travelers to Mexico, Guatemala, and India from 2006 to 2008. Antimicrobial Agents Chemother 2011;55:874–8.
34. Steffen R, Tornieporth N, Clemens SA, et al. Epidemiology of travelers' diarrhea: details of a global survey. J Travel Med 2004;11:231–7.
35. Pitzinger B, Steffen R, Tschopp A. Incidence and clinical features of traveler's diarrhea in infants and children. Pediatr Infect Dis J 1991;10:719–23.
36. Stauffer WM, Konop RJ, Kamat D. Traveling with infants and young children. Part III: travelers' diarrhea. J Travel Med 2002;9:141–50.
37. Shah N, DuPont HL, Ramsey DJ. Global etiology of travelers' diarrhea: systematic review from 1973 to the present. Am J Trop Med Hyg 2009;80:609–14.
38. Adachi JA, Jiang ZD, Mathewson JJ, et al. Enteroaggregative Escherichia coli as a major etiologic agent in traveler's diarrhea in 3 regions of the world. Clin Infect Dis 2001;32:1706–9.
39. Weintraub A. Enteroaggregative Escherichia coli: epidemiology, virulence and detection. J Med Microbiol 2007;56:4–8.
40. Wong CS, Mooney JC, Brandt JR, et al. Risk factors for the hemolytic uremic syndrome in children infected with Escherichia coli O157:H7: a multivariable analysis. Clin Infect Dis 2012;55:33–41.
41. Frank C, Werber D, Cramer JP, et al. Epidemic profile of Shiga-toxin-producing Escherichia coli O104:H4 outbreak in Germany. N Engl J Med 2011;365:1771–80.
42. Koo HL, Ajami NJ, Jiang ZD, et al. Noroviruses as a cause of diarrhea in travelers to Guatemala, India, and Mexico. J Clin Microbiol 2010;48:1673–6.
43. de la Cabada Bauche J, Dupont HL. New Developments in Traveler's Diarrhea. Gastroenterol Hepatol 2011;7:88–95.

44. Tate JE, Burton AH, Boschi-Pinto C, et al. 2008 estimate of worldwide rotavirus-associated mortality in children younger than 5 years before the introduction of universal rotavirus vaccination programmes: a systematic review and meta-analysis. Lancet Infect Dis 2012;12:136–41.
45. Okhuysen PC. Traveler's diarrhea due to intestinal protozoa. Clin Infect Dis 2001; 33:110–4.
46. Jiang ZD, Dupont HL, Brown EL, et al. Microbial etiology of travelers' diarrhea in Mexico, Guatemala, and India: importance of enterotoxigenic Bacteroides fragilis and Arcobacter species. J Clin Microbiol 2010;48:1417–9.
47. Kollaritsch H, Paulke-Korinek M, Wiedermann U. Traveler's Diarrhea. Infect Dis Clin North Am 2012;26:691–706.
48. Qadri F, Svennerholm AM, Faruque AS, et al. Enterotoxigenic Escherichia coli in developing countries: epidemiology, microbiology, clinical features, treatment, and prevention. Clin Microbiol Rev 2005;18:465–83.
49. Victora CG, Bryce J, Fontaine O, et al. Reducing deaths from diarrhoea through oral rehydration therapy. Bull World Health Organ 2000;78:1246–55.
50. World Health Organization. Dept. of Child and Adolescent Health and Development. The treatment of diarrhoea: a manual for physicians and other senior health workers. 4th edition. Geneva (Switzerland): Dept. of Child and Adolescent Health and Development, World Health Organization; 2005. p. 44.
51. DuPont HL. Therapy for and prevention of traveler's diarrhea. Clin Infect Dis 2007; 45(Suppl 1):S78–84.
52. Mackell S. Traveler's diarrhea in the pediatric population: etiology and impact. Clin Infect Dis 2005;41(Suppl 8):S547–52.
53. Kaplan MA, Prior MJ, McKonly KI, et al. A multicenter randomized controlled trial of a liquid loperamide product versus placebo in the treatment of acute diarrhea in children. Clin Pediatr 1999;38:579–91.
54. Ansdell VE, Ericsson CD. Prevention and empiric treatment of traveler's diarrhea. Med Clin North Am 1999;83:945–73, vi.
55. Figueroa-Quintanilla D, Salazar-Lindo E, Sack RB, et al. A controlled trial of bismuth subsalicylate in infants with acute watery diarrheal disease. N Engl J Med 1993;328:1653–8.
56. Feldman S, Chen SL, Pickering LK, et al. Salicylate absorption from a bismuth subsalicylate preparation. Clin Pharmacol Ther 1981;29:788–92.
57. Hochedez P, Caumes E. Common skin infections in travelers. J Travel Med 2008; 15:252–62.
58. Freedman DO, Weld LH, Kozarsky PE, et al. Spectrum of disease and relation to place of exposure among ill returned travelers. N Engl J Med 2006;354:119–30.
59. Caumes E, Carriere J, Guermonprez G, et al. Dermatoses associated with travel to tropical countries: a prospective study of the diagnosis and management of 269 patients presenting to a tropical disease unit. Clin Infect Dis 1995;20:542–8.
60. Lederman ER, Weld LH, Elyazar IR, et al. Dermatologic conditions of the ill returned traveler: an analysis from the GeoSentinel Surveillance Network. Int J Infect Dis 2008;12:593–602.
61. O'Brien BM. A practical approach to common skin problems in returning travellers. Trav Med Infect Dis 2009;7:125–46.
62. Malavige GN, Ranatunga PK, Velathanthiri VG, et al. Patterns of disease in Sri Lankan dengue patients. Arch Dis Child 2006;91:396–400.
63. Herbinger KH, Siess C, Nothdurft HD, et al. Skin disorders among travellers returning from tropical and non-tropical countries consulting a travel medicine clinic. Trop Med Int Health 2011;16:1457–64.

64. Zanger P, Nurjadi D, Schleucher R, et al. Import and spread of Panton-Valentine Leukocidin-positive Staphylococcus aureus through nasal carriage and skin infections in travelers returning from the tropics and subtropics. Clin Infect Dis 2012;54:483–92.
65. Feldmeier H, Schuster A. Mini review: hookworm-related cutaneous larva migrans. Eur J Clin Microbiol Infect Dis 2012;31:915–8.
66. Pavli A, Maltezou HC. Leishmaniasis, an emerging infection in travelers. Int J Infect Dis 2010;14:e1032–9.
67. Ansart S, Perez L, Jaureguiberry S, et al. Spectrum of dermatoses in 165 travelers returning from the tropics with skin diseases. Am J Trop Med Hyg 2007;76:184–6.
68. Monsel G, Caumes E. Recent developments in dermatological syndromes in returning travelers. Curr Opin Infect Dis 2008;21:495–9.
69. Machado PR, Penna G. Miltefosine and cutaneous leishmaniasis. Curr Opin Infect Dis 2012;25:141–4.
70. Davis RF, Johnston GA, Sladden MJ. Recognition and management of common ectoparasitic diseases in travelers. Am J Clin Dermatol 2009;10:1–8.
71. Jensenius M, Fournier PE, Raoult D. Rickettsioses and the international traveler. Clin Infect Dis 2004;39:1493–9.
72. Patel S, Sethi A. Imported tropical diseases. Dermatol Ther 2009;22:538–49.
73. Meltzer E, Percik R, Shatzkes J, et al. Eosinophilia among returning travelers: a practical approach. Am J Trop Med Hyg 2008;78:702–9.
74. Lipner EM, Law MA, Barnett E, et al. Filariasis in travelers presenting to the GeoSentinel Surveillance Network. PLoS Negl Trop Dis 2007;1(3):e88.
75. Chen LH, Wilson ME, Davis X, et al. Illness in long-term travelers visiting GeoSentinel clinics. Emerg Infect Dis 2009;15:1773–82.
76. Nicolls DJ, Weld LH, Schwartz E, et al. Characteristics of schistosomiasis in travelers reported to the GeoSentinel Surveillance Network 1997-2008. Am J Trop Med Hyg 2008;79:729–34.
77. Libman MD, MacLean JD, Gyorkos TW. Screening for schistosomiasis, filariasis, and strongyloidiasis among expatriates returning from the tropics. Clin Infect Dis 1993;17:353–9.
78. Seybolt LM, Christiansen D, Barnett ED. Diagnostic evaluation of newly arrived asymptomatic refugees with eosinophilia. Clin Infect Dis 2006;42:363–7.
79. Ustianowski A, Zumla A. Eosinophilia in the returning traveler. Infect Dis Clin North Am 2012;26:781–9.
80. Rivas P, Aguilar-Duran S, Lago M. Lung nodules, fever, and eosinophilia in a traveler returning from Madagascar. Am J Trop Med Hyg 2012;86:2–3.
81. Oermann CM, Panesar KS, Langston C, et al. Pulmonary infiltrates with eosinophilia syndromes in children. J Pediatr 2000;136:351–8.
82. Bierman WF, Wetsteyn JC, van Gool T. Presentation and diagnosis of imported schistosomiasis: relevance of eosinophilia, microscopy for ova, and serology. J Travel Med 2005;12:9–13.
83. Checkley AM, Chiodini PL, Dockrell DH, et al. Eosinophilia in returning travellers and migrants from the tropics: UK recommendations for investigation and initial management. J Infect 2010;60:1–20.
84. Piper-Jenks N, Horowitz HW, Schwartz E. Risk of hepatitis E infection to travelers. J Travel Med 2000;7:194–9.

Index

Note: Page numbers of article titles are in **boldface** type.

Pediatr Clin N Am 60 (2013) 529–543
http://dx.doi.org/10.1016/S0031-3955(13)00011-4

F

G

H

N

Q

R

S

V

W